Emerging Topics in Statistics and Biostatistics

Yuhlong Lio • Ding-Geng Chen •
Hon Keung Tony Ng • Tzong-Ru Tsai
Editors

Bayesian Inference and Computation in Reliability and Survival Analysis

Springer

Editors
Yuhlong Lio
Department of Mathematical Sciences
University of South Dakota
Vermillion, SD, USA

Ding-Geng Chen
College of Health Solutions
Arizona State University
Phoenix, AZ, USA

Hon Keung Tony Ng
Department of Mathematical Sciences
Bentley University
Waltham, MA, USA

Tzong-Ru Tsai
Department of Statistics
Tamkang University
New Taipei City, Taiwan

ISSN 2524-7735 ISSN 2524-7743 (electronic)
Emerging Topics in Statistics and Biostatistics
ISBN 978-3-030-88657-8 ISBN 978-3-030-88658-5 (eBook)
https://doi.org/10.1007/978-3-030-88658-5

This Springer imprint is published by the registered company Springer Nature Switzerland AG
The registered company address is: Gewerbestrasse 11, 6330 Cham, Switzerland

Preface

Bayesian frameworks and methods have been successfully applied to solve practical problems in reliability and survival analysis, which have a wide range of real-world applications in medical and biological sciences, social and economic sciences, and engineering. Bayesian analysis is one of the important tools for statistical modeling and inference. Because of the complexity of the Bayesian framework, numerous Bayesian computation techniques have been developed in the past decades. This book focuses on the recent development of Bayesian computation technologies with emphasis on the applications to reliability and survival modeling.

Our aim in creating this book is to bring together experts engaged in the research on Bayesian computation with applications in reliability and survival analysis to present and discuss issues of important recent advances in the area. The topics covered in the book are timely and have a high potential to impact and influence biostatistics, engineering, medical sciences, statistics, and other related areas.

Outline of This Book Volume

This book volume brings together 16 chapters that are categorized as follows: Reliability Data Analysis (Part I), Stochastic Processes in Reliability Analysis (Part II), and Biomedical Data Analysis (Part III). All the chapters have undergone a thorough review process.

Part I of this book includes the following four chapters:

The chapter "A Bayesian Approach for Step-Stress-Accelerated Life Tests for One-Shot Devices Under Exponential Distributions" introduces the procedure to collect failures for the one-shot device under the step stress accelerated life test with multiple stress levels. Under exponential distributions with cumulative exposure models, Ling and Hu present the likelihood function for the observed failures collected from step-stress accelerated life test with multiple stress levels for one-shot devices and use two priors, normal prior, and Jeffry prior to address Bayesian inference through the Markov-Chain Monte-Carlo method via Metropolis-Hastings algorithm.

The chapter "Bayesian Estimation of Stress-Strength Parameter for Moran-Downton Bivariate Exponential Distribution Under Progressive Type II Censoring" introduces many useful simulation procedures for the Bayesian estimations of the stress-strength quantity $\delta = \Pr(X < Y)$ by utilizing correlated progressively type-II censored sample collected from Moran-Downton bivariate exponential distribution. An easy way to generate the progressively type-II censored sample from Moran-Downton bivariate exponential distribution and Markov-Chain Monte-Carlo procedure via Metropolis-Hastings algorithm is also introduced for Bayesian estimation.

The chapter "Bayesian Computation in a Birnbaum-Saunders Reliability Model with Applications to Fatigue Data" introduces a Bayesian methodology to compare two treatments and evaluate reliability based on the Birnbaum-Saunders distribution by utilizing inverse gamma and gamma distributions as priors. The strengths of 6061-T6 aluminum pieces, in terms of fatigue life and under two stress levels, are used for application purposes. Some open problems are also addressed.

The chapter "A Competing Risk Model Based on a Two-Parameter Exponential Family Distribution Under Progressive Type II Censoring" introduces a competing risks model with two dependent failure causes whose latent failure times follow Marshall-Olkin bivariate exponential family distribution. Maximum likelihood estimation (MLE) and Bayesian estimation methods for the model parameters are discussed under the progressive type-II censoring scheme. Some regular conditions are provided for the existence and uniqueness of MLE. A Markov-Chain Monte Carlo process is proposed for Bayesian estimation method. Since the possible flaw of MLE method, a simulation study for the Bayesian estimations of model parameters as well as lifetime percentiles under two loss functions is conducted. A dataset regarding the effect of laser treatment to delay the onset of blindness from the patient under the diabetic retinopathy study was used for application illustration.

Part II of this book includes the following four chapters:

The chapter "Bayesian Computations for Reliability Analysis in Dynamic Environments" discusses different modeling strategies for the evolution of the dynamic environment and develops Bayesian analysis of the models using Markov chain Monte Carlo methods and data augmentation techniques. The developed methods are illustrated using data from software testing, railroad track maintenance, and power outages from a repairable system for illustrations.

The chapter "Bayesian Analysis of Stochastic Processes in Reliability" provides an overview of the Bayesian modeling of some stochastic processes used in the context of reliability. The author starts with a survey of various forms of intensity functions and then reviews the applications of the Bayesian techniques for the inference of various types of stochastic processes.

The chapter "Bayesian Analysis of a New Bivariate Wiener Degradation Process" proposes a new bivariate Wiener degradation model to describe the unit-to-unit variation and dependence simultaneously and derives the closed forms for the reliability functions of the system and residual lifetime. Then the statistical inference is conducted by data augmentation and Bayesian methods.

The chapter "Bayesian Estimation for Bivariate Gamma Processes with Copula" discusses the bivariate gamma processes that have been proposed to model two-degradation paths observed from ADT under the independent assumption and also extends the processes by utilizing Clayton, Frank and Gumbel copulas to describe the possible dependence characteristics. Bayesian analysis using Markov-Chain Monte-Carlo method has been proposed to deal with high dimensional parameter estimation and model comparison. The related software is also included.

Part III of this book includes the following eight chapters:

The chapter "Review of Statistical Treatment for Oncology Dose-Escalation Trial with Prolonged EvaluationWindow or Fast Enrollment" starts with the review of three classes of methodologies for oncology dose-escalation trial design. The chapter also gives a comprehensive outline of the various statistical extensions of these methods to address the statistical challenges caused by the prolonged safety evaluation window or, equivalently, the fast enrollment rate. The methods under discussion can play a valuable role in improving the accuracy of optimal dose identification without sacrificing patient safety or significantly prolonging the trial duration

The chapter "A Bayesian Approach for the Analysis of Tumorigenicity Data from Sacrificial Experiments Under Weibull Lifetimes" describes a Bayesian inference on the onset time of tumors based on tumorigenicity data from sacrificial experiments. Authors set up tumorigenicity experiments with serial sacrifice. Assuming the tumor onset time has a Weibull distribution with log-linear link functions of covariates as scale and shape parameters, the Bayesian estimation procedure has been established by utilizing three priors, which include Laplace distribution, normal distribution with non-informative prior for the variance and beta distribution, as well as two prior beliefs.

The chapter "Bayesian Sensitivity Analysis in Survival and Longitudinal Trials with Missing Data" reviews sensitivity analysis methods and strategies for handling missing data for survival analysis and longitudinal trials by using control-based imputation and delta-adjusted strategies under informative censoring or missing-not-at-random from a Bayesian perspective. Applications to clinical trials are presented for illustration and future potential approach is also introduced.

The chapter "Bayesian Analysis for Clustered Data under a Semi-Competing Risks Framework" utilizes an illness-death model under a semi-competing risks framework that can characterize some nonterminal events such as relapse and a terminal event such as death. A full Bayesian approach is used to analyze diverse survival data including clustered data to account for patients' transitions within a time of interest. Metropolis-Hastings algorithm within Gibbs chains is used to obtain the estimates for regression coefficients in which R packages are employed for implementation.

The chapter "Survival Analysis for the Inverse Gaussian Distribution: Natural Conjugate and Jeffrey's Priors" focuses on the use of the Bayesian method to analyze survival data that follow inverse Gaussian distribution by utilizing the natural conjugate and Jeffrey's priors to estimate both unknown inverse Gaussian parameters as well as the average remaining time of the censored units. Because the closed-form of posteriors is not tractable due to censored data, the Gibbs sampling procedure is used. An extensive simulation study is conducted to assess the effects of natural conjugate hyperparameter settings at different levels of skewness as well as compare the behavior of the two priors.

The chapter "Bayesian Inferences for Panel Count Data and Interval-Censored Data with Nonparametric Modeling of the Baseline Functions" discusses a novel unified Bayesian approach to analyze the real-life applications where both panel count data and interval-censored data are generated for study subjects under periodic follow-ups. Interval-censored data are studied when the exact times of the events are of interest, and these exact times are not directly observed but are only known to fall within some intervals formed by the observation times. Panel count data are under investigation when the exact times of the recurrent events are not of interest but the counts of the recurrent events occurring within the time intervals are available and of interest. Specifically, this unified Bayesian approach is developed for analyzing panel count data under the gamma frailty Poisson process model and interval-censored data under Cox's proportional hazards model and the proportional odds model. The baseline functions in these models share the same property of being nondecreasing positive functions and are modeled nonparametrically by assigning a Gamma process prior. Efficient Gibbs samplers are developed for the posterior computation under these three models for the two types of data. The proposed methods are evaluated in a simulation study and illustrated by three real-life data applications.

The chapter "Bayesian Approach for Interval-Censored Survival Data with Time-Varying Coefficients" discusses a Bayesian approach to analyze the interval-censored failure time data, which are commonly obtained in medical and epidemiological studies. In this chapter, the authors present a Bayesian approach for correlated interval-censored data under a dynamic Cox regression model with piecewise constant coefficients. The dimensions of coefficients are automatically determined by the reversible jump Markov chain Monte Carlo algorithm. Two real datasets are used to demonstrate the applicability of these methods.

The chapter "Bayesian Approach for Joint Modeling Longitudinal Data and Survival Data Simultaneously in Public Health Studies" overviews the joint modeling through the harmonization of longitudinal data and time-to-event data by using Bayesian approach. Using a dataset from an HIV/AIDS study, which contains time-to-death due to AIDS and longitudinal CD4 measurements and was collected by a randomized clinical trial to compare the efficacy and the safety of two antiretroviral drugs given to patients who had failed or were intolerant of zidovudine therapy, this chapter demonstrates the merits of the joint-modeling of longitudinal continuous data and time-to-event data simultaneously over the separated linear mixed-effects modeling for longitudinal data and survival analysis for time-to-event data.

List of Reviewers

Dr. Ding-Geng Chen College of Health Solutions, Arizona State University, Phoenix, AZ, USA; Department of Statistics, University of Pretoria, South Africa

Dr. Jorge Figueroa-Zúñiga, Departamento de Ing. Estadística, Universidad de Concepci6n, Chile

Dr. Yuhlong Lio Department of Mathematical Sciences, The University of South Dakota, Vermillion, SD, USA

Dr. Man Ho Ling, Department of Mathematics and Information Technology, The Education University of Hong Kong, China

Dr. Hon Keung Tony Ng Department of Mathematical Sciences, Bentley University, Waltham, MA, USA

Dr. Tzong-Ru Tsai Department of Statistics, Tamkang University, New Taipei City, Taiwan

Dr. Min Wang Department of Management Science and Statistics, University of Texas at San Antonio, TX, USA

Jeffrey R. Wilson Department of Economics, Arizona State University, Phoenix, AZ, USA

Dr. Lili Yu Department of Biostatistics, Epidemiology, and Environmental Health Sciences, Jiann-Ping Hsu College of Public Health, Georgia Southern University. GA, USA.

Acknowledgments

We are deeply grateful to those who have supported us in the process of creating this book. We thank the contributors to this book for their enthusiastic involvement and their kindness in sharing their professional knowledge and expertise. Our sincere gratitude goes to all the chapter reviewers for their expert reviews of the book chapters, which led to a substantial improvement in the quality of this book. We thank all the reviewers for providing thoughtful and in-depth evaluations of the chapters contained in this book. We gratefully acknowledge the professional support of Laura Aileen Briskman from Springer who made the publication of this book a reality. We acknowledge the support and encouragement received from the editor-in-chief of the Springer Book Series in Emerging Topics in Statistics and Biostatistics, Professor Ding-Geng Chen.

The work of Professor Ding-Geng Chen is based upon research supported by the National Research Foundation, South Africa (South Africa DST-NRF-SAMRC SARChI Research Chair in Biostatistics, Grant number 114613). Opinions expressed and conclusions arrived at are those of the authors and are not necessarily to be attributed to the NRF.

We welcome readers' comments, including notes on typos or other errors, and look forward to receiving suggestions for improvements to future editions. Please send comments and suggestions to any of the editors.

Vermillion, SD, USA	Yuhlong Lio
Phoenix, AZ, USA	Ding-Geng Chen
Waltham, MA, USA	Hon Keung Tony Ng
New Taipei City, Taiwan	Tzong-Ru Tsai
May 2022	

Contents

Part III Biomedical Data Analysis

Contributors

Atilla Ay George Washington University, Washington, DC, USA

Narayanaswamy Balakrishnan Department of Mathematics and Statistics, McMaster University, Hamilton, ON, Canada

Ding-Geng Chen College of Health Solutions, Arizona State University, Phoenix, AZ, USA
Department of Statistics, University of Pretoria, Pretoria, South Africa

Fang Chen SAS Institute Inc, Cary, NC, USA

Raj S. Chhikara University of Houston, Houston, TX, USA

Erin P. Eifert University of Houston, Houston, TX, USA

Evans Gouno Universite Bretagne Sud, LMBA, Vannes, France

Yewon Han Department of Applied Mathematics, Hanyang University, Ansan, South Korea

Sehwa Hong Department of Applied Statistics, University of Suwon, Suwon, South Korea

Xuwen Hu Department of Statistics, Seoul National University, Seoul, South Korea

Kalanka P. Jayalath University of Houston, Houston, TX, USA

Jinheum Kim Department of Applied Statistics, University of Suwon, Suwon, South Korea

Seong W. Kim Department of Applied Mathematics, Hanyang University, Ansan, South Korea

Henry Laniado Department of Mathematical Sciences, Universidad Eafit, Medellín, Colombia

Vıctor Leiva School of Industrial Engineering, Pontificia Universidad, Catolica de Valparaiso, Valparaiso, Chile

Yu-Jau Lin Applied Mathematics Department, Chung Yuan Christian University, Taoyuan City, Taiwan

Xiaoyan Lin Department of Statistics, University of South Carolina, Columbia, SC, USA

Man Ho Ling Department of Mathematics and Information Technology, The Education University of Hong Kong, Hong Kong, China

Yuhlong Lio Department of Mathematical Sciences, The University of South Dakota, Vermillion, SD, USA

G. Frank Liu Merck & Co., Inc., North Wales, PA, USA

Rong Liu Global Biometrics and Data Science, Bristol Myers Squibb, New York, NY, USA

Hon Keung Tony Ng Department of Mathematical Sciences, Bentley University, Waltham, MA, USA

Fabrizio Ruggeri CNR-IMATI, Milano, Italy

Hon Yiu So Department of Mathematics and Statistics, Oakland University, Rochester, MI, USA

Refik Soyer George Washington University, Washington, DC, USA

Tzong-Ru Tsai Department of Statistics, Tamkang University, New Taipei, Taiwan

Liang Wang School of Mathematics, Yunnan Normal University, Kunming, P. R. China

Lianming Wang Department of Statistics, University of South Carolina, Columbia, SC, USA

Lu Wang Department of Mathematics, Western New England University, Springfield, MA, USA

Xin Wei Global Biometrics and Data Science, Bristol Myers Squibb, New York, NY, USA

Jeffrey R. Wilson Department of Economics, Arizona State University, Phoenix, AZ, USA

Ancha Xu Department of Statistics, Zhejiang Gongshang University, Zhejiang, China

Bin Zhang Division of Biostatistics and Epidemiology, Cincinnati Children's Hospital Medical Center, Cincinnati, OH, USA

Yue Zhang Department of Bioinformatics and Biostatistics, School of Life Sciences and Biotechnology, Shanghai Jiao Tong University, Shanghai, PR China

About the Editors

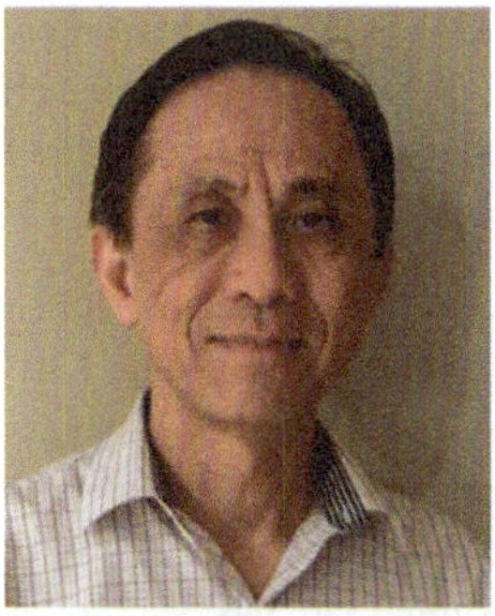

Yuhlong Lio is a professor in the Department of Mathematical Sciences at the University of South Dakota, Vermillion, SD, USA. He is an associate editor of professional journals, including the *Journal of Statistical Computation and Simulation.* His research interests include reliability, quality control, censoring methodology, kernel smoothing estimate, and accelerated degradation data modeling. Dr. Lio has written more than 100 refereed publications.

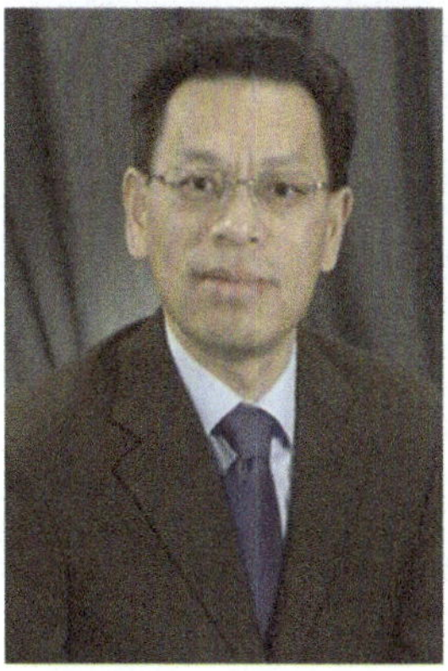

Ding-Geng Chen is an elected fellow of the American Statistical Association and currently the executive director of Biostatistics Initiative in the College of Health Solutions at Arizona State University. He was the Wallace H. Kuralt Distinguished Professor of Biostatistics at the University of North Carolina at Chapel Hill, USA; Extraordinary Professor at the University of Pretoria, South Africa; Professor of Biostatistics at the University of Rochester; and the Karl E. Peace endowed eminent scholar chair in biostatistics at Georgia Southern University. He is also a senior consultant for biopharmaceuticals and government agencies with extensive expertise in clinical trial biostatistics and public health statistics. Professor Chen has written more than 200 refereed publications and co-authored/co-edited 33 books on clinical trial methodology, meta-analysis, causal inference, and public health statistics.

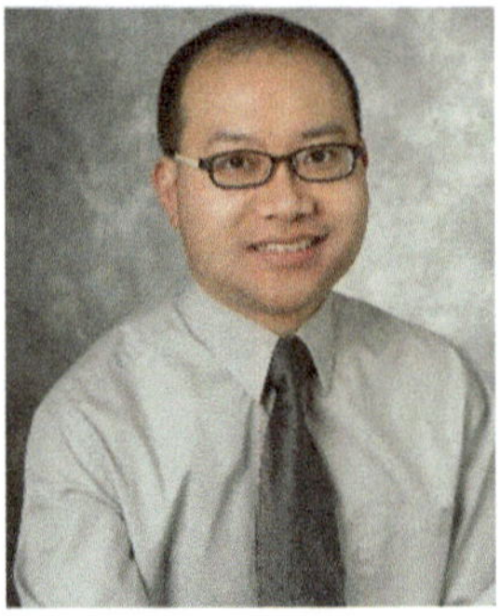

Hon Keung Tony Ng is a Professor with the Department of Mathematical Sciences, Bentley University, Waltham, MA, USA. He is an associate editor of *Communications in Statistics*, *Computational Statistics*, *IEEE Transactions on Reliability*, *Journal of Statistical Computation and Simulation*, *Naval Research Logistics*, *Sequential Analysis*, and *Statistics and Probability Letters*. His research interests include reliability, censoring methodology, ordered data analysis, nonparametric methods, and statistical inference. He has published more than 150 research papers in refereed journals. He is the co-author of the book *Precedence-Type Tests and Applications* and co-editor of *Ordered Data Analysis, Modeling and Health Research Methods*. Professor Ng is a fellow of the American Statistical Association, an elected senior member of IEEE, and an elected member of the International Statistical Institute.

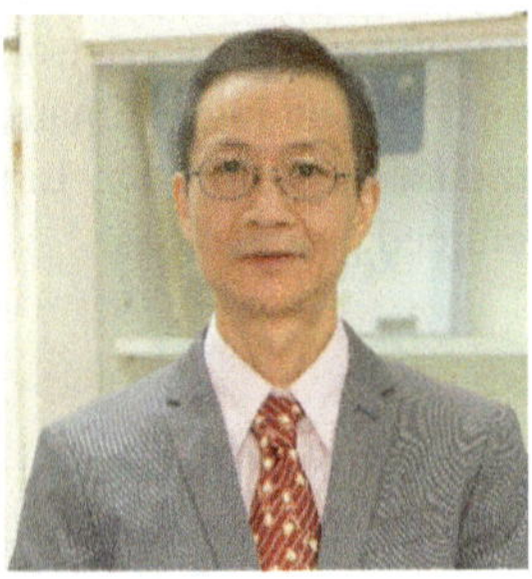

Tzong-Ru Tsai is a professor in the Department of Statistics at Tamkang University in New Taipei City, Taiwan. He is also the dean of the College of Business and Management at Tamkang University. His main research interests include quality control, reliability analysis, and machine learning. He has served as a consultant with extensive expertise in statistical quality control and experimental design for many companies in the past years. He is an associate editor of the *Journal of Statistical Computation and Simulation* and serves in the editorial boards of *Mathematics* and *International Journal of Reliability, Quality and Safety Engineering*. Dr. Tsai has written more than 100 refereed publications.

Part I
Reliability Data Analysis

A Bayesian Approach for Step-Stress-Accelerated Life Tests for One-Shot Devices Under Exponential Distributions

Man Ho Ling and Xuwen Hu

Abstract In practice, accelerated life tests are commonly used to collect failure time data within a short period of time by elevating stress levels. In this chapter, step-stress-accelerated life tests with multiple stress levels are considered for one-shot devices that can be used only once. As the exact failure times of one-shot devices cannot be observed from accelerated life tests, a Bayesian approach incorporating with prior information provides some useful inference on the reliability. To extrapolate the reliability under normal operating conditions from elevated stress levels, cumulative exposure models with exponential distributions are adopted. The Markov Chain Monte Carlo method via Metropolis–Hastings algorithm is performed to estimate the model parameters, the reliability, and the mean lifetime. Finally, comprehensive simulation studies for normal (subjective) and Jeffreys (objective) priors are carried out to evaluate the performance of the Bayesian estimation in terms of bias and root mean square error. A real data on samples of grease-based magnetorheological fluids is analyzed for illustration of the Bayesian estimation.

1 Introduction

Units that can be used once only are called one-shot devices, for instance airbags of vehicles, rockets, and missiles. One-shot devices cannot be used again after their intended functions perform. Researchers can only observe whether a device

M. Ho Ling (✉)
Department of Mathematics and Information Technology, The Education University of Hong Kong, Hong Kong, China
e-mail: amhling@eduhk.hk

X. Hu
Department of Statistics, Seoul National University, Seoul, South Korea

Y. Lio et al. (eds.), *Bayesian Inference and Computation in Reliability and Survival Analysis*, Emerging Topics in Statistics and Biostatistics,
https://doi.org/10.1007/978-3-030-88658-5_1

functions at the inspection time in a life test, instead of its actual lifetime. Many researchers have recently studied one-shot devices/systems [8–10, 25, 28, 30, 32–34]. For a book length account of methods and analysis of one-shot device testing data, interested readers may refer to the recent book by Balakrishnan, Ling, and So [4].

With the rapid change of technology, high-reliable products with long lifetimes are in high demand and accelerated life tests (ALTs) have received much attention in reliability studies. ALTs are usually run under higher-than-normal stress levels to shorten the lifetimes of devices. The accelerating factors include humidity, voltage, current, and temperature. Under ALTs, the experimental time and the cost of conducting experiments can be reduced. Meeker et al. [23] considered accelerated degradation models to predict the lifetime of products at normal temperature. Step-stress ALTs (SSALTs) are one of the most popular ALTs in practice; see, for example [26, 27]. Zheng et al. [35] considered SSALTs with four elevated levels of temperature (333K, 339K, 345K, 351K) to collect grease-based magnetorheological fluid (G-MRF) samples for predicting the lifetime of G-MRF at the normal operating temperature of 293K. In SSALTs, each unit is initially placed at a higher-than-normal stress level with a pre-specified inspection time. Subsequently, some of the units are randomly selected and tested and the stress level will immediately increase. The remaining units are subject to the elevated stress levels for another pre-specified period of time. If the stress levels are more than two, the process of selecting units and increasing stress levels will be repeated for the remaining units. SSALTs with only one increase in the stress level are called simple SSALTs. For SSALTs, there are three fundamental models for the effect of increased stress levels on the lifetime distribution: The tampered random variable model [12], the cumulative exposure model [26, 27], and the tampered failure rate model [6]. Ling [19] considered exponential distributions with the cumulative exposure models and developed the expectation–maximization algorithm for finding the maximum likelihood estimates of the model parameters as well as optimal designs of simple SSALTs for one-shot devices. In this chapter, a Bayesian approach is presented for analyzing one-shot device testing data collected from SSALTs with multiple stress levels. In line with [19], the exponential distributions with the cumulative exposure models are considered. Moreover, the performance of the Bayesian estimation with different priors, namely normal and Jeffreys priors, is compared with the maximum likelihood estimation in terms of bias and root mean square error.

The Bayesian approach is one of the most popular statistical techniques for estimation when the likelihood function is complicated. This method is especially useful and efficient for estimation when we have limited information on lifetime. Also, Bayesian estimation incorporating prior information can provide us with more useful inference. Therefore, the Bayesian approach becomes a mainstream estimation method in reliability studies over the past several decades. Marta and Wailera [21] analyzed the reliability for complex systems in a Bayesian framework.

Coolen and Newby [11] discussed Bayesian reliability analysis when a range of possible probabilities from an expert for events of interest were considered. Yates and Mosleh [31] estimated the reliability of aerospace systems by using Bayesian estimation method. Fan et al. [14] described a Bayesian framework to analyze the reliability of electro-explosive devices with several priors. LeSage [17] presented the process of estimating the dependent variable in spatial autoregressive models through Bayesian estimation method. Ling et al. [18] presented remaining useful life estimation under degradation data for prognostic and system health management in a Bayesian framework. Hamada et al. [15] provide concrete concepts of the Bayesian approach and numerous methods and techniques for analyzing reliability data from a Bayesian perspective.

The rest of this chapter is organized as follows. Section 2 presents the one-shot devices testing data under exponential distributions with cumulative exposure models. The maximum likelihood estimation method and a Bayesian framework will be described in Sects. 3 and 4. Two priors for the Bayesian estimation are also presented. In Sect. 5, comprehensive simulation studies are conducted to evaluate the performance of the Bayesian estimation method with those two priors in terms of bias and root mean square error (RMSE). In Sect. 6, a real data on samples of grease-based magnetorheological fluids is analyzed for illustration of the Bayesian estimation. Finally, some concluding remarks are made in Sect. 7.

2 Model Description

Consider SSALTs with $I \geq 2$ stress levels, $x_1, x_2, \ldots, x_I$, for one-shot devices. K devices are exposed to stress level x_1, K_1 devices are tested at inspection time τ_1, and the number of failures is recorded as n_1. Meanwhile, the remaining devices $K - K_1$ are subject to an increased stress level x_2 and K_2 devices are tested at inspection time τ_2. The number of failures, n_2, is recorded. Similarly, for $i = 3, 4, \ldots, I$, in the i-th cycle, the remaining devices $K - \sum_{m=1}^{i-1} K_m$ are subject to an increased stress level x_i, K_i devices are tested at inspection time τ_i, and the number of failures, n_i, is recorded. It is noting that $K = \sum_{m=1}^{I} K_m$. Finally, one-shot devices testing data under SSALTs with I stress levels are denoted as $\mathbf{z} = \{\tau_i, K_i, n_i, x_i, i = 1, 2, \ldots, I\}$.

Suppose the lifetimes of the devices follow exponential distributions. Let $\tau_0 = 0$. The corresponding cumulative hazard function under cumulative exposure models is derived as

$$H(t) = \sum_{m=1}^{i-1} \alpha_m(\tau_m - \tau_{m-1}) + \alpha_i(t - \tau_{i-1}), \quad \tau_{i-1} < t \leq \tau_i, \tag{1}$$

where α_i is the rate parameter under the tests. Hence, the associated reliability at inspection time τ_i is therefore

$$p_i = \exp(-H(\tau_i)) = \exp\left(-\sum_{m=1}^{i} \alpha_m(\tau_m - \tau_{m-1})\right). \tag{2}$$

Furthermore, it is assumed that the rate parameter is related to the stress levels in a log-linear from [29], i.e.,

$$\alpha_i = \exp(a_0 + a_1 x_i). \tag{3}$$

For notational convenience, we let $\theta = (a_0, a_1)$ as the model parameters to be estimated. Since the lifetimes of devices are independent, the joint likelihood function of $\theta = (a_0, a_1)$ is then given by

$$L(\theta) = \prod_{i=1}^{I} (1 - p_i)^{n_i} p_i^{K_i - n_i}. \tag{4}$$

3 Maximum Likelihood Estimation

Maximum likelihood estimation method is one of the popular methods for the estimation of model parameters, and it relies on the maximization of likelihood function of an assumed model based on observed data. Likelihood inference on one-shot device testing data has been discussed extensively for many prominent lifetime distributions; see [1–3, 19]. In our settings, we first consider the log-likelihood function

$$\ell(\theta) = \ln(L(\theta)) = \sum_{i=1}^{I} n_i \ln(1 - p_i) + (K_i - n_i) \ln(p_i). \tag{5}$$

The likelihood function and the log-likelihood function get maximized when the following equations simultaneously hold:

$$\frac{\partial \ell(\theta)}{\partial a_0} = \sum_{i=1}^{I} \left(\frac{n_i}{1 - p_i} - \frac{K_i - n_i}{p_i} \right) p_i H(\tau_i) = 0, \tag{6}$$

$$\frac{\partial \ell(\theta)}{\partial a_1} = \sum_{i=1}^{I} \left(\frac{n_i}{1 - p_i} - \frac{K_i - n_i}{p_i} \right) p_i H(\tau_i) x_i = 0. \tag{7}$$

However, a closed-form solution is not available, and in such a case, optimization methods, for example, Newton–Raphson method, can be employed for obtaining the maximum likelihood estimates. In one-shot device testing, all the failure times are either left- or right-censored. An expectation–maximization (EM) algorithm [22] that is known to be a convenient and efficient method for estimating model parameters in the presence of censoring can also be applied for the estimation. The EM algorithm involves two steps in each iteration of the numerical method of maximizing the likelihood function: expectation-step (E-step) in which the censored data are approximated by their expected values, and maximization-step (M-step) in which the likelihood function, with imputed values replacing the censored data, gets maximized. Interested readers may refer to [19] for SSALTs with $I = 2$ in detail.

4 Bayesian Approach

The maximum likelihood estimation provides accurate estimation only when the sample size is sufficiently large. On the other hand, for life tests with small sample sizes, Bayesian approaches are alternative for estimation [5]. Here, we intend to estimate the model parameters $\theta = \{a_0, a_1\}$ from the Bayesian perspective.

Let $\pi(\theta)$ be the joint prior density of θ. Given the observed data $\mathbf{z}$, the joint posterior density is given by

$$\pi(\theta|\mathbf{z}) = \frac{L(\theta)\pi(\theta)}{\int L(\theta)\pi(\theta)d\theta} = \frac{q(\theta)}{\int q(\theta)d\theta}. \tag{8}$$

It is observed that the denominator is not in a closed form and thus the posterior distribution cannot be analyzed numerically. The posterior distribution of the model parameters θ can then be approximated by using Markov Chain Monte Carlo (MCMC) methods via Metropolis–Hastings algorithm [16, 24]. The Metropolis–Hastings algorithm proceeds as follows: In the m-th step of the iterative procedure:

Step 1: Generate θ^* from a proposal distribution based on $\theta^{(m)} = \left(a_0^{(m)}, a_1^{(m)}\right)$.

Step 2: Compute the acceptance probability $p = \min\left(1, q(\theta^*)/q(\theta^{(m)})\right)$.

Step 3: Set $\theta^{(m+1)} = \begin{cases} \theta^* & \text{with probability } p, \\ \theta^{(m)} & \text{with probability } 1 - p. \end{cases}$

Suppose $M \geq 100{,}000$ iterated samples of θ are obtained, $\{\theta^{(m)}, m = 1, 2, \ldots, M\}$, by using the above procedure. We then usually discard the first $D = 1000$ (say) samples as burn-in and sample one value in every $B = 100$ (say) iterations after the burn-in to reduce autocorrelation between the iterated samples in the MCMC sample. This way, we will end up with $R = \lfloor (M - D)/B \rfloor$ samples to approximate the posterior distribution, where $\lfloor a \rfloor$ denotes the floor function of a. Now, there is a sequence of posterior samples of θ, say $\theta^{(r)}, r = 1, 2, \ldots, R$, generated from Metropolis–Hastings algorithm. Subsequently, based on the posterior samples, the

Bayesian estimates of the model parameters, the reliability, and the mean lifetime under normal operating condition x_0 are given by

$$\hat{a}_0 = \frac{1}{R}\sum_{r=1}^{R} a_0^{(r)} \tag{9}$$

$$\hat{a}_1 = \frac{1}{R}\sum_{r=1}^{R} a_1^{(r)} \tag{10}$$

$$\hat{p}(t) = \frac{1}{R}\sum_{r=1}^{R} \exp\left(-\alpha_0^{(r)} t\right) \tag{11}$$

$$\hat{\mu} = \frac{1}{R}\sum_{r=1}^{R} \frac{1}{\alpha_0^{(r)}}, \tag{12}$$

where $\alpha_0^{(r)} = \exp\left(a_0^{(r)} + a_1^{(r)} x_0\right)$.

In the Bayesian framework, the prior information, $\pi(\theta)$, plays an important role in getting the posterior distribution, especially when lifetime information is limited. Here, we consider two different priors, including normal (subjective) prior and Jeffreys (objective) prior. It is noting that subjective priors are usually suggested by experts or past experiments.

4.1 Normal Prior

Fan et al. [14] compared three different subjective priors, namely exponential, normal, and beta priors, for Bayesian estimation for one-shot device testing data collected from constant-stress ALTs through extensive simulation studies and realized that normal prior is the best among those priors for the estimation. Therefore, it is natural to consider normal prior for one-shot device testing data collected from SSALTs. The normal prior assumes that there are errors between actual values of the parameters and the belief priors. Here, the error is denoted as ϵ_i, and it is assumed that

$$\hat{p}_i = p_i + \epsilon_i, \quad i = 1, 2, \ldots, I, \tag{13}$$

and ϵ_i are i.i.d. normal random variables with a mean of 0 and a variance of σ^2, say $N(0, \sigma^2)$. Let $\hat{\mathbf{p}} = \{\hat{p}_i, i = 1, 2, \ldots, I\}$. Given σ^2, the conditional likelihood function of θ is

$$\pi(\theta|\mathbf{z}, \hat{\mathbf{p}}, \sigma^2) \propto \prod_{i=1}^{I} \frac{1}{\sqrt{\sigma^2}} \exp\left(-\frac{(p_i - \hat{p}_i)^2}{2\sigma^2}\right) \tag{14}$$

$$= \left(\sigma^2\right)^{-\frac{I}{2}} \exp\left(-\frac{\sum_{i=1}^{I}(p_i - \hat{p}_i)^2}{2\sigma^2}\right). \tag{15}$$

Because the σ^2 is unknown, we adopt the most common prior,

$$\pi(\sigma^2) \propto \frac{1}{\sigma^2}, \quad \sigma^2 > 0. \tag{16}$$

Therefore, the joint prior density of θ is given by

$$\pi_N(\theta|\mathbf{z}, \hat{\mathbf{p}}) \propto \int_0^\infty \pi(\theta|\mathbf{z}, \hat{\mathbf{p}}, \sigma^2)\pi(\sigma^2)d\sigma^2 \tag{17}$$

$$\propto \int_0^\infty (\sigma^2)^{-\frac{I+2}{2}} \exp\left(-\frac{1}{2\sigma^2}\sum_{i=1}^{I}(p_i - \hat{p}_i)^2\right)d\sigma^2 \tag{18}$$

$$\propto \left(\sum_{i=1}^{I}(p_i - \hat{p}_i)^2\right)^{-I/2}. \tag{19}$$

Consequently, the posterior density of θ becomes

$$\pi(\theta|\mathbf{z}, \hat{\mathbf{p}}) = \prod_{i=1}^{I}(1 - p_i)^{n_i} p_i^{K_i - n_i} \left(\sum_{i=1}^{I}(p_i - \hat{p}_i)^2\right)^{-I/2}. \tag{20}$$

Instead of being suggested by experts for $\hat{p}_i$'s, from Eqs. (2) and (3), we can obtain $\hat{p}_i$'s from the observed data $\mathbf{z}$ as follows:

$$\ln(-\ln(p_i) + \ln(p_{i-1})) - \ln(\tau_i - \tau_{i-1}) = a_0 + a_1 x_i, \quad i = 1, 2, \ldots, I. \tag{21}$$

We can further obtain the least-square estimates of $\theta = (a_0, a_1)$ by setting

$$y_i = \ln\left(-\ln\left(1 - \frac{n_i}{K_i}\right) + \ln\left(1 - \frac{n_{i-1}}{K_{i-1}}\right)\right) - \ln(\tau_i - \tau_{i-1}) \tag{22}$$

for $i = 1, 2, \ldots, I$, and solving the system of equations

$$\begin{bmatrix} y_1 \\ y_2 \\ \vdots \\ y_I \end{bmatrix} = \begin{bmatrix} 1 & x_1 \\ 1 & x_2 \\ \vdots & \vdots \\ 1 & x_I \end{bmatrix} \begin{bmatrix} a_0 \\ a_1 \end{bmatrix}. \tag{23}$$

Let $\hat{a}_0^{LSE}$ and $\hat{a}_1^{LSE}$ be the respective least-square estimates. Finally, $\hat{p}_i$'s can also be obtained from $\hat{a}_0^{LSE}$ and $\hat{a}_1^{LSE}$, i.e.,

$$\hat{p}_i = \exp\left(-\sum_{j=1}^{i} \exp\left(\hat{a}_0^{LSE} + \hat{a}_1^{LSE} x_j\right)(\tau_j - \tau_{j-1})\right). \tag{24}$$

4.2 *Jeffreys Prior*

Jeffreys prior is an objective prior that comes from the Fisher information matrix. This prior is also useful and commonly used in Bayesian approaches when we have no information about the model parameters. Jeffreys prior is the square root of the determinant of the Fisher information matrix. In one-shot device testing data under SSALTs, the Fisher information is given by

$$\mathbf{I} = -E\left[\frac{\partial^2 \ell(\theta)}{\partial a_p \partial a_q}\right] \tag{25}$$

$$= \sum_{i=1}^{I} \left(\frac{\partial p_i}{\partial a_p}\right)\left(\frac{\partial p_i}{\partial a_q}\right)\left(\frac{K_i}{p_i} + \frac{K_i}{1-p_i}\right), \quad p = 0, 1, q = 0, 1, \tag{26}$$

and Jeffreys prior is therefore

$$\pi_J(\theta) = \sqrt{Det(\mathbf{I})} \propto \prod_{i=1}^{I} \frac{\alpha_i}{\sqrt{1-p_i}}. \tag{27}$$

It turns out that the joint posterior density of (a_0, a_1) is given by

$$\pi(\theta|\mathbf{z}, \hat{\mathbf{p}}) = \prod_{i=1}^{I} (1-p_i)^{n_i - 1/2} p_i^{K_i - n_i} \alpha_i. \tag{28}$$

5 Simulation Study

In this section, we conduct simulation studies to compare the maximum likelihood estimates and the Bayesian estimates incorporating with normal and Jeffreys priors for SSALTs with $I = \{2, 3\}$ stress levels for various sample sizes $K = \{50, 100, 200\}$. The pair of values of the unknown parameters is set to be $(a_0, a_1) = (-5.5, 0.05)$. First we consider simple SSALTs with two stress levels $x = \{35, 55\}$ and inspection times $\tau = \{15, 30\}$. In simple SSALTs for one-shot devices [19], it is assumed that 80% of the devices are tested at the first inspection time. Then the stress level is increased immediately, and the remaining devices are tested at the second inspection time. Afterward, SSALTs with three stress levels $x = \{35, 45, 55\}$ and inspection times $\tau = \{10, 20, 30\}$ are considered. In this setup, the allocations of devices tested at the first, second, and last inspections are 75%, 20%, and 5%, respectively.

Here, the MCMC method is used to approximate the posterior distribution of the model parameters $\theta = (a_0, a_1)$. Metropolis–Hastings algorithm [16] incorporating normal distributions for the model parameters is employed to simulate $M = 100{,}000$ random samples iteratively. Then, the first $D = 1000$ iterative samples are discarded, and one sample in every $B = 100$ iterative sample is randomly selected to reduce the autocorrelation among the posterior samples. Consequently, we obtain $R = 990$ posterior samples to approximate the joint posterior distribution of the model parameters $\theta = (a_0, a_1)$. Furthermore, the reliability under the normal operating condition $x_0 = 25$ at a mission time can be estimated.

Table 1 presents bias and RMSE of the estimates of a_0 and a_1. Generally speaking, bias and RMSE decrease when the sample size increases. It is observed that the maximum likelihood estimation method works well only when the sample sizes are sufficiently large. In addition, when the sample size is large enough, $\hat{p}_i$'s are close to the respective reliability p_i, and thus $\hat{p}_i$'s provide important information on the reliability. It is therefore realized that normal prior generally outperforms Jeffreys prior in terms of bias and RMSE. It is surprising that, under the exponential distributions, we observe that the bias and RMSE for $I = 3$ are greater than those for $I = 2$ when the sample size K is fixed. It indicates that SSALTs with more stress levels have less statistical efficiency of the estimation of the model parameters.

Moreover, it is of great interest in evaluating the performance of the estimation of the reliability and the mean lifetime under the normal operating condition. Tables 2 and 3 present bias and RMSE of the estimates of the reliability at different mission

Table 1 Bias and RMSE of the estimates of the model parameters for different methods with various sample sizes for SSALTs with $I = \{2, 3\}$ stress levels

		$I = 2$				$I = 3$			
		$a_0 = -5.5$		$a_1 = 0.05$		$a_0 = -5.5$		$a_1 = 0.05$	
K	Method	Bias	RMSE	Bias	RMSE	Bias	RMSE	Bias	RMSE
50	MLE	−0.1059	2.2558	0.0027	0.0625	1.0884	8.9315	−0.0329	0.2516
	π_N	−0.0294	1.4961	0.0000	0.0374	0.4422	1.5815	−0.0110	0.0357
	π_J	−0.3229	2.1024	0.0085	0.0565	−2.0100	3.2855	0.0531	0.0847
100	MLE	−0.0337	0.9429	0.0004	0.0250	0.0413	2.7551	−0.0024	0.0750
	π_N	0.0188	0.9776	−0.0011	0.0238	0.0150	1.2587	0.0012	0.0302
	π_J	−0.0704	1.0809	0.0015	0.0272	−0.8696	1.8782	0.0231	0.0490
200	MLE	−0.0036	0.6232	0.0001	0.0161	−0.0085	1.2609	−0.0001	0.0329
	π_N	0.0403	0.6279	−0.0013	0.0148	−0.0540	0.9047	0.0032	0.0223
	π_J	−0.0198	0.7400	0.0005	0.0184	−0.3252	1.1444	0.0086	0.0298

Table 2 Bias and RMSE of the estimates of the reliability at different mission times and the mean lifetime under the normal operating condition for different methods with various sample sizes for SSALTs with $I = 2$ stress levels

$I = 2$		$p(10) = 0.8671$		$p(20) = 0.7518$		$p(30) = 0.6519$		$\mu = 70.1054$	
K	Method	Bias	RMSE	Bias	RMSE	Bias	RMSE	Bias	RMSE
50	MLE	−0.0123	0.0894	−0.0134	0.1254	−0.0101	0.1487	17.3643	68.5893
	π_N	−0.0159	0.0823	−0.0189	0.1229	−0.0161	0.1479	24.5436	160.0178
	π_J	−0.0246	0.0910	−0.0265	0.1328	−0.0188	0.1558	68.6334	271.1758
100	MLE	−0.0050	0.0451	−0.0067	0.0742	−0.0062	0.0930	5.0178	30.8023
	π_N	−0.0084	0.0583	−0.0103	0.0879	−0.0093	0.1074	7.4580	33.5800
	π_J	−0.0135	0.0598	−0.0163	0.0930	−0.0134	0.1123	16.1128	46.3670
200	MLE	−0.0025	0.0278	−0.0036	0.0476	−0.0037	0.0611	1.6924	15.9847
	π_N	−0.0054	0.0358	−0.0080	0.0605	−0.0085	0.0769	2.4602	20.3021
	π_J	−0.0079	0.0408	−0.0106	0.0670	−0.0100	0.0834	6.6181	23.8042

Table 3 Bias and RMSE of the estimates of the reliability at different mission times and the mean lifetime under the normal operating condition for different methods with various sample sizes for SSALTs with $I = 3$ stress levels

$I = 3$		$p(10) = 0.8671$		$p(20) = 0.7518$		$p(30) = 0.6519$		$\mu = 70.1054$	
K	Method	Bias	RMSE	Bias	RMSE	Bias	RMSE	Bias	RMSE
50	MLE	−0.0543	0.2226	−0.0447	0.2471	−0.0267	0.2601	78.4813	328.9704
	π_N	−0.0513	0.1236	−0.0725	0.1807	−0.0777	0.2065	7.3117	68.6431
	π_J	0.0170	0.0864	0.0443	0.1383	0.0734	0.1767	733.5855	10347
100	MLE	−0.0240	0.1253	−0.0259	0.1664	−0.0202	0.1886	24.7547	109.6319
	π_N	−0.0213	0.0798	−0.0302	0.1252	−0.0318	0.1508	6.9939	42.3457
	π_J	0.0037	0.0685	0.0161	0.1094	0.0316	0.1372	65.9641	136.7232
200	MLE	−0.0068	0.0616	−0.0080	0.1009	−0.0059	0.1255	9.9092	37.8818
	π_N	−0.0106	0.0503	−0.0157	0.0829	−0.0172	0.1036	3.1028	28.1661
	π_J	−0.0025	0.0507	0.0012	0.0821	0.0079	0.1023	21.7381	45.8657

times $t = \{10, 20, 30\}$ and the mean lifetime under normal operating condition $x_0 = 25$. It is realized that the maximum likelihood estimation method outperforms the Bayesian approach with normal and Jeffreys priors for the estimation of the reliability and the mean lifetime under SSALTs with $I = 2$. However, for SSALTs with three stress levels, Jeffreys prior generally yields less bias and RMSE of the estimates of the reliability. In general, under the exponential distributions, introducing more stress levels does not improve the statistical efficiency of the estimation of the reliability and the mean lifetime, except for normal prior for the estimation of the mean lifetime when sample size $K = 50$. It may indicate that SSALTs with more stress levels are recommended for the estimation of the mean lifetime only when the sample size is not sufficiently large. Otherwise, simple SSALTs with two stress levels are highly recommended.

6 Data Analysis

In this section, we present an application of the Bayesian estimation for samples of grease-based magnetorheological fluids (G-MRFs) presented in [35]. Twenty G-MRF samples were collected from a SSALT with four higher-than-normal stress levels. In this test, the failure of each G-MRF sample is defined as its viscosity or shear stress has decreased by more than 10%. However, the exact failure times cannot be observed. We can only observe whether the viscosity and shear stress cross the thresholds at the inspection time. This results in one-shot device testing data. The data on 20 G-MRFs samples are presented in Table 4. As the inverse power law [13] is commonly used to develop a relationship between the temperature and the lifetime distribution, we consider $x_0 = -1/293, x_1 = -1/333, x_2 = -1/339, x_3 = -1/345, x_4 = -1/351$. For the Bayesian estimation, we set $M = 1{,}000{,}000$, $D = 10{,}000$, $B = 100$ to obtain $R = 99{,}900$ posterior samples to approximate the joint posterior distribution of the model parameters. Trace plots and histograms of posterior samples of the parameters of interest generated from Metropolis–Hastings algorithm for normal and Jeffreys priors are presented in Figs. 1 and 2. The maximum likelihood estimates and the Bayesian estimates of the model parameters, the reliability at mission time $t = 20{,}000$ h, and the mean lifetime under normal operating condition of $x_0 = 293K$ are presented

Table 4 Data on G-MRF samples under SSALTs with four stress levels

Temperature (K)	Inspection time (h)	No. of samples	No. of failures
333	864	5	1
339	1512	5	1
345	1944	5	2
351	2160	5	2

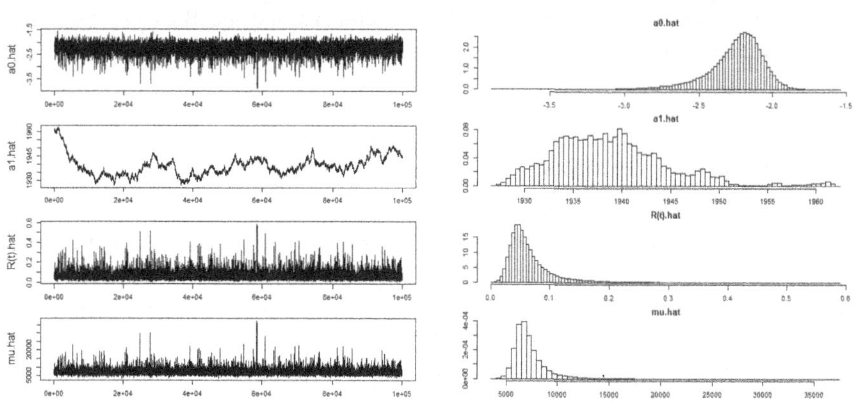

Fig. 1 Trace plots (left) and histograms (right) of posterior samples of $a_0, a_1, R(t)$, and μ generated from Metropolis–Hastings algorithm for normal prior

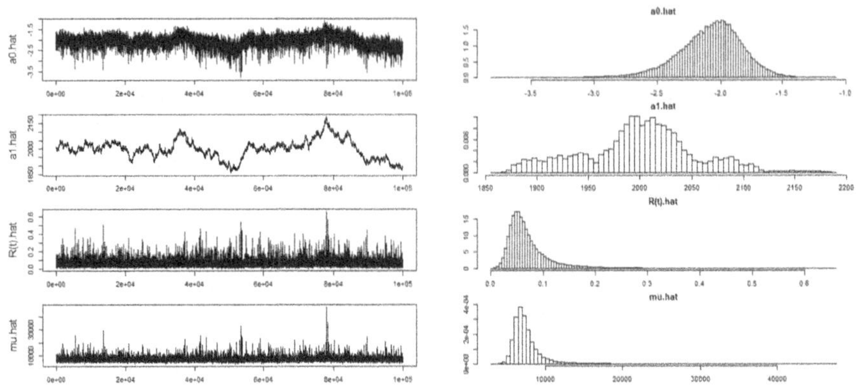

Fig. 2 Trace plots (left) and histograms (right) of posterior samples of $a_0, a_1, R(t)$ and μ generated from Metropolis–Hastings algorithm for Jeffreys prior

Table 5 Estimates of the model parameters $(\hat{a}_0, \hat{a}_1)$, the reliability at mission time $t = 20{,}000$ h, $\hat{p}(t)$, and the mean lifetime, $\hat{\mu}$, under the normal operating condition of $x_0 = 293K$ for data presented in Table 4

Method	$\hat{a}_0$	$\hat{a}_1$	$\hat{p}(t)$	$\hat{\mu}$
MLE	−0.3832	2703	0.2612	14897
π_N	−2.2562	1938	0.0666	7304
π_J	−2.0807	1999	0.0723	7546

in Table 5. In addition, the potential scale reduction factor (PSRF) proposed by Brooks and Gelman [7] is useful to measure the convergence of posterior samples. In general, values of the factor below 1.1 are acceptable. The values of the factor for the posterior samples of $\theta = (a_0, a_1)$ under normal and Jeffreys priors are (1.001, 1.090) and (1.002, 1.005), respectively. Moreover, as the number of samples is small, the maximum likelihood estimates and the Bayesian estimates of the parameters of interest are not similar.

7 Concluding Remarks

In this chapter, we have studied SSALTs for one-shot devices in a Bayesian framework with normal (subjective) and Jeffreys (objective) priors. The exponential distributions with cumulative exposure models are considered in this chapter. The Metropolis–Hastings algorithm is employed to approximate the joint posterior density of the model parameters $\theta = (a_0, a_1)$. Simulation studies were carried out to evaluate the performance of the Bayesian estimation of the model parameters, the reliability, and the mean lifetime under the normal operating condition in terms of bias and RMSE. The numerical results suggest normal prior for the estimation of the parameters of interest. Besides, simple SSALTs with two stress levels are recommended for exponential distributions as SSALTs with more stress levels may not possess a higher statistical efficiency of the estimation.

Moreover, it is of great interest to extend the exponential distributions to more general and flexible distributions with scale and shape parameters, namely Weibull, gamma, log-normal distributions for SSALTs with $I \geq 2$ stress levels. These distributions are also widely used in reliability studies. However, if both scale and shape parameters are related to the stress levels, there are 4 model parameters in the joint posterior density to be estimated. Jeffreys prior involves the determinant of a 4-by-4 matrix, and thus it might not be easy to derive. Instead, normal prior is easier to be implemented for those flexible distributions.

Besides, the development of optimal designs of SSALTs is another important topic in reliability studies. The simulation results show that simple SSALTs with two stress levels have a higher statistical efficiency of the estimation than SSALTs with three stress levels in the considered situations. However, decision variables, including the number of stress levels (I), stress levels (x_i), inspection times (τ_i), and allocation of the devices (K_i), can greatly affect the statistical efficiency of the estimation. In line with [20], it is therefore important to develop optimal designs of SSALTs with more than two stress levels for one-shot devices.

Acknowledgments This work was supported by a grant from the Research Grants Council of the Hong Kong Special Administrative Region, China (Project No. [T32-101/15-R]), and the Education University of Hong Kong (Ref. IDS-2 2019, MIT/SGA05/19-20).

References

1. Balakrishnan, N., Ling, M.H.: EM algorithm for one-shot device testing under the exponential distribution. Comp. Stat. Data Anal. **56**, 502–509 (2012)
2. Balakrishnan, N., Ling, M.H.: Expectation maximization algorithm for one shot device accelerated life testing with Weibull lifetimes, and variable parameters over stress. IEEE Trans. Reliab. **62**, 537–551 (2013)
3. Balakrishnan, N., Ling, M.H.: Gamma lifetimes and one-shot device testing analysis. Reliab. Eng. Syst. Saf. **126**, 54–64 (2014)
4. Balakrishnan, N., Ling, M.H., So, H.Y.: Accelerated Life Testing of One-Shot Devices: Data Collection and Analysis. John Wiley & Sons, Hoboken (2021)
5. Berger, J.O.: Statistical Decision Theory and Bayesian Analysis (2nd edn.) Springer, New York (1985)
6. Bhattacharyya, G.K., Soejoeti, Z.A.: A tampered failure rate model for step-stress accelerated life test. Commun. Stat. Theory Methods **18**, 1627–1643 (1989)
7. Brooks, S.P., Gelman, A.: General methods for monitoring convergence of iterative simulations. J. Comput. Graph. Stat. **7**, 434–455 (1998)
8. Cheng, Y., Elsayed, E.A.: Reliability modeling and prediction of systems with mixture of units. IEEE Trans. Reliab. **65**, 914–928 (2016)
9. Cheng, Y., Elsayed, E.A.: Reliability modeling of mixtures of one-shot units under thermal cyclic stresses. Reliab. Eng. Syst. Safe. **167**, 58–66 (2017)
10. Cheng, Y., Elsayed, E.A.: Reliability modeling and optimization of operational use of one-shot units. Reliab. Eng. Syst. Safe. **176**, 27–36 (2018)

11. Coolen, F., Newby, M.: Bayesian reliability analysis with imprecise prior probabilities. Reliab. Eng. Syst. Safe. **43**, 75–85 (1994)
12. DeGroot, M.H., Goel, P.K.: Bayesian estimation and optimal design in partially accelerated life test. Nav. Res. Logist. **26**, 223–235 (1979)
13. Escobar, L.A., Meeker, W.Q.: A review of accelerated test model. Stat. Sci. **21**, 552–577 (2006)
14. Fan, T.H., Balakrishnan, N., Chang, C.C.: The Bayesian approach for highly reliable electro-explosive devices using one-shot device testing. J. Stat. Comput. Simul. **79**, 1143–1154 (2009)
15. Hamada, M.S., Wilson, A., Reese, C.S., Martz, H.: Bayesian Reliability. Springer Science & Business Media, Berlin (2008)
16. Hastings, W.K. Monte Carlo sampling methods using Markov chains and their application. Biometrika **57**, 97–109 (1970)
17. LeSage, J.P.: Bayesian estimation of limited dependent variable spatial autoregressive models. Geogr. Anal. **32**, 19–35 (2010)
18. Ling, M.H., Ng, H.K.T., Tsui, K.L.: Bayesian and likelihood inferences on remaining useful life in two-phase degradation models under gamma process. Reliab. Eng. Syst. Safe. **184**, 77–85 (2019)
19. Ling, M.H.: Optimal design of simple step-stress accelerated life tests for one-shot devices under exponential distributions. Probab. Eng. Inf. Sci. **33**, 121–135 (2019)
20. Ling, M.H., Hu, X.W.: Optimal design of simple step-stress accelerated life tests for one-shot devices under Weibull distributions. Reliab. Eng. Syst. Safe. **193**, 106630 (2020)
21. Martza, H.F., Wailera, R.A.: Bayesian reliability analysis of complex series/parallel systems of binomial subsystems and components. Technometrics **32**, 407–416 (1990)
22. McLachlan, G.J., Krishnan, T.: The EM Algorithm and Extensions (2nd edn.) John Wiley & Sons, Hoboken, (2008)
23. Meeker, W.Q., Escobar, L.A. Lu, C.J.: Accelerated degradation tests: modeling and analysis. Technometrics **40**, 89–99 (1998)
24. Metropolis, N., Rosenbluth, A.W., Rosenbluth, M.N., Teller, A.H., Teller, E.: Equation of state calculations by fast computing machines. J. Chem. Phys. **21**, 1087–1092 (1953)
25. Mun, B.M., Lee, C., Jang, S.G., Ryu, B.T., Bae, S.J.: A Bayesian approach for predicting functional reliability of one-shot devices. Int. J. Ind. Eng. Comput. **26**, 71–82 (2019)
26. Nelson, W.B.: Accelerated life testing – step-stress models and data analyses. IEEE Trans. Reliab. **29**, 103–108 (1980)
27. Nelson, W.B.: Accelerated Modeling - Statistical Models, Test Plans, and Data analyses. John Wiley & Sons, Hoboken (2009)
28. Sharma, R., Upadhyay, S.K.: A hierarchical Bayes analysis for one-shot device testing experiment under the assumption of exponentiality. Commun. Stat. Simul. Comput. **47**, 1297–1314 (2018)
29. Wang, W.D., Kececioglu, D.B.: Fitting the Weibull log-linear model to accelerated life-test data. IEEE Trans. Reliab. **49**, 217–223 (2000)
30. Wu, S.J., Hsu, C.C., Huang, S.R.: Optimal designs and reliability sampling plans for one-shot devices with cost considerations. Reliab. Eng. Syst. Safe. **197**, 106795 (2020)
31. Yates, S.W., Mosleh, A.: A Bayesian approach to reliability demonstration for aerospace systems. In: Reliability and Maintainability Symposium, pp. 611–617 (2006)
32. Yun, W.Y., Han, Y.J., Kim, H.W.: Simulation-based inspection policies for a one-shot system in storage over a finite time span. Commun. Stat. Simul. Comput. **43**, 1979–2003 (2014)
33. Zhao, Q.Q., Yun, W.Y.: Determining the inspection intervals for one-shot systems with support equipment. Reliab. Eng. Syst. Safe. **169**, 63–75 (2018)
34. Zhao, Q.Q., Yun, W.Y.: Storage availability of one-shot system under periodic inspection considering inspection error. Reliab. Eng. Syst. Safe. **186**, 120–133 (2019)
35. Zheng, J., Li, Y., Wang, J., Shiju, E., Li, X.: Accelerated thermal aging of grease-based magnetorheological fluids and their lifetime prediction. Mat. Res. Exp. **5**, 085702 (2018).

Bayesian Estimation of Stress–Strength Parameter for Moran–Downton Bivariate Exponential Distribution Under Progressive Type II Censoring

Yu-Jau Lin, Yuhlong Lio, Hon Keung Tony Ng, and Liang Wang

Abstract In the stress–strength model, the estimation of the probability $\delta = \Pr(X < Y)$ is one of the important issues. In this chapter, Bayesian estimation of δ under correlated progressively type II censored sample from the Moran–Downton bivariate exponential (DBVE) distribution is investigated. The Markov-Chain Monte Carlo (MCMC) method is applied to find the Bayesian estimate of δ. An extensive simulation study is conducted to demonstrate the performance of the developed methods. Finally, the proposed approach is applied to a bivariate data set for illustration.

1 Introduction

In the context of reliability and medical studies, stress–strength models have received much attention for many years. The stress–strength models can also be applied to different fields such as engineering, medicine, quality control, and so on. Among them, the quantity $\delta = \Pr(X < Y)$ is of interest, where X and Y are random variables that represent lifetimes. For example, in biometry, let X and Y represent the remaining lifetimes when patients are treated with drug A and

Y.-J. Lin (✉)
Applied Mathematics Department, Chung Yuan Christian University, Taoyuan City, Taiwan
e-mail: yujaulin@cycu.edu.tw

Y. Lio
Department of Mathematical Sciences, University of South Dakota, Vermillion, SD, USA
e-mail: Yuhlong.Lio@usd.edu

H. K. T. Ng
Department of Mathematical Sciences, Bentley University, Waltham, MA, USA
e-mail: ngh@mail.smu.edu

L. Wang
School of Mathematics, Yunnan Normal University, Kunming, P. R. China
e-mail: liang610112@163.com

Y. Lio et al. (eds.), *Bayesian Inference and Computation in Reliability and Survival Analysis*, Emerging Topics in Statistics and Biostatistics,
https://doi.org/10.1007/978-3-030-88658-5_2

drug B, respectively. Then, the question about the probability $\delta \geq 1/2$ is crucial because it can be used to choose the treatment for a patient in between drug A and drug B. In engineering and reliability studies, δ may represent the probability that the strength of a component Y exceeds the stress X for external factors. When X and Y are independent [8] provided an interesting connection between δ and the classical Mann–Whitney statistic. Since then, the estimation of δ has received considerable attention in the statistical literature and has been investigated under various distributions and life test settings, for example [1, 3, 12, 14, 20, 22–24, 30, 31, 33, 35–37] under complete random samples. The monograph presented by Kotz et al. [21] provided an excellent review of the development of the estimation of $\delta = \Pr(X < Y)$ up to the year 2003. Because the subject could be lost or have a long lifetime due to the technology advancement, collecting a random sample of lifetimes from the life test experiment could be difficult. Recently, more research work has adopted many different methodologies to accommodate this drawback. For example [18] studied the statistical inference of δ under truncated exponentially distributed data. Saracoglu and Kuş [32] investigated statistical inference for δ based on progressively censored data. Lio and Tsai [26] discussed estimates of δ for Burr-XII distribution based on progressively first failure-censored samples. Saracoglu et al. [34] studied the estimation problem of δ based on progressively type II censored samples from two independent exponential distributions. Genç [14] also studied the estimation of δ based on left-censored sample from Topp–Leone distributions. Note that all these aforementioned papers assumed X and Y are independent.

To shorten the time needed and/or to save the cost of a life testing experiment, censoring is one of the commonly used techniques, and a progressive type II censoring scheme with a fixed number of observed failures can be considered. The progressive type II censoring can be implemented as follows. Suppose n items are placed on the life test at the same initial time, and a prefixed value $m < n$ is the number of observed failures. Then, at the time of the jth failure, R_j surviving items are randomly removed from the experiment for $j = 1, 2, \cdots, m$, where $R_j, j = 1, 2, \cdots, m$ are pre-specified values with $\sum_{j=1}^{m} R_j = n - m$. Statistical inference and reliability analysis based on progressively type II censored samples have long been studied. For comprehensive reviews of the theory and applications of progressive censoring, the readers may refer to the review papers by Balakrishnan [4], the articles by Cramer [9] and Ng [29], and the two books on progressive censoring by Balakrishnan and Aggarwala [5] and Balakrishnan and Cramer [3].

If the random vector (X, Y) follows the three-parameter Moran–Downton bivariate exponential (DBVE) distribution with parameters μ_1, μ_2, and ρ, denoted as DBVE(μ_1, μ_2, ρ), the joint probability density function (PDF) is given by

$$f(x, y) = \frac{\mu_1 \mu_2}{1-\rho} \exp\left\{-\frac{\mu_1 x + \mu_2 y}{1-\rho}\right\} I_0 \left\{\frac{2(\mu_1 x \mu_2 y \rho)^{1/2}}{1-\rho}\right\}, \tag{1}$$

where $\mu_1 > 0$, $\mu_2 > 0$, $0 \leq \rho < 1$, and $I_0(z) = \sum_{r=0}^{\infty} (z/2)^{2r}/(r!)^2$ is the modified Bessel function of the first kind of order zero. In the DBVE distribution, $1/\mu_1$ and

$1/\mu_2$ are the marginal means of X and Y, respectively, and ρ is the *correlation* coefficient of X and Y. The DBVE distribution is useful in reliability theory for modeling the lifetimes of two dependent components. More details of the DBVE distribution will be discussed in Sect. 2. Based on the PDF of the DBVE distribution in Eq. (1), the stress–strength, $\delta = \Pr(X < Y)$, involves a double integral that consists of a Bessel function of first kind that can be represented as an infinite series. In this chapter, we study the statistical inference of δ based on progressively type II censored samples from the DBVE model.

The rest of this chapter is organized as follows. More details of the DBVE model and the likelihood function based on a progressively type II censored sample from the DBVE distribution are presented in Sect. 2. The Bayesian estimation of δ will be discussed in Sect. 3. A Monte Carlo simulation study to evaluate the performance of the estimation method is provided in Sect. 4. In Sect. 5, a numerical example generated from a real-world example is used to illustrate the methodology discussed in this chapter. Finally, concluding remarks are given in Sect. 6.

2 Model and Notations

Let $(X_i, Y_i), i = 1, 2, \cdots, n$, be independent and identically distributed random vectors that follow the DBVE(μ_1, μ_2, ρ) distribution with joint PDF in Eq. (1). The joint PDF of the DBVE(μ_1, μ_2, ρ) distribution was originally derived in a different form by Moran [28], and the form in Eq. (1) was derived by Downton [11] in a reliability context. Hence, this distribution is commonly called the Moran–Downton bivariate exponential distribution. The DBVE distribution can be considered as a special case of the bivariate gamma distribution proposed by Kibble [19]. It can be shown that X has a marginal exponential distribution with mean $1/\mu_1$, Y has a marginal exponential distribution with mean $1/\mu_2$, and ρ is the correlation coefficient between X and Y. The estimation of the parameter ρ has been studied by many authors. For example [2] derived the method of moment estimator for ρ through equating a population of mixed moments and sample mixed moments and suggested a modified method of moment estimator through a standard bias reduction method. They also suggested a bias-reduced estimator based on the sample correlation coefficient. Balakrishnan and Ng [7] modified the estimation procedures of [2] and derived an improved method of moment estimator by using the standard bias reduction method as well as the Jackknife method. These aforementioned estimation procedures for ρ were based on a complete sample.

An alternative way to express the joint PDF of the DBVE(μ_1, μ_2, ρ) distribution can be obtained by expanding the series $I_0(z)$ as

$$f(x, y) = \sum_{k=0}^{\infty} \pi(k, \rho) g_{k+1}(x; \mu_1/(1-\rho)) g_{k+1}(y; \mu_2/(1-\rho)), \quad (2)$$

where $g_{k+1}(x; b)$ is the PDF of a gamma random variable with a rate parameter b and a shape parameter $k+1$, denoted as Gamma($k+1, b$), i.e.,

$$g_{k+1}(x; b) = \frac{b^{k+1}}{\Gamma(k+1)} x^k e^{-bx}, x > 0,$$

where $\Gamma(z) = \int_0^\infty x^{z-1} e^{-x} dx$ is the complete gamma function, and $\pi(k, \rho) = (1-\rho)(\rho)^k, k = 0, 1, 2, \ldots$ is the probability mass function of a geometric random variable. Let K be the random variable that has a probability mass function $\pi(k, \rho)$. Then, conditional on $K = k$, X and Y are independent gamma random variates with the common shape parameter $k+1$ and rate parameters $\mu_1/(1-\rho)$ and $\mu_2/(1-\rho)$, respectively. This property has been used in the computer algorithm for generating random variates from the DBVE(μ_1, μ_2, ρ) distribution (see, for example [11]).

Based on the PDF in Eq. (2), the stress–strength parameter $\delta = \Pr(X < Y)$ can be derived as

$$\begin{aligned}
\delta &= \int_0^\infty \int_x^\infty \sum_{k=0}^\infty (1.0-\rho)\rho^k g_{k+1}\left(x, \frac{\mu_1}{1.0-\rho}\right) g_{k+1}\left(y, \frac{\mu_2}{1.0-\rho}\right) dy dx \\
&= \sum_{k=0}^\infty (1.0-\rho)\rho^k \int_0^\infty \int_x^\infty \frac{b_1^{k+1}}{\Gamma(k+1)} x^k e^{-b_1 x} \frac{b_2^{k+1}}{\Gamma(k+1)} y^k e^{-b_2 y} dy dx \\
&= \sum_{k=0}^\infty (1.0-\rho)\rho^k \int_0^\infty \frac{b_1^{k+1}}{\Gamma(k+1)} x^k e^{-b_1 x} \int_x^\infty \frac{b_2^{k+1}}{\Gamma(k+1)} y^k e^{-b_2 y} dy dx \\
&= \sum_{k=0}^\infty (1.0-\rho)\rho^k \int_0^\infty \frac{b_1^{k+1}}{\Gamma(k+1)} x^k e^{-b_1 x} e^{-b_2 x} \sum_{i=0}^k \frac{b_2^i x^i}{\Gamma(i+1)} dx \\
&= \sum_{k=0}^\infty (1.0-\rho)\rho^k \frac{b_1^{k+1}}{\Gamma(k+1)} \sum_{i=0}^k \frac{b_2^i}{\Gamma(i+1)} \int_0^\infty x^{k+i} e^{-(b_1+b_2)y} dx \\
&= \sum_{k=0}^\infty (1.0-\rho)\rho^k \frac{b_1^{k+1}}{\Gamma(k+1)} \sum_{i=0}^k \frac{b_2^i}{\Gamma(i+1)} \frac{\Gamma(i+k+1)}{(b_1+b_2)^{i+k+1}} \\
&= \sum_{k=0}^\infty \frac{(1.0-\rho)\rho^k}{\Gamma(k+1)} \frac{b_1^{k+1}}{(b_1+b_2)^{k+1}} \sum_{i=0}^k \frac{\Gamma(i+k+1)}{\Gamma(i+1)} \frac{b_2^i}{(b_1+b_2)^i} \\
&= \frac{(1.0-\rho)b_1}{b_1+b_2} \sum_{k=0}^\infty \frac{\rho^k b_1^k}{\Gamma(k+1)(b_1+b_2)^k} \sum_{i=0}^k \frac{\Gamma(i+k+1)}{\Gamma(i+1)} \frac{b_2^i}{(b_1+b_2)^i} \\
&= \frac{(1.0-\rho)\mu_1}{\mu_1+\mu_2} \sum_{k=0}^\infty \frac{\rho^k \mu_1^k}{\Gamma(k+1)(\mu_1+\mu_2)^k} \sum_{i=0}^k \frac{\Gamma(i+k+1)}{\Gamma(i+1)} \frac{\mu_2^i}{(\mu_1+\mu_2)^i},
\end{aligned} \tag{3}$$

where

$$b_1 = \frac{\mu_1}{1.0 - \rho}, \quad b_2 = \frac{\mu_2}{1.0 - \rho}, \text{ and } \frac{b_1}{b_1 + b_2} = \frac{\mu_1}{\mu_1 + \mu_2}.$$

For a given random sample of size n, $(X_i, Y_i), i = 1, 2, \cdots, n$, from the DBVE$(\mu_1, \mu_2, \rho)$, we denote $\underline{t}_{i:n} = (X_{i:n}, Y_{[i:n]}), i = 1, 2, \ldots, n$, where $X_{1:n} \leq X_{2:n} \leq \cdots \leq X_{n:n}$ are the order statistics of the X sample $X_1, X_2, \ldots, X_n$ and $Y_{[i:n]}$ is the corresponding value of Y associated with $X_{i:n}$. Prior to the experiment, a prefixed number of pairs to be observed $(m < n)$ and the progressive censoring scheme $(R_1, R_2, \cdots, R_m)$ are provided. Considering the ordering based on the X sample, at the jth ordered observed pair $(X_{j:m:n}, Y_{[j:m:n]})$, $R_j > 0$ randomly selected pairs from unobserved pairs are removed from the experiment, where $X_{j:m:n} < X_{j+1:m:n}$ for $j = 1, 2, \cdots, m-1$. The observed m pairs, $(X_{j:m:n}, Y_{[j:m:n]}), j = 1, 2, \cdots, m$, are called progressively censored samples of size m from n systems under a progressively type II censored life test with censoring scheme $(R_1, R_2, \cdots, R_m)$. Let $D = \{(X_{j:m:n}, Y_{[j:m:n]}, R_j), j = 1, 2, \cdots, m\}$, be the observed progressively type II censored sample. The likelihood function based on the progressively type II censored sample D can be expressed as

$$L(\mu_1, \mu_2, \rho; D) \propto \left\{ \left(\frac{\mu_1\mu_2}{1-\rho}\right)^m \exp\left[-\sum_{j=1}^{m} \frac{\mu_1 X_{j:m:n} + \mu_2 Y_{[j:m:n]}}{1-\rho}\right] \prod_{j=0}^{m} I_0 \right.$$
$$\left. \times \left[\frac{2(\mu_1 X_{j:m:n}\mu_2 Y_{[i:m:n]})^{1/2}}{1-\rho}\right]\right\} \times \prod_{j=1}^{m} \exp(-R_j \mu_1 X_{j:m:n}). \tag{4}$$

When $R_j = 0$ for $j = 1, 2, \cdots, m-1$ and $R_m = n - m$, the progressively type II censored sample reduces to the conventional type II right-censored sample. Based on the conventional type II right-censored sample, He and Nagaraja [16] developed the method of moment estimators for the correlation parameter ρ by generalizing the estimators proposed by Al-Saadi and Young [2] and Balakrishnan and Ng [7]. Lin et al. [25] studied the Bayesian estimation of the parameters μ_1, μ_2, and ρ based on a type II right-censored sample.

3 Bayesian Framework

Under the Bayesian framework, we consider that the unknown parameters μ_1, μ_2, and ρ are independent, $\mu_l, l = 1, 2$, has a prior gamma distribution with PDF

$$g_l(\mu_l; \alpha_l, \lambda_l) = \frac{1}{\Gamma(\alpha_l)\lambda_l^{\alpha_l}} \mu_l^{\alpha_l - 1} \exp\left(-\frac{\mu_l}{\lambda_l}\right), \quad \mu_l > 0, \tag{5}$$

where $\alpha_l > 0$ and $\lambda_l > 0$ are hyper-parameters, and ρ has a prior beta distribution with probability density function,

$$h(\rho;\beta_1,\beta_2)=\frac{\Gamma(\beta_1+\beta_2)}{\Gamma(\beta_1)\Gamma(\beta_2)}\rho^{\beta_1-1}(1-\rho)^{\beta_2-1},\quad 0<\rho\leq 1, \tag{6}$$

where $\beta_1 > 0$ and $\beta_2 > 0$ are hyper-parameters. It should be mentioned that Iliopoulos et al. [17] and [25] also used the same independent priors for the population parameters in the DBEV distribution.

Combining Eqs. (4), (5), and (6), the joint posterior PDF of μ_1, μ_2, and ρ, based on a progressively type II right-censored sample, can be expressed as

$$\begin{aligned}\Pi(\mu_1,\mu_2,\rho|D)\propto&\left\{\left(\frac{\mu_1\mu_2}{1-\rho}\right)^m\exp\left[-\sum_{j=1}^{m}\frac{\mu_1X_{j:m:n}+\mu_2Y_{[j:m:n]}}{1-\rho}\right]\prod_{j=0}^{m}I_0\right.\\&\left.\times\left[\frac{2(\mu_1X_{j:m:n}\mu_2Y_{[i:m:n]})^{1/2}}{1-\rho}\right]\right\}\prod_{j=1}^{m}\exp(-R_j\mu_1X_{j:m:n})\\&\times g_1(\mu_1;\alpha_1,\lambda_1)g_2(\mu_2;\alpha_2,\lambda_2)h(\rho;\beta_1,\beta_2).\end{aligned} \tag{7}$$

Hence, the marginal posterior PDFs of μ_1, μ_2, and ρ given the progressively type II right-censored data D are, respectively,

$$\Pi_1(\mu_1|D)=\int\int\Pi(\mu_1,\mu_2,\rho|D)d\mu_2d\rho, \tag{8}$$

$$\Pi_2(\mu_2|D)=\int\int\Pi(\mu_1,\mu_2,\rho|D)d\mu_1d\rho, \tag{9}$$

and

$$\Pi_3(\rho|D)=\int\int\Pi(\mu_1,\mu_2,\rho|D)d\mu_1d\mu_2. \tag{10}$$

Additionally, the full conditional posterior PDF of μ_1, given μ_2 and ρ, is

$$\begin{aligned}\Pi_1(\mu_1|\mu_2,\rho,D)\propto&\left(\frac{\mu_1}{1-\rho}\right)^m\exp\left(-\sum_{i=1}^{m}\frac{\mu_1X_{i:m:n}}{1-\rho}\right)\prod_{i=1}^{m}I_0\\&\times\left\{\frac{2(\mu_1X_{i:m:n}\mu_2Y_{[i:m:n]}\rho)^{1/2}}{1-\rho}\right\}\\&\times\prod_{i=1}^{m}\exp(-R_i\mu_1X_{j:m:n})g_1(\mu_1;\alpha_1,\lambda_1),\end{aligned} \tag{11}$$

the full conditional posterior probability density function of μ_2, given μ_1 and ρ, is

$$\Pi_2(\mu_2|\mu_1, \rho, D) \propto \left(\frac{\mu_2}{1-\rho}\right)^m \exp\left(-\sum_{i=1}^{m} \frac{\mu_2 Y_{[i:m:n]}}{1-\rho}\right) \prod_{i=1}^{m} I_0 \times \left\{\frac{2(\mu_1 X_{i:m:n} \mu_2 Y_{[i:m:n]}\rho)^{1/2}}{1-\rho}\right\} \times g_2(\mu_2; \alpha_2, \lambda_2), \tag{12}$$

and the full conditional posterior probability density function of ρ, given μ_1 and μ_2, is

$$\Pi_3(\rho|\mu_1, \mu_2, D) \propto \left(\frac{\mu_1\mu_2}{1-\rho}\right)^m \exp\left(-\sum_{i=1}^{m} \frac{\mu_1 X_{i:m:n} + \mu_2 Y_{[i:m:n]}}{1-\rho}\right) \prod_{i=1}^{m} I_0 \times \left\{\frac{2(\mu_1 X_{i:m:n} \mu_2 Y_{[i:m:n]}\rho)^{1/2}}{1-\rho}\right\} \times h(\rho; \beta_1, \beta_2). \tag{13}$$

All these posterior PDFs for the parameters μ_1, μ_2, and ρ are not in closed forms, and numerical integration may not be applied to approximate their values either. Hence, in order to obtain the Bayesian estimates, Markov-Chain Monte Carlo (MCMC) method through the application of the Metropolis–Hastings (M–H) algorithm [15, 27]) via the Gibbs scheme [13] can be utilized to draw the samples of μ_1, μ_2, and ρ, respectively.

3.1 A Markov-Chain Monte Carlo (MCMC) Process

The Markov chain $\{\theta^{(\ell)}, \ell = 1, 2, \ldots\}$ of a given parameter, θ, can be constructed by applying the Metropolis–Hastings (M–H) algorithm stated as follows. Let $q(\theta^{(*)}|\theta^{(\ell-1)})$ be a proposed conditional transition probability density function for $\theta^{(*)}$, given $\theta^{(\ell-1)}$. Given the current state value, $\theta^{(\ell-1)}$, of the parameter θ, $\theta^{(*)}$ is a candidate value of the parameter θ in the next state that can be generated by $q(\theta^{(*)}|\theta^{(\ell-1)})$. Then, $\theta^{(*)}$ is accepted as the value of the next state, $\theta^{(\ell)}$, with a probability of $\min\left\{1, \frac{\Pi(\theta^{(*)}|D)q(\theta^{(\ell)}|\theta^{(*)})}{\Pi(\theta^{(\ell)}|D)q(\theta^{(*)}|\theta^{(\ell)})}\right\}$. If $\theta^{(*)}$ is rejected as the value of the next state, then the next state $\theta^{(\ell)} = \theta^{(\ell-1)}$. In this chapter, we let $q_1(\mu_1^{(b)}|\mu_1^{(a)})$, $q_2(\mu_2^{(b)}|\mu_2^{(a)})$, and $q_3(\rho^{(b)}|\rho^{(a)})$ be the transition probabilities from $\mu_1^{(a)}$ to $\mu_1^{(b)}$, from $\mu_2^{(a)}$ to $\mu_2^{(b)}$, and from $\rho^{(a)}$ to $\rho^{(b)}$, respectively. The Markov chain for $\{\mu_1^{(\ell)}, \mu_2^{(\ell)}, \rho^{(\ell)}\}$ can be generated through the following iterative process:

1. Generate $\mu_1^{(*)}$ from $q_1(\mu_1^{(*)}|\mu_1^{(\ell)})$ and generate u_1 from uniform distribution over $(0, 1)$ interval independently, and set

$$\mu_1^{(\ell+1)} = \begin{cases} \mu_1^{(*)} \text{ if } u_1 \le \min\left\{1, \frac{\Pi_1(\mu_1^{(*)}|D,\mu_2^{(\ell)},\rho^{(\ell)})q_1(\mu_1^{(\ell)}|\mu_1^{(*)})}{\Pi_1(\mu_1^{(\ell)}|D,\mu_2^{(\ell)},\rho^{(\ell)})q_1(\mu_1^{(*)}|\mu_1^{(\ell)})}\right\}, \\ \mu_1^{(\ell)} \text{ otherwise.} \end{cases}$$

2. Generate $\mu_2^{(*)}$ from $q_2(\mu_2^{(*)}|\mu_2^{(\ell)})$ and generate u_2 from uniform distribution over $(0, 1)$ interval independently, and set

$$\mu_2^{(\ell+1)} = \begin{cases} \mu_2^{(*)} \text{ if } u_2 \le \min\left\{1, \frac{\Pi_2(\mu_2^{(*)}|D,\mu_1^{(\ell+1)},\rho^{(\ell)})q_2(\mu_2^{(\ell)}|\mu_2^{(*)})}{\Pi_2(\mu_2^{(\ell)}|D,\mu_1^{(\ell+1)},\rho^{(\ell)})q_2(\mu_2^{(*)}|\mu_2^{(\ell)})}\right\}, \\ \mu_2^{(\ell)} \text{ otherwise.} \end{cases}$$

3. Generate $\rho^{(*)}$ from $q_3(\rho^{(*)}|\rho^{(\ell)})$ and generate u_3 from uniform distribution over $(0, 1)$ interval independently, and set

$$\rho^{(\ell+1)} = \begin{cases} \rho^{(*)} \text{ if } u_3 \le \min\left\{1, \frac{\Pi_3(\rho^{(*)}|D,\mu_1^{(\ell+1)},\mu_2^{(\ell)})q_3(\rho^{(\ell)}|\rho^{(*)})}{\Pi_3(\rho^{(\ell)}|D,\mu_1^{(\ell+1)},\mu_2^{(\ell+1)})q_3(\rho^{(*)}|\rho^{(\ell)})}\right\}, \\ \rho^{(\ell)} \text{ otherwise.} \end{cases}$$

Starting with initial values, $\mu_1^{(0)}$, $\mu_2^{(0)}$, and $\rho^{(0)}$, the above iterative process is running through a huge number of periods (says, N). The empirical distributions of μ_1, μ_2, and ρ could be described by the realizations of μ_1, μ_2, and ρ after a burn-in period, N_b. The Bayes estimators of μ_1, μ_2, and ρ can be approximated based on the values of $\left\{\mu_1^{(\ell)}|\ell = N_b + 1, \ldots, N\right\}$, $\left\{\mu_2^{(\ell)}|\ell = N_b + 1, \ldots, N\right\}$, and $\left\{\rho^{(\ell)}|j = N_b + 1, \ldots, N\right\}$, respectively. For instance, if we consider the squared error loss, then the Bayesian estimates of μ_1, μ_2, and ρ are the means of $\left\{\mu_1^{(\ell)}|\ell = N_b + 1, \ldots, N\right\}$, $\left\{\mu_2^{(\ell)}|\ell = N_b + 1, \ldots, N\right\}$, and $\left\{\rho^{(\ell)}|\ell = N_b + 1, \ldots, N\right\}$, respectively; and if we consider the absolute value of error loss, then the Bayesian estimates of μ_1, μ_2, and ρ are the medians of the empirical distributions of $\left\{\mu_1^{(\ell)}|\ell = N_b + 1, \ldots, N\right\}$, $\left\{\mu_2^{(\ell)}|\ell = N_b + 1, \ldots, N\right\}$, and $\left\{\rho^{(j)}|\ell = N_b + 1, \ldots, N\right\}$, respectively. It should be mentioned that $\Pi_1(\mu_1|D, \mu_2, \rho)$, $\Pi_2(\mu_2|D, \mu_1, \rho)$, and $\Pi_3(\rho^{(*)}|D, \mu_1, \mu_2)$ can be replaced by $\Pi(\mu_1, \mu_2, \rho; D)$ during the implementation of Metropolis–Hastings algorithm. When the MCMC process is implemented based on non-informative priors (i.e., $g_l(\mu_l; \alpha_l, \lambda_l) \propto C$ for $l = 1, 2$ and $h(\rho; \beta_1, \beta_2) \propto C$, where C is a constant), the MCMC process will approach to the maximum likelihood estimates for the parameters μ_1 and μ_2 and ρ (see, for example [5]).

3.2 Plug-In Bayesian Estimate of δ

Under the Gibbs sampling scheme, the parameters, μ_1, μ_2 and ρ, are alternately updated by assuming the other parameters are fixed. The latent variable δ can be approximated by the MCMC samplers as the empirical distribution. Specifically, at the j-th Gibbs iteration, after $\mu_1^{(j)}$, $\mu_2^{(j)}$, and $\rho^{(j)}$ are generated by the procedure described in Sect. 3.1, the realization $\delta^{(j)}$ of δ can be calculated by plugging the parameters $\mu_1^{(j)}$, $\mu_2^{(j)}$, and $\rho^{(j)}$ into its closed-form formula in Eq. (3). If the loss function is the square error loss function, then the Bayesian estimate of δ is the sample mean of $\{\delta^{(\ell)}\}$ after the burn-in period N_b, i.e.,

$$\widehat{\delta} \approx \frac{1}{N - N_b} \sum_{j=N_b+1}^{N} \delta^{(j)}.$$

If the loss function is the absolute value of different loss function, then the Bayesian estimate of δ is the sample median of the empirical distribution of $\{\delta^{(\ell)}\}$ after the burn-in period N_b.

3.3 Mean-Value Monte Carlo Method

Instead of using the double sums of infinite series in Eq. (3), the latent parameter δ can be viewed as an expectation and approximated by the mean-value Monte Carlo method (as know as crude Monte Carlo method) using the proportion of $(X_i < Y_i)$ in a large random sample of (X_i, Y_i) from the DBVE distribution. Specifically,

$$\delta = \mathrm{E}(\mathbb{I}_{\{X<Y\}}) = \int_0^{\infty}\int_0^{y} \frac{\mu_1\mu_2}{1-\rho} \exp\left\{-\frac{\mu_1 x + \mu_2 y}{1-\rho}\right\} I_0\left\{\frac{2(\mu_1 x \mu_2 y \rho)^{1/2}}{1-\rho}\right\} dxdy,$$

where $\mathbb{I}_{\{A\}}$ is an indicator function defined as

$$\mathbb{I}_{\{A\}} = \begin{cases} 1, & \text{if } A \text{ is true;} \\ 0, & \text{otherwise.} \end{cases}$$

By the weak law of large number, δ can be approximated by using Monte Carlo simulation method as

$$\frac{1}{N_1}\sum_{k=1}^{N_1} \mathbb{I}_{\{X_k<Y_k\}} \longrightarrow \delta = \mathrm{E}(\mathbb{I}_{\{X<Y\}}) \text{ when } N_1 \to \infty. \tag{14}$$

Hence, at the j-th Gibbs iteration, the sample point of $\delta^{(j)}$ can be approximated by the mean of $\mathbb{I}_{\{X_k<Y_k\}}$, $k = 1, 2, \cdots, N_1$, where (X_k, Y_k) are generated from DBVE$(\mu_1^{(j)}, \mu_1^{(j)}, \rho^{(j)})$. The Bayesian estimate of δ is the mean of empirical distribution from $\delta^{(j)}$ after burn-in period N_b if the loss function is the square error loss function. If the error loss function is an absolute value of error, then the Bayesian estimate of δ is the median of the empirical distribution from $\delta^{(j)}$ after burn-in period N_b.

3.4 Importance Sampling Estimation

The quantity of interest, $\delta = \Pr(X < Y)$, can also be estimated by importance sampling technique, especially when the true value of δ is small (says, < 0.1) or stable estimates cannot be obtained based on the closed form of δ and the Monte Carlo method. For important sampling, suppose we can easily generate a bivariate sample (X_i^*, Y_i^*), $i = 1, 2, \ldots, n$, from a distribution with joint PDF $g^*(x, y)$ with the same support as the DBVE distribution (i.e., $x > 0$ and $y > 0$); then δ can be expressed as

$$\begin{aligned}
\delta = \mathrm{E}(\mathbb{I}_{\{X<Y\}}) &= \int_0^\infty \int_0^y f(x, y)dxdy \\
&= \int_0^\infty \int_0^y \left[\frac{f(x, y)}{g^*(x, y)}\right] g^*(x, y)dxdy \\
&= \mathrm{E}\left[\mathbb{I}_{\{X^*<Y^*\}} \frac{f(X^*, Y^*)}{g^*(X^*, Y^*)}\right].
\end{aligned}$$

Hence, δ can be approximated by

$$\frac{1}{N_2}\sum_{k=1}^{N_2} \mathbb{I}_{\{x_k^*<y_k^*\}} \frac{f(x_k^*, y_k^*)}{g^*(x_k^*, y_k^*)} \longrightarrow \delta = \mathrm{E}\left[\mathbb{I}_{\{X^*<Y^*\}} \frac{f(X^*, Y^*)}{g^*(X^*, Y^*)}\right] \text{ when } N_2 \to \infty. \tag{15}$$

A possible choice of the distribution $g^*(x, y)$ for the purpose of estimating δ for the DBVE(μ_1, μ_2, ρ) distribution is $g^*(x, y) = g(x)g(y)$, where $g(x) = \mu_1 \exp(-\mu_1 x)$, $x > 0$, and $g(y) = \mu_2 \exp(-\mu_2 y)$, $y > 0$.

4 Monte Carlo Simulation Study

In this section, a Monte Carlo simulation study is conducted to investigate the performance of the proposed estimation procedures for the parameters, μ_1, μ_2, ρ, and δ based on progressively type II censored sample D from DBVE$(\mu_1, \mu_2,$

ρ) distribution. We generate the progressively type II censored samples from the DBVE(μ_1, μ_2, ρ) distribution with different settings of (μ_1, μ_2, ρ), sample sizes $(n, m) = (20, 5), (30, 15), (50, 20), (50, 30)$, and different censoring schemes. Two types of prior distributions that include non-informative and informative priors are used. The informative priors used for the study have prior distributions to be gamma distributions for μ_1 and μ_2 and the prior distribution for ρ to be beta distribution with parameters not equal to 1. Moreover, informative priors have been selected to have a mean equal to the corresponding parameters and variance equal to 0.5. The non-informative prior distributions used for the study have all priors proportional to constant (Tables 1 and 2).

For given m, μ_1, μ_2, ρ, and progressive type II censoring scheme $(R_1, R_2, \cdots, R_m)$, a progressively type II censored sample D can be generated from the following algorithm:

Step 1. Generate an ordered random sample $\{(x_{j:n}, y_{[j:n]})\}_{j=1}^{n}$ from the target DBVE(μ_1, μ_2, ρ) distribution through Steps 2 and 3.

Step 2. Generate $(x_j, y_{[j]})$ by the following steps:

i. Generate k from geometric distribution with probability mass function $\pi(k, \rho) = (1 - \rho)(\rho)^k, k = 0, 1, 2, \ldots$.
ii. Generate x_j from Gamma $\left(k + 1, \frac{1-\rho}{\mu_1}\right)$.
iii. Generate $y_{[j]}$ Gamma $\left(k + 1, \frac{1-\rho}{\mu_2}\right)$.

Table 1 The observed progressively type II censored sample for the numerical example

X	Y	X	Y	X	Y	X	Y	X	Y	X	Y
0.75	0.75	0.85	0.85	1.38	1.38	1.65	1.65	2.05	3.98	2.58	2.58
2.98	2.98	3.43	3.43	3.88	6.43	4.22	9.48	5.52	11.27	5.78	25.98
6.42	15.08	6.42	6.42	6.85	34.58	7.05	7.05	7.23	9.68	7.78	7.78
8.98	8.98	9.05	9.05	10.15	10.15	10.35	10.35	10.57	14.28	10.85	38.07
13.8	49.75	14.58	14.58	14.58	20.57	15.53	15.53				

Table 2 Posterior means and 95% credible sets of the model parameters and the stress–strength parameter δ obtained by the plug-in method (SP), the mean-value Monte Carlo method (MC), and importance sampling (IM)

Parameter	Posterior mean	95% credible set
μ_1	0.0961	(0.0635, 0.1353)
μ_2	0.0594	(0.0386, 0.0847)
ρ	0.8391	(0.7054, 0.9254)
$\hat{\delta}_{SP}$	0.7458	(0.6201, 0.8353)
$\hat{\delta}_{MC}$	0.7603	(0.5900, 0.9000)
$\hat{\delta}_{IM}$	0.7604	(0.5144, 1.0000)

Step 3. Set $j = j + 1$, if $j \leq n$, and then go to Step 2; otherwise, move to Step 4 to obtain the progressively type II censored sample.

Step 4. Put $(x_j, y_{[j]})$, $j = 1, 2, 3, \cdots, n$ in ascending order according to x_j, $j = 1, 2, 3, \cdots, n$. At the j-th failure, $x_{j:m:n}$, δ_j $(j = 1, 2, \cdots, m)$ survival pairs are randomly removed. Then, $(x_{j:m:n}, y_{[j:m:n]})$, $j = 1, 2, \cdots, m$, is the progressively type II censored sample:

Given a simulated progressively type II censored sample, $N = 15{,}000$ MCMC for μ_1, μ_2, ρ, and δ are generated with burn-in period $N_b = 5000$. For the mean-value Monte Carlo method and importance sampling method described in Sects. 3.3 and 3.4, respectively, $N_1 = N_2 = 200$ samples are used to obtain an estimate of δ. The Monte Carlo simulation is run for 1000 times to obtain 1000 Bayesian estimates for μ_1, μ_2, ρ, and δ. The mean squared errors (MSE) and biases are calculated of the 1000 Bayesian estimates for μ_1, μ_2, ρ, and δ are computed. The simulation results are presented in Tables A.1, A.2, A.3, A.4, A.5, A.6, A.7, A.8, A.9, A.10, A.11, and A.12 in Appendix. From Tables A.1, A.2, A.3, A.4, A.5, A.6, A.7, A.8, A.9, A.10, A.11, and A.12, generally, informative prior could provide more accurate estimates than non-informative prior for a given simulation setting. However, when ρ is close to 0 or 1, informative prior does not necessarily provide more accurate estimates than the non-informative prior for a given simulation setting. When the number of test items increases, the more accurate the estimates provided by non-informative and information priors.

5 Numerical Example

In this section, a real data set obtained from the matches of the American Football League (National Football League) on three consecutive weekends in 1986. The data set was analyzed by Csorgo and Welsch [10] using the Marshall–Olkin bivariate exponential model. The sample size is $n = 42$. In the bivariate data set (X, Y), the variable X represents the game time to the first points scored by kicking the ball between goal posts and Y represents the game time by moving the ball into the end zone. For illustrative purpose, we obtain a progressively type II censored sample based on this data set with $m = 28$ and progressive censoring scheme $(R_1, R_2, \cdots, R_{28}) = (1, 0, 1, 0, 1, 0, \cdots, 1, 0)$. The smallest observation, $x_{1:28:42} = 0.75$, was the first observation. With $R_1 = 1$, an observation was randomly removed. The smallest observation of the rest test items, $x_{2:28:42} = 0.85$, was observed. With $\delta_2 = 0$, no test item was removed. After $x_{3:28:42} = 1.38$ was observed, an observation was randomly removed since $R_3 = 1$. The process continued until the last observation $x_{28:28:42} = 15.53$. The value $R_{28} = 0$ indicates no observation was left. The corresponding values $y_{[i:28:42]}$, $i = 1, 2, \cdots, 28$ were collected accordingly. The observed progressively type II censored sample is presented in Table 1.

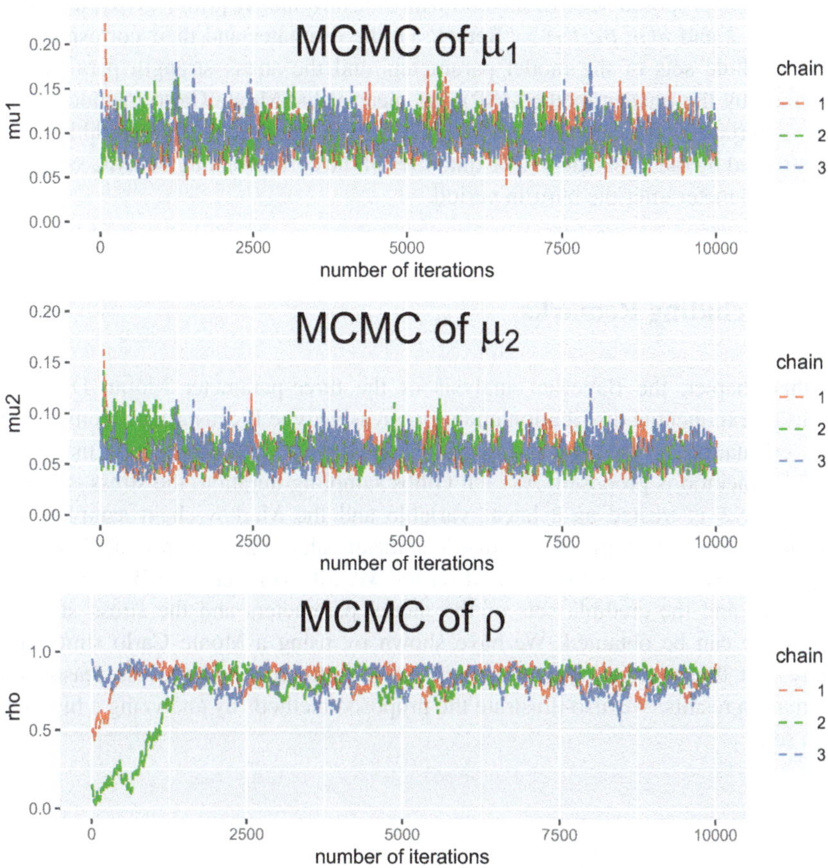

Fig. 1 The trace plots of MCMC samplers for the parameters μ_1, μ_2, and ρ

We use three different sets of initial values of μ_1, μ_2, and ρ for the Bayesian computation in order to obtain the MCMC samplers of the three parameters in the DBVE distribution:

- Chain 1: $\mu_1^{(0)} = 0.5$, $\mu_2^{(0)} = 0.5$, $\rho^{(0)} = 0.5$.
- Chain 2: $\mu_1^{(0)} = 0.05$, $\mu_2^{(0)} = 0.05$, $\rho^{(0)} = 0.15$.
- Chain 3: $\mu_1^{(0)} = 0.15$, $\mu_2^{(0)} = 0.05$, $\rho^{(0)} = 0.95$.

The trace plots of MCMC samplers for the parameters μ_1, μ_2, and ρ are presented in Fig. 1. The trace plots in Fig. 1 look stationary after the burn-in period around 2000 iterations.

Using the proposed MCMC method with non-informative priors: $g_i(\mu_i; \alpha_i, \lambda_i) \propto 1$, $i = 1, 2$ and $h(\rho; \beta_1, \beta_2) = \text{Beta}(1, 1)$, the estimates and their corresponding 95% credible sets of the model parameters and the stress–strength parameter δ obtained by the plug-in method (SP), the mean-value Monte Carlo method (MC), and importance sampling (IM) are summarized in Table 2. A 95% credible set is constructed by the 2.5% and 97.5% quantiles of the corresponding MCMC samplers of the parameter after the burn-in period.

6 Concluding Remarks

In this chapter, the Bayesian analysis of the three-parameter Moran–Downton bivariate exponential distribution under progressive type II censoring is considered. The estimation of the stress–strength parameter $\delta = \Pr(X < Y)$ using the MCMC method is proposed. At each Gibbs sampling iteration, the stress–strength parameter δ is treated as a latent variable and the Markov-chain samplers are constructed by the plug-in formula, the mean-value Monte Carlo method, and importance sampling method. Based on the MCMC samplers, the Bayesian point estimates and the credible sets of the model parameters and the stress–strength parameter can be obtained. We have shown by using a Monte Carlo simulation study that the proposed Bayesian methods are effective and provide reasonable estimation results. We also illustrate the proposed methods by analyzing a bivariate data set.

Appendix: Monte Carlo Simulation Results

Table A.1 Estimated MSEs and biases (in parentheses) of the Bayes estimators for μ_1, μ_2, and ρ with non-informative prior distributions based on Monte Carlo simulation from $(\mu_1, \mu_2, \rho) = (0.6, 0.6, 0.2)$ and $(\mu_1, \mu_2, \rho) = (0.6, 0.6, 0.8)$

	m	Scheme	$(\mu_1, \mu_2, \rho) = (0.6, 0.6, 0.2)$			$(\mu_1, \mu_2, \rho) = (0.6, 0.6, 0.8)$		
			μ_1	μ_2	ρ	μ_1	μ_2	ρ
1	5	(0,0,0,0,15)	0.2302(0.2375)	0.1875(0.1295)	0.0514(0.1737)	0.2501(0.2622)	1.1503(0.8106)	0.1457(−0.3334)
2		(15,0,0,0,0)	0.2226(0.2265)	0.2697(0.2483)	0.0452(0.1485)	0.2518(0.3133)	0.4284(0.3989)	0.0706(−0.2003)
3		(3,3,3,3,3)	0.1837(0.2216)	0.2126(0.1542)	0.0539(0.1737)	0.2400(0.2540)	1.1811(0.7754)	0.1401(−0.3222)
4	15	(0,...,0,15)	0.0429(0.0840)	0.0348(0.0127)	0.0379(0.1424)	0.05716(0.1134)	0.3411(0.4175)	0.1096(−0.2694)
5		(15,0,...,0)	0.0467(0.0792)	0.0369(0.0644)	0.0206(0.0798)	0.0610(0.1302)	0.0624(0.1331)	0.0251(−0.1019)
6		(3,0,0,...,3,0,0)	0.0403(0.0757)	0.0419(0.0578)	0.0262(0.0970)	0.0542(0.1238)	0.0985(0.1906)	0.0420(−0.1412)
7	20	(0,...,0,30)	0.0322(0.0653)	0.0289(−0.0150)	0.0375(0.1455)	0.0355(0.0842)	0.4022(0.4842)	0.1251(−0.2970)
8		(30,0,...,0)	0.0270(0.0490)	0.0302(0.0538)	0.0175(0.0651)	0.0404(0.1087)	0.4251(0.1155)	0.0180(−0.0831)
9		(3,0,3,0,...,3,0)	0.0301(−0.0611)	0.0260(−0.0241)	0.0248(0.0970)	0.0396(0.0953)	0.1103(0.2148)	0.0464(−0.1533)
10	30	(0,...,0,20)	0.0158(0.0403)	0.0167(−0.0088)	0.0282(0.1106)	0.0188(0.0617)	0.0787(0.1852)	0.0479(−0.1537)
11		(20,0,...,0)	0.0154(0.0288)	0.0150(0.0266)	0.0142(0.0524)	0.02251(0.0675)	0.02016(0.0658)	0.0089(−0.0508)
12		(2,0,0,...,2,0,0)	0.0157(0.0360)	0.0164(0.0188)	0.0126(0.0685)	0.0195(0.0666)	0.0275(0.0871)	0.0144(−0.0703)

Table A.2 Estimated MSEs and biases (in parenthesis) of the Bayes estimators for δ with non-informative prior distributions based on Monte Carlo simulation when $(\mu_1, \mu_2, \rho) = (0.6, 0.6, 0.2)$ and true $\delta = 0.5$

	m	Scheme	Plug-in	Mean-value MC	Important sampling
			MSE (bias)	MSE (bias)	MSE (bias)
1	5	(0,0,0,0,15)	0.0321(0.0551)	0.0353(0.0644)	0.0352(0.0643)
2		(15,0,0,0,0)	0.0253(0.0008)	0.0260(0.0030)	0.0260(0.0030)
3		(3,3,3,3,3)	0.0281(0.0446)	0.0307(0.0540)	0.0307(0.0540)
4	15	(0,...,0,15)	0.0145(0.0488)	0.0151(0.0506)	0.0151(0.0505)
5		(15,0,...,0)	0.0092(0.0067)	0.0092(0.0068)	0.0092(0.0068)
6		(3,0,0,...,3,0,0)	0.0105(0.0158)	0.0105(0.0162)	0.0105(0.0162)
7	20	(0,...,0,30)	0.0146(0.0580)	0.0154(0.0599)	0.0153(0.0598)
8		(30,0,...,0)	0.0071(−0.0012)	0.0071(−0.0012)	0.0071(−0.0012)
9		(3,0,3,0,...,3,0)	0.0092(0.0259)	0.0093(0.0262)	0.0093(0.0262)
10	30	(0,...,0,20)	0.0079(0.0362)	0.0081(0.0367)	0.0081(0.0367)
11		(20,0,...,0)	0.0045(0.0010)	0.0045(0.0010)	0.0045(0.0010)
12		(2,0,0,...,2,0,0)	0.0055(0.0124)	0.0055(0.0124)	0.0055(0.0124)

Table A.3 Estimated MSEs and biases (in parenthesis) for the Bayes estimators for δ with non-informative prior distributions based on Monte Carlo simulation when $(\mu_1, \mu_2, \rho) = (0.6, 0.6, 0.8)$ and true $\delta = 0.5$

	m	Scheme	Plug-in	Mean-value MC	Important sampling
			MSE (bias)	MSE (bias)	MSE (bias)
1	5	(0,0,0,0,15)	0.0377(−0.1272)	0.0400(−0.1056)	0.0398(−0.1059)
2		(15,0,0,0,0)	0.0168(−0.0325)	0.0188(−0.0110)	0.0188(−0.0111)
3		(3,3,3,3,3)	0.0359(−0.1213)	0.0374(−0.1018)	0.0373(−0.1019)
4	15	(0,...,0,15)	0.0184(−0.0899)	0.01932(−0.0760)	0.01934(−0.0759)
5		(15,0,...,0)	0.0064(−0.0118)	0.0068(0.0005)	0.0068(0.0005)
6		(3,0,0,...,3,0,0)	0.0090(0.0310)	0.0099(−0.0174)	0.0099(−0.0174)
7	20	(0,...,0,30)	0.0229(−0.1134)	0.0238(−0.1018)	0.0238(−0.1018)
8		(30,0,...,0)	0.0055(−0.0136)	0.0058(−0.0035)	0.0058(−0.0034)
9		(3,0,3,0,...,3,0)	0.0102(−0.0480)	0.0111(−0.0357)	0.0111(−0.0357)
10	30	(0,...,0,20)	0.0087(−0.0511)	0.0092(−0.0407)	0.0092(−0.0408)
11		(20,0,...,0)	0.0038(−0.0090)	0.0039(0.0006)	0.0039(0.0005)
12		(2,0,0,...,2,0,0)	0.0042(−0.0160)	0.0046(−0.0056)	0.0046(−0.0056)

Table A.4 Estimated MSEs and biases (in parentheses) of the Bayes estimators for μ_1, μ_2, and ρ with non-informative prior distributions based on Monte Carlo simulation from $(\mu_1, \mu_2, \rho) = (0.6, 0.3, 0.2)$ and $(\mu_1, \mu_2, \rho) = (0.6, 0.3, 0.8)$

			$(\mu_1, \mu_2, \rho) = (0.6, 0.3, 0.2)$			$(\mu_1, \mu_2, \rho) = (0.6, 0.3, 0.8)$		
	m	Scheme	μ_1	μ_2	ρ	μ_1	μ_2	ρ
1	5	(0,0,0,0,15)	0.2239(0.2256)	0.0639(0.0717)	0.0557(0.1811)	0.2106(0.2486)	0.6423(0.5939)	0.1699(−0.3771)
2		(15,0,0,0,0)	0.1830(0.2001)	0.0739(0.1187)	0.0457(0.1494)	0.2537(0.3054)	0.1046(0.1929)	0.0730(−0.2047)
3		(3,3,3,3,3)	0.1420(0.0968)	0.0283(−0.0176)	0.0875(0.2474)	0.1117(0.0830)	0.1885(0.2452)	0.0998(−0.2582)
4	15	(0,...,0,15)	0.0474(0.0878)	0.0087(0.0024)	0.0411(0.1484)	0.05525(0.1126)	0.0681(0.1894)	0.1042(−0.2675)
5		(15,0,...,0)	0.0433(0.0777)	0.0090(−0.0338)	0.0242(−0.0929)	0.0565(0.1305)	0.0145(0.0687)	0.0257(−01044)
6		(3,0,0,...,3,0,0)	0.0303(0.0179)	0.0073(−0.0047)	0.0343(0.1237)	0.0429(0.0648)	0.0184(0.0641)	0.0337(−0.1184)
7	20	(0,...,0,30)	0.0304(0.0632)	0.0064(−0.0146)	0.0398(0.1509)	0.0332(0.0755)	0.0935(0.2323)	0.1158(−0.2862)
8		(30,0,...,0)	0.0244(0.0512)	0.0065(0.0263)	0.0196(0.0758)	0.0269(0.0441)	0.0071(0.0249)	0.0145(−0.0674)
9		(3,0,3,0,...,3,0)	0.0233(0.0207)	0.0054(−0.0108)	0.0328(0.1267)	0.0245(0.046)	0.0169(0.0667)	0.0345(−0.1166)
10	30	(0,...,0,20)	0.0179(0.0448)	0.0038(−0.0028)	0.0267(0.1080)	0.0152(0.0245)	0.0132(0.0586)	0.0373(−0.1234)
11		(20,0,...,0)	0.0146(0.0306)	0.0039(0.0174)	0.0144(0.0542)	0.0184(0.0628)	0.0047(0.0325)	0.0079(−0.0522)
12		(2,0,0,...,2,0,0)	0.0147(0.0164)	0.0036(−0.0008)	0.0203(0.0796)	0.0156(0.0298)	0.0054(0.0261)	0.0116(−0.0560)

Table A.5 Estimated MSEs and biases (in parenthesis) for the Bayes estimators of δ with non-informative prior distributions based on Monte Carlo simulation when $(\mu_1, \mu_2, \rho) = (0.6, 0.3, 0.2)$ and true $\delta = 0.6838$

			Plug-in	Mean-value MC	Important sampling
	m	Scheme	MSE (bias)	MSE (bias)	MSE (bias)
1	5	(0,0,0,0,15)	0.0217(0.0225)	0.0242(0.0345)	0.0241(0.0344)
2		(15,0,0,0,0)	0.0194(−0.0078)	0.0200(−0.0040)	0.0200(−0.0040)
3		(3,3,3,3,3)	0.0210(0.0425)	0.0247(0.0589)	0.0247(0.0589)
4	15	(0,...,0,15)	0.0095(0.0425)	0.0103(0.0449)	0.0102(0.0449)
5		(15,0,...,0)	0.0066(0.0063)	0.0067(0.0065)	0.0067(0.0065)
6		(3,0,0,...,3,0,0)	0.0080(0.0203)	0.0082(0.0213)	0.0082(0.0213)
7	20	(0,...,0,30)	0.0093(0.0508)	0.0099(0.0527)	0.0099(0.0526)
8		(30,0,...,0)	0.0050(0.0038)	0.0050(0.0039)	0.0050(0.0039)
9		(3,0,3,0,...,3,0)	0.0070(0.0294)	0.0071(0.0299)	0.0071(0.0299)
10	30	(0,...,0,20)	0.0057(0.0321)	0.0058(0.0325)	0.0058(0.0325)
11		(20,0,0,..,0)	0.0033(0.0016)	0.0033(0.0016)	0.0033(0.00162)
12		(2,0,0,...,2,0,0)	0.0045(0.0144)	0.0045(0.0145)	0.0450(0.0145)

Table A.6 Estimated MSEs and biases (in parenthesis) for the Bayes estimators of δ with non-informative prior distributions based on Monte Carlo simulation when $(\mu_1, \mu_2, \rho) = (0.6, 0.3, 0.8)$ and true $\delta = 0.8101$

			Plug-in	Mean-value MC	Important sampling
	m	Scheme	MSE (bias)	MSE (bias)	MSE (bias)
1	5	(0,0,0,0,15)	0.1088(−0.2943)	0.1038(−0.2781)	0.1038(−0.2782)
2		(15,0,0,0,0)	0.0248(−0.1186)	0.0197(−0.0817)	0.0197(−0.0817)
3		(3,3,3,3,3)	0.0718(−0.2262)	0.0622(−0.1849)	0.0622(−0.1853)
4	15	(0,...,0,15)	0.0368(−0.1657)	0.0347(−0.1465)	0.0347(−0.1465)
5		(15,0,...,0)	0.0066(−0.0604)	0.0054(−0.0370)	0.0054(−0.037)
6		(3,0,0,...,3,0,0)	0.0135(−0.0894)	0.0113(−0.0589)	0.0113(−0.0589)
7	20	(0,...,0,30)	0.0509(−0.1986)	0.0488(−0.1813)	0.0488(−0.1813)
8		(30,0,...,0)	0.0047(−0.0497)	0.0039(−0.0255)	0.0039(−0.0255)
9		(3,0,3,0,...,3,0)	0.0144(−0.0935)	0.0127(−0.0656)	0.0127(−0.0656)
10	30	(0,...,0,20)	0.0138(−0.0898)	0.0130(−0.0680)	0.0130(−0.0680)
11		(20,0,...,0)	0.0027(−0.0370)	0.0022(−0.0201)	0.0022(−0.0201)
12		(2,0,0,...,2,0,0)	0.0049(−0.0511)	0.0043(−0.0279)	0.0043(−0.0279)

Table A.7 Estimated MSEs and biases (in parentheses) of the Bayes estimators for μ_1, μ_2, and ρ with informative prior distributions based on Monte Carlo simulation from $(\mu_1, \mu_2, \rho) = (0.6, 0.6, 0.2)$ and $(\mu_1, \mu_2, \rho) = (0.6, 0.6, 0.8)$

	m	Scheme	$(\mu_1, \mu_2, \rho) = (0.6, 0.6, 0.2)$			$(\mu_1, \mu_2, \rho) = (0.6, 0.6, 0.8)$		
			μ_1	μ_2	ρ	μ_1	μ_2	ρ
1	5	(0,0,0,0,15)	0.0970(0.0853)	0.0663(0.0529)	0.0043(0.0109)	0.0776(0.0620)	0.0628(0.0440)	0.0063(−0.0112)
2		(15,0,0,0,0)	0.0915(0.0765)	0.0971(0.0868)	0.0052(0.0085)	0.0523(0.0317)	0.0622(0.0441)	0.0081(−0.0210)
3		(3,3,3,3,3)	0.0959(0.0825)	0.0792(0.0768)	0.0045(0.0156)	0.0736(0.0514)	0.0667(0.0495)	0.0072(−0.0175)
4	15	(0,...,0,15)	0.0210(−0.0030)	0.0514(0.0909)	0.0038(−0.0124)	0.0285(0.0247)	0.0396(0.0622)	0.0086(−0.0387)
5		(15,0,...,0)	0.0205(0.0002)	0.0382(0.0688)	0.0072(0.0045)	0.0244(0.0264)	0.0240(0.0318)	0.0067(−0.0275)
6		(3,0,0,...,3,0,0)	0.0291(0.0363)	0.0275(0.0353)	0.0063(0.0017)	0.0270(0.0250)	0.0299(0.0476)	0.0076(−0.0341)
7	20	(0,...,0,30)	0.0185(−0.0041)	0.0695(−0.2590)	0.0754(0.2458)	0.0187(0.0220)	0.0353(0.0599)	0.0083(−0.0395)
8		(30,0,...,0)	0.0159(−0.0241)	0.0418(−0.1959)	0.0087(0.0220)	0.0169(0.0123)	0.0198(0.0258)	0.0054(−0.0223)
9		(3,0,3,0,...,3,0)	0.0169(−0.0154)	0.0516(−0.2212)	0.0313(0.1354)	0.0181(0.0155)	0.0442(0.0782)	0.0096(−0.0445)
10	30	(0,...,0,20)	0.0113(−0.0013)	0.0186(0.0462)	0.0046(−0.0106)	0.0104(0.0083)	0.0292(0.0714)	0.0095(−0.0496)
11		(20,0,...,0)	0.0112(−0.0022)	0.0151(0.0328)	0.0065(−0.0064)	0.0125(0.0128)	0.0145(0.0277)	0.0043(−0.0199)
12		(2,0,0,...,2,0,0)	0.0109(−0.0021)	0.0176(0.0372)	0.0063(−0.0089)	0.0126(0.0045)	0.0194(0.0326)	0.0058(−0.0280)

Table A.8 Estimated MSEs and biases (in parenthesis) for the Bayes estimators of δ with informative prior distributions based on Monte Carlo simulation when $(\mu_1, \mu_2, \rho) = (0.6, 0.6, 0.2)$ and true $\delta = 0.5$

	m	Scheme	Plug-in MSE (bias)	Mean-value MC MSE (bias)	Important sampling MSE (bias)
1	5	(0,0,0,0,15)	0.0172(0.0171)	0.0172(−0.0727)	0.0172(0.0172)
2		(15,0,0,0,0)	0.0165(0.0002)	0.0165(0.0002)	0.0165(0.0002)
3		(3,3,3,3,3)	0.0192(0.0073)	0.0193(0.0074)	0.0193(0.0074)
4	15	(0,...,0,15)	0.0093(−0.0291)	0.0093(−0.0291)	0.0093(−0.0291)
5		(15,0,...,0)	0.0079(−0.0253)	0.0079(−0.0253)	0.0079(−0.0253)
6		(3,0,0,...,3,0,0)	0.0085(0.0031)	0.0085(0.0074)	0.0085(0.0031)
7	20	(0,...,0,30)	0.0361(0.1746)	0.0370(0.1764)	0.0370(0.1765)
8		(30,0,...,0)	0.0126(0.0914)	0.0126(0.0914)	0.0126(0.0914)
9		(3,0,3,0,...,3,0)	0.0206(0.1250)	0.0207(0.1252)	0.0207(0.1252)
10	30	(0,...,0,20)	0.0048(−0.0150)	0.0048(−0.0150)	0.0048(−0.0150)
11		(20,0,0,..,0)	0.0044(−0.0145)	0.0044(−0.0145)	0.0044(−0.0145)
12		(2,0,0,...,2,0,0)	0.0044(−0.0138)	0.0044(−0.0138)	0.0044(−0.0138)

Table A.9 Estimated MSEs and biases (in parenthesis) for the Bayes estimators of δ with informative prior distributions based on Monte Carlo simulation when $(\mu_1, \mu_2, \rho) = (0.6, 0.6, 0.8)$ and true $\delta = 0.5$

	m	Scheme	Plug-in MSE (bias)	Mean-value MC MSE (bias)	Important sampling MSE (bias)
1	5	(0,0,0,0,15)	0.0243(−0.0313)	0.0366(0.0462)	0.0361(0.0453)
2		(15,0,0,0,0)	0.0186(−0.0417)	0.0220(0.0008)	0.0219(0.0008)
3		(3,3,3,3,3)	0.0246(−0.0366)	0.0337(0.0269)	0.0335(0.0266)
4	15	(0,...,0,15)	0.0125(−0.0291)	0.0159(0.0009)	0.0159(0.0009)
5		(15,0,...,0)	0.0072(−0.0225)	0.0075(−0.0037)	0.0075(−0.0037)
6		(3,0,0,...,3,0,0)	0.0097(−0.0291)	0.0109(−0.0079)	0.0109(−0.0079)
7	20	(0,...,0,30)	0.0107(−0.0211)	0.0152(0.0107)	0.0152(0.0107)
8		(30,0,...,0)	0.0061(−0.0247)	0.0061(−0.0088)	0.0061(−0.0088)
9		(3,0,3,0,...,3,0)	0.0102(−0.0396)	0.0120(−0.0184)	0.0120(−0.0184)
10	30	(0,...,0,20)	0.0084(−0.0387)	0.0096(−0.0224)	0.0096(−0.0225)
11		(20,0,...,0)	0.0044(−0.0232)	0.0044(−0.0110)	0.0044(−0.0110)
12		(2,0,0,...,2,0,0)	0.0053(−0.0275)	0.0056(−0.0136)	0.0056(−0.0136)

Table A.10 Estimated MSEs and biases (in parentheses) of the Bayes estimators for μ_1, μ_2, and ρ with informative prior distributions based on Monte Carlo simulation from $(\mu_1, \mu_2, \rho) = (0.6, 0.3, 0.2)$ and $(\mu_1, \mu_2, \rho) = (0.6, 0.3, 0.8)$

	m	Scheme	$(\mu_1, \mu_2, \rho) = (0.6, 0.3, 0.2)$			$(\mu_1, \mu_2, \rho) = (0.6, 0.3, 0.8)$		
			μ_1	μ_2	ρ	μ_1	μ_2	ρ
1	5	(0,0,0,0,15)	0.0422(−0.0867)	0.1076(0.1656)	0.0030(−0.0183)	0.0765(0.0553)	0.0314(0.0584)	0.0070(−0.0193)
2		(15,0,0,0,0)	0.0388(−0.0665)	0.0785(0.1358)	0.0054(0.0031)	0.0698(0.0492)	0.0197(0.0336)	0.0095(−0.0293)
3		(3,3,3,3,3)	0.0381(−0.0822)	0.0841(0.1389)	0.0029(−0.0142)	0.0845(0.0587)	0.0255(0.0435)	0.0070(−0.0203)
4	15	(0,...,0,15)	0.0301(0.0373)	0.0067(0.0172)	0.0050(0.0136)	0.0241(0.0258)	0.0133(0.0419)	0.0097(−0.0472)
5		(15,0,...,0)	0.0280(0.0266)	0.0069(0.0208)	0.0065(−0.0004)	0.0264(0.0296)	0.0067(0.0175)	0.0066(−0.0269)
6		(3,0,0,...,3,0,0)	0.0299(0.0332)	0.0069(0.0143)	0.0054(0.0025)	0.0270(0.0302)	0.0082(0.0226)	0.0079(−0.0325)
7	20	(0,...,0,30)	0.0226(0.0299)	0.0048(0.0098)	0.0048(0.0110)	0.0158(−0.0025)	0.0211(0.0779)	0.0152(−0.0778)
8		(30,0,...,0)	0.0231(0.0249)	0.0049(0.0111)	0.0069(−0.0029)	0.0160(−0.0039)	0.0050(0.0076)	0.0054(−0.0232)
9		(3,0,3,0,...,3,0)	0.0191(0.0216)	0.0057(0.0121)	0.0062(0.0080)	0.0151(0.0046)	0.0091(0.0372)	0.0086(−0.0443)
10	30	(0,...,0,20)	0.0121(−0.0101)	0.0043(0.0218)	0.0045(−0.0074)	0.0122(0.0047)	0.0075(0.0322)	0.0093(−0.0464)
11		(20,0,...,0)	0.0109(−0.0120)	0.0040(0.0173)	0.0070(−0.0071)	0.0112(−0.0035)	0.0030(0.0060)	0.0039(−0.0149)
12		(2,0,0,...,2,0,0)	0.0110(−0.0179)	0.0045(0.0183)	0.0066(−0.0078)	0.0118(0.0067)	0.0040(0.0150)	0.0054(−0.0258)

Table A.11 Estimated MSEs and biases (in parenthesis) for the Bayes estimators of δ with informative prior distributions based on Monte Carlo simulation when $(\mu_1, \mu_2, \rho) = (0.6, 0.3, 0.2)$ and true $\delta = 0.6838$

			Plug-in	Mean-value MC	Important sampling
	m	Scheme	MSE (bias)	MSE (bias)	MSE (bias)
1	5	(0,0,0,0,15)	0.0381(−0.1347)	0.0381(−0.1347)	0.0381(−0.1347)
2		(15,0,0,0,0)	0.0302(−0.1152)	0.0302(−0.1151)	0.0302(−0.1151)
3		(3,3,3,3,3)	0.0326(−0.1226)	0.0326(−0.1226)	0.0326(−0.1226)
4	15	(0,...,0,15)	0.0064(−0.0038)	0.0064(−0.0038)	0.0064(−0.0038)
5		(15,0,...,0)	0.0057(−0.0128)	0.0057(−0.0127)	0.0057(−0.0127)
6		(3,0,0,...,3,0,0)	0.0060(−0.0044)	0.0060(−0.0044)	0.0060(−0.0043)
7	20	(0,...,0,30)	0.0050(0.0013)	0.0050(0.0014)	0.0050(0.0014)
8		(30,0,...,0)	0.0042(−0.0050)	0.0042(−0.0050)	0.0042(−0.0050)
9		(3,0,3,0,...,3,0)	0.0054(−0.0033)	0.0054(−0.0033)	0.0054(−0.0033)
10	30	(0,...,0,20)	0.0043(−0.0226)	0.0043(−0.0226)	0.0043(−0.0226)
11		(20,0,0,..,0)	0.0036(−0.0212)	0.0036(−0.0212)	0.0036(−0.0212)
12		(2,0,0,...,2,0,0)	0.0045(−0.0234)	0.0045(−0.0234)	0.0045(−0.0234)

Table A.12 Estimated MSEs and biases (in parenthesis) for the Bayes estimators of δ with informative prior distributions based on Monte Carlo simulation when $(\mu_1, \mu_2, \rho) = (0.6, 0.3, 0.8)$ and true $\delta = 0.8101$

			Plug-in	Mean-value MC	Important sampling
	m	Scheme	MSE (bias)	MSE (bias)	MSE (bias)
1	5	(0,0,0,0,15)	0.0436(−0.1602)	0.0260(0.0664)	0.0260(−0.0671)
2		(15,0,0,0,0)	0.0206(−0.1051)	0.0117(−0.0303)	0.0117(−0.0305)
3		(3,3,3,3,3)	0.0350(−0.1389)	0.0226(−0.0445)	0.0225(−0.0528)
4	15	(0,...,0,15)	0.0143(−0.0878)	0.0117(−0.045)	0.0117(−0.0453)
5		(15,0,...,0)	0.0056(−0.0521)	0.0035(−0.0135)	0.0036(−0.0135)
6		(3,0,0,...,3,0,0)	0.0075(−0.0617)	0.0057(−0.0209)	0.0057(−0.0209)
7	20	(0,...,0,30)	0.02357(−0.1262)	0.0201(−0.0917)	0.0201(−0.0917)
8		(30,0,...,0)	0.0047(−0.0498)	0.0032(−0.0170)	0.0032(−0.0170)
9		(3,0,3,0,...,3,0)	0.0107(−0.0800)	0.0088(−0.0480)	0.0088(−0.0480)
10	30	(0,...,0,20)	0.0087(−0.0701)	0.0076(−0.0415)	0.0076(−0.0415)
11		(20,0,...,0)	0.0029(−0.0395)	0.0021(−0.0123)	0.0021(−0.123)
12		(2,0,0,...,2,0,0)	0.0042(−0.0471)	0.0036(−0.0202)	0.0036(−0.0202)

Acknowledgments H. K. T. Ng's work was supported by a grant from the Simons Foundation (#709773 to Tony Ng). L. Wang's work is supported by the National Natural Science Foundation of China (No. 12061091) and the Yunnan Fundamental Research Projects (No. 202101AT070103).

References

1. Ali, M., Woo, J., Pal, M.: Inference on reliability $P(Y < X)$ in two-parameter exponential distributions. Int. J. Stat. Sci. **3**, 119–125 (2004)
2. Al-Saadi, S.D., Young, D.H.: Estimators for the correlation coefficient in a bivariate exponential distribution. J. Stat. Comput. Simul. **11**, 13–20 (1980)
3. Bai, D.S., Hong, Y.W.: Estimation of $P(X < Y)$ in the exponential case with common location parameter. Commun. Stat. Theory Methods **21**, 269–282 (1992)
4. Balakrishnan, N.: Progressive censoring methodology: an appraisal (with Discussions). Test **16**, 211–296 (2007)
5. Balakrishnan, N., Aggarwala, R.: Progressive Censoring: Theory, Methods, and Applications. Birkhäuser, Boston (2000)
6. Balakrishnan, N., Cramer, E.: The Art of Progressive Censoring. Applications to Reliability and Quality. Birkhäuser, New York (2014)
7. Balakrishnan, N., Ng, H.K.T.: Improved estimation of the correlation coefficient in a bivariate exponential distribution. J. Stat. Comput. Simul. **68**, 173–184 (2001)
8. Birnbaum, Z.W.: On a use of Mann-Whitney statistics. In: Proceedings of the Third Berkley Symposium in Mathematics, Statistics and Probability, vol. 1, pp. 13–17 (1956)
9. Cramer, E.: Progressive censoring schemes. In: Balakrishnan, N., Colton, T., Everitt, B., Piegorsch, W., Ruggeri, F., Teugels, J.L. (eds.) Wiley StatsRef: Statistics Reference Online (2017). https://doi.org/10.1002/9781118445112.stat01760.pub2
10. Csorgo, S., Welsh, A.H.: Testing for exponential and Marshall-Olkin distribution. J. Stat. Plan. Infer. **23**, 287–300 (1989)
11. Downton, F.: Bivariate exponential distributions in reliability theory. J. R. Stat. Soc. Ser. B **32**, 408–417 (1970)
12. Enis, P., Geisser, S.: Estimation of probability that $Y > X$. J. Am. Stat. Assoc. **66**, 162–168 (1971)
13. Geman, S., Geman, D.: Stochastic relaxation, Gibbs distributions and the Bayesian restoration of images. IEEE Trans. Pattern Anal. Mach. Intell. **6**, 721–741 (1984)
14. Genç, A.I.: Estimation of $P(X > Y)$ with Topp-Leone distribution. J. Stat. Comput. Simul. **83**, 326–339 (2013)
15. Hastings, W.K.: Monte Carlo sampling methods using Markov chains and their applications. Biometrika **57**, 97–109 (1970)
16. He, Q., Nagaraja, H.N.: Correlation estimation in the Downton's bivariate exponential distribution using incomplete samples. J. Stat. Comput. Simul. **81**, 531–546 (2011)
17. Iliopoulos, G., Karlis, D., Ntzoufras, I.: Bayesian estimation in Kibble's bivariate gamma distribution. Can. J. Stat. **33**(4), 571–589 (2005)
18. Jiang, L., Wong, A.C.M.: A note on inference for $P(X < Y)$ for right truncated exponentially distribution data. Stat. Papers **19**, 637–651 (2008)
19. Kibble, W.F.: A two-variate gamma type distribution. Sankhyã **5**, 137–150 (1941)
20. Kim, C., Chung, Y.: Bayesian estimation of $P(Y < X)$ from Burr type X model containing spurious observations. Stat. Papers **47**, 643–651 (2006)
21. Kotz, S., Lumelskii, Y., Pensky, M.: The Stress-strength Model and Its Generalization: Theory and Applications. World Scientific, Singapore (2003)
22. Kundu, D., Gupta, R.D.: Estimation of $R = P(Y < X)$ for the generalized exponential distribution. Metrika **61**, 291–308 (2005)

23. Kundu, D., Gupta, R.D.: Estimation of $R = P(Y < X)$ for Weibull distribution. IEEE Trans. Reliab. **55**, 270–280 (2006)
24. Kundu, D., Raqab, M.Z.: Estimation of $R = P(Y < X)$ for three parameter Weibull distribution. Stat. Probab. Lett. **79**, 1839–1846 (2009)
25. Lin, Y.J., Lio, Y.L., Ng, H.K.T.: Bayesian estimation of Moran-Downton bivariate exponential distribution based on censored samples. J. Stat. Comput. Simul. **83**, 837–852 (2013)
26. Lio, Y.L., Tsai, T.-R.: Estimation of $\delta = P(X < Y)$ for Burr XII distribution based on the progressively first failure-censored samples. J. Appl. Stat. **39**(2), 309–322 (2012)
27. Metropolis, N., Rosenbluth, A.W., Rosenbluth, M.N., Teller, A.H. and Teller, E.: Equations of state calculations by fast computing machines. J. Chem. Phys. **21**, 1087–1091 (1953)
28. Moran, P.A.P.: Testing for correlation between non-negative variates. Biometrika. **54**, 385–394 (1967)
29. Ng, H.K.T. Progressively censored data analysis. In: Balakrishnan, N., Colton, T., Everitt, B., Piegorsch, W., Ruggeri, F., Teugels, J.L. (eds.) Wiley StatsRef: Statistics Reference Online (2021) https://doi.org/10.1002/9781118445112.stat01761.pub2
30. Raqab, M.Z., Madi, M.T., Kundu, D.: Estimation of $R = P(Y < X)$ for the 3-parameter generalized exponential distribution. Commun. Stat. Theory Methods. **37**, 2854–2864 (2008)
31. Saracoglu, B., Kaya, M.F.: Maximum likelihood estimation and confidence intervals of system reliability for Gompertz distribution in stress-strength models. Selcuk J. Appl. Math. **8**, 25–36 (2007)
32. Saracoglu, B., Kuş, C.: Estimation of the stress-strength reliability under progressive censoring for Gompertz distribution. In: Proceedings of the Sixth Symposium of Statistics Days, Ondokuz Mayis University, Samsun, pp. 464–471 (2008)
33. Saracoglu, B., Kaya, M.F., Abd-Elfattah, A.M.: Comparison of estimators for stress-strength reliability in Gompertz case. Hacettepe J. Math. Stat. **38**, 339–349 (2009)
34. Saracoglu, B., Kinaci, I., Kundu, D.: On estimation of $R = P(Y < X)$ for exponential distribution under progressive type-II censoring. J. Stat. Comput. Simul. **82**, 729–744 (2012)
35. Surles, J.G., Padgett, W.J.: Inference for $P(Y < X)$ in the Burr type X model. J. Appl. Stat. Sci. **7**, 225–238 (1998)
36. Surles, J.G., Padgett, W.J.: Inference for reliability and stress-strength for a scaled Burr Type X distribution. Lifetime Data Anal. **7**, 187–200 (2001)
37. Tong, H.: A note on the estimation of $P(Y < X)$ in the exponential case. Technometrics **16**, 625 (1974)

Bayesian Computation in a Birnbaum–Saunders Reliability Model with Applications to Fatigue Data

Víctor Leiva, Fabrizio Ruggeri, and Henry Laniado

Abstract The Birnbaum–Saunders distribution has been widely considered and applied to reliability studies. This chapter uses such a distribution to analyze the effect of two treatments and evaluate reliability. Bayesian computation is considered for inferring on the parameters of the Birnbaum–Saunders reliability model analyzed in this work. The methodology is applied to real fatigue data with the aid of the R software.

1 Introduction

Birnbaum and Saunders [9] introduced a distribution that later took their names and nowadays keeps attracting a lot of interest in many fields; see the recent works in [5, 6, 14, 23] for thorough reviews. The Birnbaum–Saunders distribution is widely used to model fatigue life. Its origin stems from considering fatigue in materials provoked by vibrations in commercial aircrafts. In particular, it describes the time spent until the extension of a crack exceeds a threshold producing the failure of materials. These materials are exposed to fatigue produced by cumulative damage generated from cyclical stress and tension; see [24]. The Birnbaum–Saunders distribution has been largely applied to reliability studies; see [3, 7, 8, 19, 25, 32, 33, 37, 38, 40, 43, 46, 50].

V. Leiva (✉)
School of Industrial Engineering, Pontificia Universidad Católica de Valparaíso, Valparaíso, Chile
e-mail: victor.leiva@pucv.cl;

F. Ruggeri
CNR-IMATI, Milano, Italy
e-mail: fabrizio@mi.imati.cnr.it

H. Laniado
Department of Mathematical Sciences, Universidad Eafit, Medellín, Colombia
e-mail: hhlaniado@eafit.edu.co

Y. Lio et al. (eds.), *Bayesian Inference and Computation in Reliability and Survival Analysis*, Emerging Topics in Statistics and Biostatistics,
https://doi.org/10.1007/978-3-030-88658-5_3

Many of the previous works have been analysis of reliability with censored and fatigue data, where other well-known distributions as gamma and Weibull are also used to model the lifetime of system devices. Note that the comparisons between coherent systems are useful for deciding what is the optimal configuration of their components in some stochastic sense. In particular, the analysis of the reliability of parallel and series systems has great practical interest, since these kinds of systems are often implemented in industrial processes, manufacturing and safety. For example, in [22], the authors considered combinations of parallel and series systems with components and reserves following both different distributions. The main result of that study was obtaining the best configuration of new and used components in a combined parallel and series system, in order to reach an optimal reliability. Later the result was improved in [51] by imposing a stronger stochastic criterion. However, despite its usefulness, the Birnbaum–Saunders distribution applied to the coherent system reliability as parallel or series systems is an aspect that it has not been extensively examined. Nevertheless, a recent work [2] discussed stochastic comparisons of lifetimes of parallel and series systems with just two components having generalized Birnbaum–Saunders distributions.

Although the main applications of the Birnbaum–Saunders distribution lie naturally in engineering, it has also been successfully applied to several other fields of knowledge such as agriculture, air contamination, bioengineering, business, economics, environment, finance, food and textile industries, forestry, human and tree mortality, informatics, insurance, inventory management, medicine, neurology, nutrition, pharmacology, psychology, queuing theory, toxicology, water quality, and wind energy; see details in [23]. For a compendium with diverse tools for statistical quality control based on the Birnbaum–Saunders distribution, see [27, 29].

The Birnbaum–Saunders distribution possesses interesting properties and is useful for modeling data that take values greater than zero. It is unimodal, has asymmetry to the right (positively skewed), and its shape and scale are addressed by its two parameters. The Birnbaum–Saunders failure rate has an upside-down bathtub shape, but, depending on the values of its parameters, other shapes can also be obtained; see [4]. In addition, the Birnbaum–Saunders distribution is closely related to the normal distribution. Specifically, a Birnbaum–Saunders distributed random variable is considered as a transformation of a standard normal distributed random variable; see [20, pp. 651–663] and [23]. The skewed shape of its density function permits us to state its median as a more appropriate centrality indicator than its mean. It is worth mentioning that its scale parameter is also the median of the model, similarly, although in an asymmetrical framework, to the Gaussian distribution where one of the parameters coincide with its mean and median. Other standard life distributions often employed in parametric reliability, such as the gamma, inverse Gaussian, log-normal, and Weibull models, do not share the relation between one parameter and mean/median, at least in their most used forms. Furthermore, the correspondence between one parameter and the median will be exploited in comparing the effects of two treatments through the median in the present work.

Bayesian methods for the Birnbaum–Saunders distribution have been considered by a number of authors. By using Jeffreys and reference priors, Bayesian inference was performed in [1] for the parameters of the Birnbaum–Saunders distribution. A similar approach, also relying on Gibbs sampling, was considered in [54]. Markov Chain Monte Carlo methods were also used in [47] to infer about Birnbaum–Saunders log-linear models, whereas Birnbaum–Saunders non-linear regressions were considered in [16]. Birnbaum–Saunders and Weibull-accelerated life models were compared in [48], whereas Birnbaum–Saunders–Student-t models with censored data were analyzed in [10]. Some recent works on Bayesian methods for Birnbaum–Saunders models are due to [26, 36, 45, 52].

The study of the mechanical properties of different types of materials is very important to assess reliability of devices and structures. Quite a number of works are available in the literature on this topic. Crack propagation in train wheels, due to load, was studied in [30, 41], whereas reliability of wood plastic composites in extrusion processes was analyzed in [13]. Reliability of mortar projectiles and multi-body mechanisms based on dynamic properties were studied, respectively, in [12, 53]. Nano-materials have become more and more relevant in many applications and, simultaneously, there has been an increased interest on their mechanical performance. As an example, the mechanical properties of a polymeric bone cement when incorporating different types of mesoporous silica nano-particles were compared in [26]. Other factors such as creep, fatigue, fracture, and surface, along with interface, phase, and thermal stabilities, are considered to increase the reliability of modern materials; see [39]. In most of those applications, the Weibull distribution has been used, but the Birnbaum–Saunders distribution has proved to be very effective, as shown in [26].

Stemming from the successful application in [26], we are now considering a different case study to show the efficacy of the approach therein, based on combining Bayesian methods and the Birnbaum–Saunders distribution to analysis of reliability. In the current study, we are going to consider the fatigue life of aluminum pieces expressed by cycles until the failure occurs. We are in a completely different setup with respect to the case study in [26]. It is not just the difference in material (bone cement and aluminum) but also the physical experiment (insertion of nano-particles and cycles) and the mathematical nature of the quantity of interest (continuous [hardness] and integer [cycles]). The common aspects are the evaluation of the effect of two treatments and the Bayesian methods, although elicitation of priors is different between these two works.

In addition to this introduction, the rest of this chapter is organized as follows. Section 2 provides background on the Birnbaum–Saunders distribution and how it arises mathematically; see [23, pp. 1–11] for more details. Then, in Sect. 3, we briefly present the results in [26] about the Bayesian comparison of two treatments using the Birnbaum–Saunders distribution. Section 4 applies the methodology to fatigue data sets under two treatments by using the R software; see www.R-project.org and [42]. Finally, Sect. 5 gives some discussion, conclusions, and ideas for future work on this topic.

2 The Birnbaum–Saunders Distribution

In this section, we present background on the Birnbaum–Saunders distribution and properties, features, and main moments.

If a random variable T follows the Birnbaum–Saunders distribution with shape ($\alpha > 0$) and scale ($\beta > 0$) parameters, then the notation $T \sim \text{BS}(\alpha, \beta)$ is used. The density function of T is expressed as

$$f_T(t; \alpha, \beta) = \phi(A(t; \alpha, \beta))a(t; \alpha, \beta), \quad t > 0, \tag{1}$$

where ϕ is the standard normal density function and $a(t; \alpha, \beta)$, the derivative of $A(t; \alpha, \beta)$, is given by

$$a(t; \alpha, \beta) = \frac{1}{2\alpha\beta}\left(\left(\frac{\beta}{t}\right)^{\frac{1}{2}} + \left(\frac{\beta}{t}\right)^{\frac{3}{2}}\right).$$

The Birnbaum–Saunders cumulative distribution function can be obtained from the density function defined in (1) and expressed as

$$F_T(t; \alpha, \beta) = \Phi(A(t; \alpha, \beta)), \quad t > 0, \tag{2}$$

where Φ is a standard normal cumulative distribution function and

$$A(t; \alpha, \beta) = \frac{1}{\alpha}\left(\left(\frac{t}{\beta}\right)^{\frac{1}{2}} - \left(\frac{\beta}{t}\right)^{\frac{1}{2}}\right).$$

Let $T \sim \text{BS}(\alpha, \beta)$. Then, we have the following properties, features as well as the mean, variance, and coefficients of variation (CV), skewness (CS), and kurtosis (CK):

(A1) $kT \sim \text{BS}(\alpha, k\beta)$, with $k > 0$.
(A2) $1/T \sim \text{BS}(\alpha, 1/\beta)$.
(A3) $V^2 = (T/\beta + \beta/T - 2)/\alpha^2 \sim \chi^2(1)$.
(A4) $\text{E}(T) = \beta\left(1 + \frac{\alpha^2}{2}\right)$.
(A5) $\text{Var}(T) = \beta^2\alpha^2\left(1 + \frac{5\alpha^2}{4}\right)$.
(A6) $\text{CV}(T) = \frac{\alpha\left(5\alpha^2 + 4\right)^{1/2}}{(2 + \alpha^2)}$.
(A7) $\text{CS}(T) = \frac{4\alpha(11\alpha^2 + 6)}{(5\alpha^2 + 4)^{3/2}}$.
(A8) $\text{CK}(T) = 3 + \frac{6\alpha^2(40 + 93\alpha^2)}{(4 + 5\alpha^2)^2}$.

(A9) For $Z \sim \mathrm{N}(0,\ 1)$, we have

$$T = \beta \left(\frac{\alpha Z}{2} + \left(\left(\frac{\alpha Z}{2} \right)^2 + 1 \right)^{1/2} \right)^2 .$$

(A10) From the transformation in (A9) and its monotonicity, it follows

$$Z = \frac{1}{\alpha} \xi \left(\frac{T}{\beta} \right),$$

where $\xi(y) = y^{1/2} - y^{-1/2} = 2 \sinh(\log(y^{1/2}))$, for $y > 0$.

Remark 2.1 From (A1), note that the Birnbaum–Saunders distribution belongs to the scale family, which is parametrized by a positive scale parameter. Then, for any random variable T whose distribution belongs to such a family, the distribution of kT, with $k > 0$, also belongs to this family.

Remark 2.2 From (A2), note that the Birnbaum–Saunders distribution belongs to the closed under reciprocation family. For any random variable T whose distribution belongs to such a family, the distribution of $1/T$ also belongs to this family.

Properties (A1)–(A10) are useful for different purposes. From (A9), note that a random variable with Birnbaum–Saunders distribution is a transformation of another random variable with N(0, 1) distribution. This property allows us to easily obtain the quantile function of the Birnbaum–Saunders distribution as

$$t(q; \alpha, \beta) = F^{-1}(q; \alpha, \beta) = \beta \left(\frac{\alpha\, z(q)}{2} + \left(\left(\frac{\alpha\, z(q)}{2} \right)^2 + 1 \right)^{1/2} \right)^2 , 0 < q < 1, \tag{3}$$

where $z(q)$ is the N(0, 1) quantile function (or $q \times 100$th quantile) and F^{-1} is the inverse function of F given in (2). From (3), note that $t(0.5) = \beta$, that is, β is also the median or 50th percentile of the Birnbaum–Saunders distribution.

Maximum likelihood estimators for the Birnbaum–Saunders model parameters are unique and can be easily obtained, solving numerically the corresponding estimating equations. For details about this maximum likelihood estimation, see [8, 23].

3 Bayesian Computation and Reliability Model

In this section, we provide a brief illustration of the Bayesian model presented in [26], to which we refer for a thorough illustration. The Bayesian approach performs inference on a parameter of interest, $\boldsymbol{\theta}$, through the Bayes theorem. This allows us to combine prior opinion (expressed through a prior distribution on $\boldsymbol{\theta}$) and experimental evidence (provided by the likelihood function) to get an updated opinion (given by the posterior distribution), which can be used to estimate the parameter, make decisions, and forecast.

In the case of the Birnbaum–Saunders distribution, the parameter of interest is $\boldsymbol{\theta} = (\alpha, \beta)^\top$. Prior distributions are chosen for both parameters. The choice of a functional form and the elicitation of its parameters based on experts' opinions is a complex task, and we prefer to provide just few explanatory details. The functional form should have properties corresponding to the possible behavior of the parameter, for example, non-negativity, unimodality, and symmetry. The parameters should be chosen to match experts' opinions about, say, mean or median, the parameter. In the case of the parameter α, an inverse gamma distribution is chosen in [26] with parameters a and b, denoted by $\mathrm{IG}(a, b)$, as the prior distribution of α^2. Observe that although the distribution of α^2 is considered, α is used because it is the Birnbaum–Saunders distribution parameter. Of course, α is the square root of a value sampled from the distribution of α^2. Note that the inverse gamma distribution, like the gamma, is very flexible besides being defined only for positive values and being unimodal. The informed choice of the parameters is typically done by finding the values matching prior opinions on mean, median, and quantiles. Sometimes, diffuse (or non-informative) priors are chosen in the absence of informed opinions: in this case the parameters are chosen to have a large variance. A gamma prior distribution would fit well also for β.

A posteriori, it is not possible to get closed forms for the distributions of α and β, but it is possible to get a sample from the posterior distribution, applying a Gibbs sampling method with a Metropolis–Hastings step. This Markov Chain Monte Carlo method [17] allows us to generate a sample from the posterior distributions of α and β recursively, actually drawing from the posterior conditional distributions of the parameters. In fact, at each step, a value is drawn from the distribution of α given β and the data, as well as one from the distribution of β given α and the data. In the former case, the simulation is easy since the posterior conditional distribution is still inverse gamma, whereas the latter conditional posterior distribution is known apart from a constant. In such case, a value of β is generated at each step from a proposal distribution and accepted or rejected according to a probability based on both proposal and conditional posterior distributions. Parameters are then estimated taking the sample mean of the generated values. It is also possible to construct $100(1-\gamma)\%$ credible intervals using the range spanned by the values sampled from the Markov Chain Monte Carlo method, when removing the smallest and largest $(\gamma/2) \times N$ values. Mathematical details of the procedures described above can be found in [26].

Given two treatments, T_1 and T_2, they can be compared considering either

$$\mathrm{P}(T_1 > T_2) \tag{4}$$

or their medians. The comparison is quite natural in the latter case when using the Birnbaum–Saunders distribution. In fact, as mentioned, its parameter β equals the median of the distribution and the medians of the two distributions are supposed to differ by a term δ. The comparison then reduces to checking if δ is zero or not.

The expression defined in (4) is what we name the Birnbaum–Saunders reliability model with the Bayesian computation carried out as indicated above in the presented section. Mathematical details on what has been illustrated here can be found in [26].

4 Application to Fatigue Data

We considered two real fatigue life data sets detailed in Table 1 and introduced in [8] to show the potential applications of the methodology for the Bayesian computation in a Birnbaum–Saunders reliability model.

The data upon analysis are related to fatigue life (T) of 6061-T6 aluminum pieces expressed by cycles ($\times 10^{-3}$) until the failure occurs. These pieces were cut parallel to the direction of rolling and oscillating at 18 cycles per seconds at two maximum stress levels corresponding to:

(a) $X_1 = 2.1$ psi ($\times 10^4$).
(b) $X_2 = 3.1$ psi ($\times 10^4$).

Table 1 Fatigue life (in cycles $\times 10^{-3}$) of aluminum pieces submitted to the maximum indicated stress level provided in [8]

2.1×10^4 psi					3.1×10^4 psi				
370	706	716	746	785	70	90	96	97	99
797	844	855	858	886	100	103	104	104	105
886	930	960	988	999	107	108	108	108	109
1000	1010	1016	1018	1020	109	112	112	113	114
1055	1085	1102	1102	1108	114	114	116	119	120
1115	1120	1134	1140	1199	120	120	121	121	123
1200	1200	1203	1222	1235	124	124	124	124	124
1238	1252	1258	1262	1269	128	128	129	129	130
1270	1290	1293	1300	1310	130	130	131	131	131
1313	1315	1330	1355	1390	131	131	132	132	132
1416	1419	1420	1420	1450	133	134	134	134	134
1452	1475	1478	1481	1485	134	136	136	137	138
1502	1505	1513	1522	1522	138	138	139	139	141
1530	1540	1560	1567	1578	141	142	142	142	142
1594	1602	1604	1608	1630	142	142	144	144	145
1642	1674	1730	1750	1750	146	148	148	149	151
1763	1768	1781	1782	1792	151	152	155	156	157
1820	1868	1881	1890	1893	157	157	157	158	159
1895	1910	1923	1924	1945	162	163	163	164	166
2023	2100	2130	2215	2268	166	168	170	174	196
2440					212				

Remark 4.1 In (a) and (b), the abbreviation "psi" is used for "pound per square inch," or, more accurately, pound-force per square inch (symbol: lbf/in2), which is a unit of pressure or of stress based on avoirdupois units, where "lbf" denotes "pound of force" or "pound-force" and "in2" denotes "square inch". Note that "psi" is the pressure resulting from a force of one pound-force applied to an area of one square inch. In the International System of Units (SI, abbreviated from the French Système International d'unitès), which is the modern form of the metric system, 1 psi is approximately equal to 6895 N/m^2, where 1 Newton/m^2 (N/m^2) = 1 Joule/m^3 (J/m^3) = 1 Pascal (P).

The sample sizes of these two treatments are $n_1 = 101$ and $n_2 = 101$ for stress levels X_1 and X_2, respectively. Thus, the total number of observations is $N = 202$ and the stress levels are $k = 2$. All pieces were tested until they failed. We wish to test if the stress level has some effect on the fatigue life.

The methodology to be used in this applications is summarized into the following steps:

(1) Collect n_i data $\boldsymbol{t}_i = (t_{i1}, \ldots, t_{in_i})^\top$ of the random variable of interest for i treatments.
(2) Carry out an exploratory analysis of the data $\boldsymbol{t}_i$ collected in Step 1 to identify distributions to be considered.
(3) Check adequacy of considered distributions in each treatment i in Step 2.
(4) Select the best distribution that describes the data in each treatment i according to Step 3.
(5) Establish prior distributions for the parameters of the selected distribution in Step 4.
(6) Estimate the treatment posterior means/medians based on the established distributions in Step 5.
(7) Compare the effects of two treatments considered in previous steps for the random variable of interest by:
    (i) Constructing 95% credible intervals for δ.
    (ii) Estimating $\mathrm{P}(\delta > 0|\boldsymbol{t}_i)$ and $\mathrm{P}(\delta \leq 0|\boldsymbol{t}_i)$ in each treatment i with the data $\boldsymbol{t}_i$.
    (iii) Determining the reliability model $\mathrm{P}(T_1 > T_2|\boldsymbol{t}_1, \boldsymbol{t}_2)$ as defined in (4).

Table 2 reports a descriptive summary of the data of both treatments. Note that, as the stress level increases, the median and mean fatigue life, as well as its variability, decrease considerably. Thus, we observe that the scale parameter β should decrease as the stress level increases. We recall that β is the scale parameter and also the median, but the mean is also in direct relation to it; see property (A4). We should detect that α, the shape parameter, it is not modified as the stress level increases.

Figure 2 shows histograms and box plots of the fatigue life data. Note that there are some atypical observations, a certain asymmetry in the distribution of the data, and that the scale of the distribution decreases as the stress level increases. Notice that the shape of the distribution is not substantially altered in the different stress

Table 2 Descriptive statistics of fatigue life (in cycles $\times 10^{-3}$) for the indicated stress level

Stress level	Minimum	First quartile	Median	Mean	Third quartile	Maximum	SD	n_i
2.1×10^4 psi	370	1115	1416	1400.84	1642	2440	391.01	101
3.1×10^4 psi	70	120	133	133.73	146	212	22.36	101

Table 3 KS p-values and BIC values of the indicated distributions and stress level for the fatigue life data

2.1×10^4 psi			3.1×10^4 psi		
Distribution	KS	BIC	Distribution	KS	BIC
Birnbaum–Saunders	0.919	1144.65	Birnbaum–Saunders	0.459	923.77
Inverse Gaussian	0.918	1144.68	Inverse Gaussian	0.457	923.80

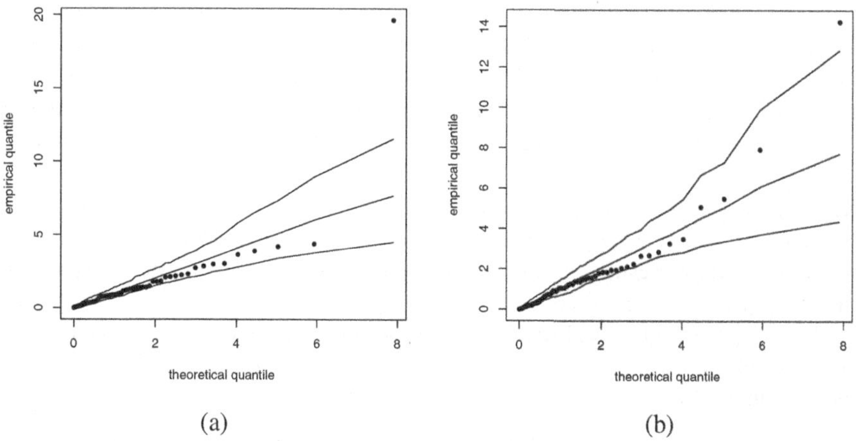

Fig. 1 QQ plots with simulated envelopes based on the Birnbaum–Saunders distribution for fatigue life data at the stress levels (**a**) 2.1×10^4 psi and (**b**) 3.1×10^4 psi

levels, supporting the fact that α, the shape parameter, it is not modified as the stress level increases.

Two life distributions that have a close connection are the Birnbaum–Saunders and inverse Gaussian models; see [21]. To analyze the fatigue life T, the Birnbaum–Saunders and inverse Gaussian distributions are proposed. We apply the Kolmogorov–Smirnov (KS) test and Bayesian information criterion (BIC) to decide which of these distributions fit the data better; see Table 3. From this table, we detect that the Birnbaum–Saunders distribution fits slightly better the data than the inverse Gaussian distribution. In addition, by Property (A3), we construct quantile versus quantile (QQ) plots with envelopes, which are shown in Fig. 1. From this figure, we note a good fit of the Birnbaum–Saunders distribution to the data.

Table 4 Bayesian estimates and 95% credible interval (CI) of the indicated parameter and treatment for the fatigue data

	α		β	
Treatment	Mean	95% CI	Mean	95% CI
2.1×10^4 psi	0.310	(0.267; 0.353)	1336.380	(1256.52; 1416.240)
3.1×10^4 psi	0.170	(0.169; 0.171)	131.819	(127.455; 136.183)

Table 5 Estimate, 95% credible interval (CI), $P(\delta > 0|\boldsymbol{t})$, $P(T_1 > T_2|\boldsymbol{t}_1, \boldsymbol{t}_2)$ for the fatigue data

Parameter	Mean	95% CI	$P(\delta \leq 0\|\boldsymbol{t})$	$P(\delta > 0\|\boldsymbol{t})$	$P(T_1 > T_2\|\boldsymbol{t}_1, \boldsymbol{t}_2)$
δ	−0.055	(−0.087; −0.023)	0.995	0.005	0.433

Table 4 reports posterior summaries of the distribution parameters for each treatment, where SD denotes standard deviation. These results are obtained by using a Gibbs sampling with a Metropolis–Hastings step for a sample of size equal to 10,000. The sample autocorrelation is monitored and no thinning is necessary. We detect that the Markov chain attains stationarity, that is, its desired posterior distribution is reached, by using graphical tools and tests. The trace plots indicate that the chains converge to their stationary distributions. The Gelman–Rubin, Raftery–Lewis, and Heidelberg–Welch tests detect convergence of the Markov chain for each parameter when comparing both stress levels. Regarding sensitivity, note that, in general, the estimates are not changing notoriously when different values of the hyperparameters are used.

We compare the fatigue life of the two treatments related to stress levels of 2.1×10^4 psi and 3.1×10^4 psi. Tables 4 and 5 report the posterior summaries from where we conclude that:

(i) The fatigue life is clearly larger as the stress level decreases, according to both the estimate of the median β provided by Table 4 and the estimate of δ when comparing both stress levels in Table 5.
(ii) The estimates of the parameters are very accurate as shown by the very narrow credible intervals; see Tables 4 and 5.
(iii) In relation to the probability $P(\delta > 0|\boldsymbol{t})$, we detect that, as the stress level increases from 2.1×10^4 psi to 3.1×10^4 psi, the fatigue life decreases significantly, as expected; see Table 5.
(iv) The slightly small value (less than 50%) of the estimate of $P(T_1 > T_2|\boldsymbol{t}_1, \boldsymbol{t}_2)$ for the treatments support the results above mentioned in item (iii); see Table 5. These estimates indicate that the fatigue life related to the low stress level is larger than the fatigue life associated with the high stress level (Fig. 2).

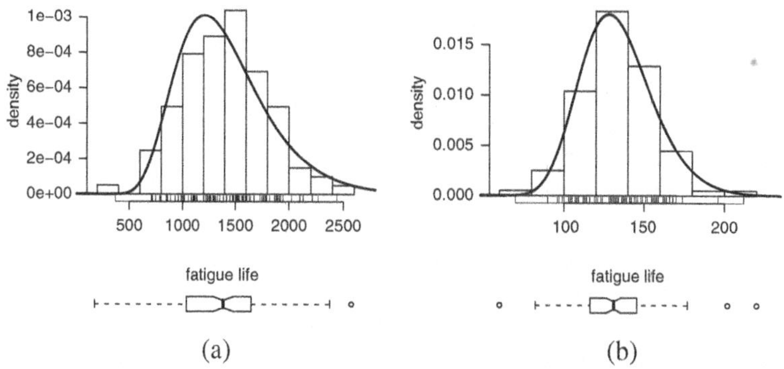

Fig. 2 Histograms with estimated BS densities and box plots for the fatigue life data at the stress levels (**a**) 2.1×10^4 psi and (**b**) 3.1×10^4 psi

5 Conclusions, Discussion, and Future Research

The present study was based on the following steps:

(i) We have presented a Birnbaum–Saunders reliability model and a literature review of its practical applications.
(ii) We have considered Bayesian computation for conducting inference on the introduced Birnbaum–Saunders reliability model.
(iii) The proposed methodology using the Birnbaum–Saunders distribution allows us to evaluate the effect of two treatments in terms of its reliability.
(iv) An algorithm that summarized the proposed methodology was provided.
(v) The methodology was implemented in the `R` software and applied to real data, comparing the Birnbaum–Saunders distribution to its natural competitor, corresponding to the inverse Gaussian distribution, showing the convenience of using the Birnbaum–Saunders distribution.
(vi) We have compared the effects of two stress levels on the fatigue life constructing credible intervals, estimating the probability of detecting difference significant statistically, and determining a reliability model.

In summary, we have applied a Birnbaum–Saunders reliability model and estimated its parameters with Bayesian methods. An empirical study with real fatigue data was performed to show the good empirical behavior of the estimators and to illustrate potential applications. Therefore, this investigation may be a knowledge addition to the tool kit of diverse practitioners, including engineers, statisticians, and data scientists.

Some open problems that arose from the present investigation are the following:

(i) Parameter estimates of censored distributions are more efficient than when censorship is not considered. Indeed, if censored cases are present and a non-censored distribution is used, evidently it is not possible to estimate the variance of the censored part. However, if censored distributions are utilized in this case, such a variance may be estimated from the data; see [15, 35].

(ii) The methodology employed in this study may be implemented in reliability analysis of engineering structures. For instance, further research may be carried out in highway designs and planning, specifically a reliability analysis to manage the time of pavement repairs. In addition, in modern building material, as concrete modified with nano-particles, reliability models can be used to determinate the performance of structures subject to different loading conditions; see [39].

(iii) In bioengineering applications, biomaterials employed in bone tissue regeneration are subject to diverse body environmental conditions and physiological loading conditions. Thus, a reliability study can be suitable to estimate the variation of mechanical responses.

(iv) A reliability study is also useful in developing smart materials, when sensors in micro- or nano-scale are embedded to measure static or dynamic mechanical performance. Thus, reliability engineering can be part of the progress and development of a variety of material applications.

(v) An extension of the present study to the multivariate case is also of practical relevance [5, 28, 34, 44].

(vi) The derivation of diagnostic techniques to detect potential influential cases is needed, which is an important tool to be used in all statistical modeling [11, 18, 31].

(vii) Robust estimation methods when outliers are present into the data set can be applied [49].

(viii) Reliability models that are based on the Birnbaum–Saunders distribution can be of great interest, due to the encouraging results shown by this distribution in the present study. For example, it is of interest to extend the results introduced in [2] to parallel and series system with multiple components and considering other stronger stochastic orders.

Therefore, the results proposed in this study promote new challenges and offer an open door to explore other theoretical and numerical issues. Research on these and other issues is in progress, and their findings will be reported in future articles.

Acknowledgments The authors thank the Editors and Reviewers for their constructive comments on an earlier version of this manuscript. This research was supported partially by project grant "Fondecyt 1200525" from the National Agency for Research and Development (ANID) of the Chilean government.

References

1. Achcar, J.A.: Inferences for the Birnbaum-Saunders fatigue life model using Bayesian methods. Comput. Stat. Data Anal. **15**, 367–380 (1993)
2. Amiri, M., Balakrishnan, N., Jamalizadeh, A.: Stochastic ordering of lifetimes of parallel and series systems comprising heterogeneous dependent components with generalized Birnbaum-Saunders distributions. Probab. Eng. Inform. Sci. 49–65 (2022)

3. Arrue, J., Arellano, R., Gomez, H.W., Leiva, V.: On a new type of Birnbaum-Saunders models and its inference and application to fatigue data. J. Appl. Stat. **47**, 2690–2710 (2020)
4. Athayde, E., Azevedo, A., Barros, M., Leiva, V.: Failure rate of Birnbaum-Saunders distributions: shape, change-point, estimation and robustness. Brazilian J. Probab. Stat. **33**, 301–328 (2019)
5. Aykroyd, R.G., Leiva, V., Marchant, C.: Multivariate Birnbaum-Saunders distributions: Modelling and applications. Risks **6**, 1–25 (2018)
6. Balakrishnan, N., Kundu, D.: Birnbaum-Saunders distribution: a review of models, analysis, and applications. Appl. Stoch. Models Bus. Ind. **35**, 4–49 (2019)
7. Barros, M., Leiva, V., Ospina, R., Tsuyuguchi, A.: Goodness-of-fit tests for the Birnbaum-Saunders distribution with censored reliability data. IEEE Trans. Reliab. **63**, 543–554 (2014)
8. Birnbaum, Z.W., Saunders, S.C.: Estimation for a family of life distributions with applications to fatigue. J. Appl. Probab. **6**, 328–347 (1969)
9. Birnbaum, Z.W., Saunders, S.C.: A new family of life distributions. J. Appl. Probab. **6**, 319–327 (1969)
10. Cancho, V.G., Ortega, E.M.M., Paula, G.A. On estimation and influence diagnostics for log-Birnbaum-Saunders Student-t regression models: full Bayesian analysis. J. Stat. Plan. Inf. **140**, 2486–2496 (2010)
11. Carrasco, J.M.F., Figueroa-Zuniga, J.I., Leiva, V., Riquelme, M, Aykroyd, R.G.: An errors-in-variables model based on the Birnbaum-Saunders and its diagnostics with an application to earthquake data. Stochastic Environ. Res. Risk Assess. **34**, 369–380 (2020)
12. Cordes, J.A., Thomas, J., Wong, R.S., Carlucci, D.: Reliability estimates for flawed mortar projectile bodies. Reliab. Eng. Syst. Safety **94**, 1887–1893 (2009)
13. Crookston, K.A., Young, T.M., Harper, D., Guess, F.M.: Statistical reliability analyses of two wood plastic composite extrusion processes. Reliab. Eng. Syst. Safety **96**, 172–177 (2011)
14. Dasilva, A., Dias, R., Leiva, V., Marchant, C., Saulo, H.: Birnbaum-Saunders regression models: a comparative evaluation of three approaches. J. Stat. Comput. Simul. **90**, 2552–2570 (2020)
15. Desousa, M., Saulo, H., Leiva, V., Santos-Neto, M.: On a new mixture-based regression model: simulation and application to data with high censoring. J. Stat. Comput. Simul. **90**(16), 2861–2877 (2020)
16. Farias, R.B.A., Lemonte, A.J.: Bayesian inference for the Birnbaum-Saunders non-linear regression model. Stat. Methods Appl. **20**, 423–438 (2011)
17. Gamerman, D., Lopes, H.: Markov Chain Monte Carlo: Stochastic Simulation for Bayesian Inference. Chapman and Hall, Boca Raton (2006)
18. Garcia-Papani, F., Leiva, V., Uribe-Opazo, M.A., Aykroyd, R.G.: Birnbaum-Saunders spatial regression models: diagnostics and application to chemical data. Chemom. Intell. Lab. Syst. **177**, 114–128 (2018)
19. Guiraud, P., Leiva, V., Fierro, R.: A non-central version of the Birnbaum-Saunders distribution for reliability analysis. IEEE Trans. Reliab. **58**, 152–160 (2009)
20. Johnson, N., Kotz, S., Balakrishnan, N.: Continuous Univariate Distributions, vol. 2. Wiley, New York (1995)
21. Kotz, S., Leiva, V., Sanhueza, A.: Two new mixture models related to the inverse Gaussian distribution. Methodol. Comput. Appl. Probab. **12**, 199–212 (2010)
22. Laniado, H., Lillo, R.E.: Allocation policies of redundancies in two-parallel-series and two-series-parallel systems. IEEE Trans. Reliab. **63**, 223–229 (2014)
23. Leiva, V.: The Birnbaum-Saunders Distribution. Academic Press, New York (2016)
24. Leiva, V., Saunders, S.C.: Cumulative damage models. In: Wiley StatsRef: Statistics Reference Online, pp. 1–10 (2015). https://doi.org/10.1002/9781118445112.stat02136.pub2
25. Leiva, V., Rojas, E., Galea, M., Sanhueza, A.: Diagnostics in Birnbaum-Saunders accelerated life models with an application to fatigue data. Appl. Stoch. Models Bus. Ind. **30**, 115–131 (2014)
26. Leiva, V., Ruggeri, F., Saulo, H., Vivanco, J.F.: A methodology based on the Birnbaum-Saunders distribution for reliability analysis applied to nano-materials. Reliab. Eng. Syst. Saf. **157**, 192–201 (2017)

27. Leiva, V., Marchant, C., Ruggeri, F., Saulo, H.: Statistical quality control and reliability analysis using the Birnbaum-Saunders distribution with industrial applications. In: Lio, Y., Ng, T.K.H., Tsai, T-R., Chen, D-G. (eds.) Statistical Quality Technologies: Theory and Practice, pp. 21–53. Springer, Cham (2019)
28. Leiva, V., Sanchez, L., Galea, M., Saulo, H.: Global and local diagnostic analytics for a geostatistical model based on a new approach to quantile regression. Stoch. Environ. Res. Risk Assess. **34**, 1457–1471 (2020)
29. Leiva, V., Saulo, H., Souza, R., Aykroyd, R.G., Vila, R.: A new BISARMA time series model for forecasting mortality using weather and particulate matter data. J. Forecast. **40**(2), 346–364 (2021)
30. Liu, Y., Liu, L., Stratman, B., Mahadevan, S.: Multiaxial fatigue reliability analysis of railroad wheels. Reliab. Eng. Syst. Saf. **93**, 456–467 (2008)
31. Liu, Y., Mao, G., Leiva, V., Liu, S., Tapia, A.: Diagnostic analytics for an autoregressive model under the skew-normal distribution. Mathematics **8**, 693 (2020)
32. Marchant, C., Leiva, V., Cysneiros, F.: A multivariate log-linear model for Birnbaum-Saunders distributions. IEEE Trans. Reliab. **65**, 816–827 (2016)
33. Marchant, C., Leiva, V., Cysneiros, F., Vivanco, J.: Diagnostics in multivariate generalized Birnbaum-Saunders regression models. J. Appl. Stat. **43**, 2829–2849 (2016)
34. Marchant, C., Leiva, V., Christakos, G., Cavieres, M.F.: Monitoring urban environmental pollution by bivariate control charts: new methodology and case study in Santiago, Chile. Environmetrics **30**, e2551 (2019)
35. Martinez-Florez, G., Leiva, V., Gomez-Deniz, E., Marchant, C.: A family of skew-normal distributions for modeling proportions and rates with zeros/ones excess. Symmetry **12**(9), 1439 (2020)
36. Moala, F.A., Achcar, J.A., Gimenez, R.: Bayesian estimation for the Birnbaum-Saunders distribution in the presence of censored data. IEEE Lat. Am. Trans. **13**, 3187–3192 (2015)
37. Owen, W., Padgett, W.: Accelerated test models for system strength based on Birnbaum-Saunders distribution. Lifetime Data Anal. **5**, 133–147 (1999)
38. Owen, W., Padgett, W.: A Birnbaum-Saunders accelerated life model. IEEE Trans. Reliab. **49**, 224–229 (2000)
39. Padmanabhan, K., Prabu, S.: Reliability of nanostructured materials. In: G. Wilde (ed.) Reliability of Nanostructured Materials, chapter 2, pp. 51–126. Elsevier, Oxford (2009)
40. Pan, Z., Balakrishnan, N.: Reliability modeling of degradation of products with multiple performance characteristics based on gamma processes. Reliab. Eng. Syst. Saf. **96**, 949–957 (2011)
41. Pievatolo, A., Ruggeri, F.: Bayesian modelling of train doors' reliability. In: O'Hagan, A., West, M. (ed.) Handbook of Applied Bayesian Analysis. Oxford University Press, Oxford (2010)
42. R Core Team: R: A Language and Environment for Statistical Computing. R Foundation for Statistical Computing, Vienna (2018)
43. Rieck, J., Nedelman, J.: A log-linear model for the Birnbaum-Saunders distribution. Technometrics **3**, 51–60 (1991)
44. Sánchez, L., Leiva, V., Galea, M., Saulo, H.: Birnbaum-Saunders quantile regression models with application to spatial data. Mathematics **8**, 1000 (2020)
45. Sun, T., Shi, Y.: Estimation for Birnbaum-Saunders distribution in simple step stress-accelerated life test with type-II censoring. Commun. Stat. Simul. Comput. **45**, 880–901 (2016)
46. Sutherland, L., Soares, C.: Review of probabilistic models of the strength of composite materials. Reliab. Eng. Syst. Saf. **56**, 183–196 (1997)
47. Tsionas, E.: Bayesian inference in Birnbaum-Saunders regression. Commun. Stat. Theory Methods **30**, 179–193 (2001)
48. Upadhyay, S., Mukherjee, B.: Bayes analysis and comparison of accelerated Weibull and accelerated Birnbaum-Saunders models. Commun. Stat. Theory Methods **39**, 195–213 (2010)
49. Velasco, H., Laniado, H., Toro, M., Leiva, V., Lio, Y.: Robust three-step regression based on comedian and its performance in cell-wise and case-wise outliers. Mathematics **8**, 1259 (2020)

50. Villegas, C., Paula, G., Leiva, V.: Birnbaum-Saunders mixed models for censored reliability data analysis. IEEE Trans. Reliab. **60**, 748–758 (2011)
51. Wang, J., Laniado, H.: A note on allocation policy in two-parallel-series and two-series-parallel systems with respect to likelihood ratio order. Stat. Probab. Lett. **102**(C), 17–21 (2015)
52. Wang, M., Sun, X., Park, C.: Bayesian analysis of Birnbaum-Saunders distribution via the generalized ratio-of-uniforms method. Comput. Stat. **31**, 207–225 (2016)
53. Wu, J., Yan, S., Zuo, M.J.: Evaluating the reliability of multi-body mechanisms: a method considering the uncertainties of dynamic performance. Reliab. Eng. Syst. Saf. **149**, 96–106 (2016)
54. Xu, A., & Tang, Y.: Reference analysis for Birnbaum-Saunders distribution. Comput. Stat. Data Anal. **54**, 185–192 (2010)

A Competing Risk Model Based on a Two-Parameter Exponential Family Distribution Under Progressive Type II Censoring

Yu-Jau Lin, Tzong-Ru Tsai, Ding-Geng Chen, and Yuhlong Lio

Abstract This chapter presents a competing risk model with two dependent failure causes whose latent failure times are Marshall–Olkin bivariate exponential family distribution that includes Burr XII, Gompertz, and Weibull distributions as special cases. Maximum likelihood estimation and Bayesian estimation methods for the model parameters are discussed. The existence and uniqueness of maximum likelihood estimates are established under some regular conditions for Weibull and Burr XII base distributions, respectively. A Markov-Chain Monte Carlo process is proposed for Bayesian estimation method. Due to the possible flaw of maximum likelihood estimation method, a Monte Carlo simulation study is only conducted to assess the performance of Bayesian estimations for model parameters, tenth percentile, median and ninety percentile lifetimes under square error, absolute error, and LINEX loss functions. A real data set is used for illustration.

1 Introduction

When the subjects under medical survival analysis or industry life testing involve multiple failure modes competing, the problem is usually refereed as the competitive

Y.-J. Lin
Applied Mathematics Department, Chung Yuan Christian University, Taoyuan City, Taiwan
e-mail: yujaulin@cycu.edu.tw

T.-R. Tsai
Department of Statistics, Tamkang University, New Taipei City, Taiwan
e-mail: tzongru@gms.tku.edu.tw

D.-G. Chen
College of Health Solutions, Arizona State University, Phoenix, AZ, USA

Department of Statistics, University of Pretoria, Pretoria, South Africa

Y. Lio (✉)
Department of Mathematical Sciences, The University of South Dakota, Vermillion, SD, USA
e-mail: Yuhlong.Lio@usd.edu

Y. Lio et al. (eds.), *Bayesian Inference and Computation in Reliability and Survival Analysis*, Emerging Topics in Statistics and Biostatistics,
https://doi.org/10.1007/978-3-030-88658-5_4

risks model. In the competitive risks model, it is assumed that a failure is associated with one of the competing failure modes. During the medical survival monitoring, subject loses happen very often. Therefore, it is common that the collected lifetimes are not complete random sample but censored sample. Many different censored samples have been generated in the medical survival analysis; for example, type I and type II censored samples mentioned by Kundu and Howlader [20] and type I interval censored data mentioned by Chen and Lio [8] as well as Lin and Lio [24]. Recent technology advancement prolongs the process of collecting a complete random sample of lifetimes in industry life test; to shorten the sampling procedure, different censoring schemes as well as step-stress life test procedures have been developed to collect lifetime information. Readers may refer to [2, 3] for more information about life test procedures used for reliability inference.

Among all censoring schemes developed in both medical survival analysis and industry life testing, the type I and type II censoring schemes have been commonly used due to their easy implementations. Placing n items on the failure test at the same initial time, labeled by $T_0 = 0$, the life test continues up to a predetermined time τ for type I censoring scheme, while the life test under the type II censoring scheme will be performed until a predetermined number $m(< n)$ of failures observed at the largest random failure time $X_{m:m:n}$. Epstein [14] introduced the type I hybrid censoring scheme where the life test would be terminated at a random time $\tau^* = \min\{X_{m:m:n}, \tau\}$, and Childs et al. [10] considered the type II hybrid censoring scheme where the life test would be terminated at the random time $\tau^{**} = \max\{X_{m:m:n}, \tau\}$. The aforementioned censoring schemes do not allow items to be removed from the life test at any other time before the terminal time. In order to allow the items removed at other time points before the terminal time and save the life test time and cost, the progressive censoring schemes have been applied to the life testing. Balakrishnan and Aggarwala [2] and Balakrishnan and Cramer [3] provided more information about progressive censoring schemes. The progressive type II censoring scheme is performed as follows, n items are placed on failure test at the same time, labeled by $T_0 = 0$, at the ith failure $X_{i:m:n}$, R_i items are randomly removed from the remaining survival items for i from $1, 2, \cdots, m$ where $R_i, i = 1, 2, \cdots, m$, and m are predetermined prior to the life testing such that $n = m + \sum_{i=1}^{m} R_i$. Combining the strategies of type II progressive censoring scheme with the hybrid type I or hybrid type II censoring scheme, Kundu and Joarder [21] studied the type I progressive hybrid censoring scheme that implemented the type II progressive censoring scheme until the random time $\tau^* = \min\{X_{m:m:n}, \tau\}$, Childs et al. [11] discussed the type II progressive hybrid censoring scheme that implemented the type II progressive censoring scheme until the random time $\tau^* = \max\{X_{m:m:n}, \tau\}$. All survival items will be removed at the terminated random time when the aforementioned progressive hybrid censoring schemes are implemented.

Recently, two new censoring schemes named as adaptive type I progressive hybrid censoring scheme (AT-I PHCS) and adaptive type II progressive hybrid censoring scheme (AT-II PHCS) have been developed, respectively. The AT-II PHCS, which was discussed by Ng et al. [29] and Balakrishnan and Kundu

[5], terminates at $X_{m:m:n}$ and has no survival items removed when the life test experiment needs to pass time τ. Lin and Huang [23] introduced the AT-I PHCS, which was shown to have a higher efficiency in estimations. The AT-I PHCS implements type II progressive censoring scheme and must terminate at a prefixed time τ. Let the number of failures just right before the termination time τ be J. If the mth failure $X_{m:m:n}$ is obtained before τ, the life time experiment will continue to observe failures without withdrawing survival items until τ. Hence, at the termination time τ, all survival items $R_J^* = n - J - \sum_{i=1}^{J} R_i$ will be removed, where $R_m = R_{m+1} = \cdots = R_J = 0$ when $m < J$; otherwise, the AT-I PHCS has the progressive censoring scheme $R_1, R_2, \cdots, R_J$.

The competitive risks models assuming independent failure models have been studied by many scholars, for example, Miyakawa [28] studied the maximum likelihood estimators and uniformly minimum variance unbiased estimators of the failure rates for the competing risks model with two failure modes based on random sample obtained from exponential distribution but the data set possibly having missing failure cause. Kundu and Basu [19] extended this work to provide the approximate and asymptotic properties of the parameter estimators, confidence intervals, and bootstrap confidence bounds. They also extended for the Weibull distribution case. Kundu et al. [22] provided the maximum likelihood estimators, uniformly minimum variance unbiased estimators, and the Bayesian estimators using the inverse Gamma prior and square error loss for the competing risks model based on progressively type II censored sample from exponential distribution. Park and Kulasekera [31] established closed-form maximum likelihood estimators for a competitive risk model that has multi-failure modes in several groups using random right-censored sample with possible missing failure causes from exponential distributions. Bunea and Mazzuchi [6] presented a Bayesian framework using gamma prior and square error loss for the competitive risk model with possible multiple competitive failure modes based on the accelerated life test data from exponential distribution. Sarhan [33] provided the maximum likelihood estimators for the competitive risk model based on type I censored sample with possible missing failure modes from the generalized exponential distributions. Balakrishnan and Han [4] derived the maximum likelihood estimators of the unknown mean parameters for the different failure causes under a cumulative exposure assumption in the competitive risk model with two failure modes whose lifetimes are exponentially distributed based on the type II censored sample collected through a simple step-stress life test. The exact distributions of the maximum likelihood estimators were obtained by utilizing conditional moment generating functions. They also compared the performance of confidence intervals using exact distribution, the asymptotic distribution as well as the parametric bootstrap method through Monte Carlo simulation. Pareek et al. [30] analyzed the competitive risks data assuming the latent failure times that are Weibull distributed under the progressive type II censoring. Cramer and Schmiedt [12] studied the maximum likelihood estimators for two failure modes competing risks model based on the progressive type II censored data from *Lomax* distributions and provided the optimal censoring scheme based on Fisher information. Xu and Tang [38] discussed the Bayesian inference based on the competitive risks sample from the accelerated life test in the presence of competing failure modes whose latent failure times are Weibull distributed. Under adaptive type I progressive hybrid censoring scheme, Ashour and Nassar [1] investigated the maximum likelihood estimation and Bayesian estimation based on squared error and LINEX loss functions with independent gamma priors for the parameters of competing risks model with two failure causes whose latent failure times are Weibull distributed with common shape parameter. Under progressive type II censoring where the failure mode could be missing and the numbers of withdrawn units at each stage are subject to a binomial distribution, Qin and Gui [32] established the maximum likelihood estimators of the parameters in a competing risks model of two independent failure modes that have Burr-XII distributions sharing with the common inner shape parameter. They proved the existence and uniqueness of the maximum likelihood estimators and provided approximated confidence intervals by using the observed Fisher information matrix and delta method. Moreover, they provided Bayes estimators and associated credible intervals under square error loss, LINEX loss, and the general entropy loss functions.

The competitive risks model under dependent failure modes has been considered through copula structure by scholars. Zheng and Klein [39, 40] treated time to death and time to censoring as the two dependent failure modes in a competing risks model and investigated the marginal distribution of two competitive failure causes under the dependence structure of a given copula. They presented an estimator of the marginal distribution based on a given copula and showed that the estimator is consistent and reduces to the Kaplan–Meier estimator under the independent copula. Escarela and Carriere [15] proposed a fully parametric copula model, called Frank's family of copulas that allows to adjust for concomitant variables and dependence parameter to assess the effects on each marginal survival model and the relationship between the causes of death, to fit and analyze the cause-specific survival times collected from a competing risks model. They also studied the identification problem, dependence structures, and flexibility in selecting marginal survival functions. Shih and Emura [34] used the generalized Farlie–Gumbel–Morgenstern copula with the Burr III marginal distribution to address the dependence of two failure modes in the competing risks model. They developed a likelihood-based inference method and asymptotic theory goodness-of-fit tests based on the closed form of sub-distribution function.

Let U_0, U_1, and U_2 be independent exponential distributions with rate parameters, λ_0, λ_1, and λ_3, respectively. Let $X = \min\{U_0, U_1\}$ and $Y = \min\{U_0, U_2\}$. Marshall and Olkin [26] established a dependent bivariate exponential distribution for X and Y that has marginal exponential distributions with rate parameters, $\lambda_0+\lambda_1$ and $\lambda_0 + \lambda_2$, respectively. When $\lambda_0 = 0$, X and Y are independent exponential distributions. Therefore, λ_0 can be associated as dependent factor between X and Y. Hereafter, this type of dependent bivariate distribution will be referred as MOB distribution. Since then, Feizjavadian and Hashemi [16] considered dependent competing risks model with two causes that have a MOB Weibull distribution via utilizing three independent Weibull distributions sharing a common shape parameter. They developed maximum likelihood and an approximated maximum likelihood estimators and constructed approximate confidence intervals using the observed Fisher information matrix and asymptotic distribution of the maximum likelihood estimators under type II progressively hybrid censoring. Shi and Wu [35] studied the maximum likelihood estimation for dependent competing risks models with two failure causes that have MOB type Gompertz distributions under type I progressively hybrid censoring scheme. Cai et al. [7] established the maximum likelihood estimators based on the expectation–maximum algorithm and Bayesian estimators incorporating with auxiliary variables for the parameters of the competing risks model that has the failure causes of the MOB Weibull distributions sharing common shape parameter. They also used the missing information principle to obtain the observed information matrix and Monte Carlo method to construct the highest posterior density credible intervals.

In this chapter, we consider the competing risks model with dependent causes that have a two-parameter exponential family distribution sharing with a common parameter under progressive type II censoring scheme. The two-parameter exponential family distribution includes Burr XII, Gompertz, and Weibull distributions as special cases. The rest of chapter is organized as follows. The competing risks models are presented in Sect. 2. Section 3 addresses the maximum likelihood estimation method. Section 4 presents Bayesian estimation method. An intensive simulation study is conducted for MOB Burr XII and MOB Weibull distributions in Sect. 5 and the application of a real example given in Sect. 6. Conclusions are addressed in Sect. 7.

2 Competitive Risk Models

A two-parameter exponential family distribution of lifetime random variable has the probability density function (PDF), cumulative distribution function (CDF), and hazard rate function that are, respectively, given as follows:

$$f(x|\beta,\lambda) = \beta g'(x;\lambda)\exp(-\beta g(x;\lambda)), \quad x \geq 0, \quad \beta \geq 0, \quad \lambda \geq 0, \tag{1}$$

$$F(x|\beta,\lambda) = 1.0 - \exp(-\beta g(x;\lambda)), \quad x \geq 0, \quad \beta \geq 0, \quad \lambda \geq 0, \tag{2}$$

and

$$h(x|\beta,\lambda) = \beta g'(x;\lambda), \quad x \geq 0, \quad \lambda > 0, \quad \beta \geq 0, \quad \lambda \geq 0, \tag{3}$$

where $g(x;\lambda)$ is an increase function of x with $g(0;\lambda) = 0$ and $\lim_{x->\infty} g(x;\lambda) = \infty$, $g'(x;\lambda)$ is the derivative of $g(x;\lambda)$ with respective to x, and $\beta > 0$ and $\lambda > 0$ are distribution parameters. For example, if $g(x;\lambda) = \ln(1+x^{\lambda})$, then it is Burr XII distribution; if $g(x;\lambda) = \lambda^{-1}(\exp(\lambda x) - 1.0)$, then it is Gompertz distribution; and if $g(x;\lambda) = x^{\lambda}$, then it is Weibull distribution.

Let the survival function of the two-parameter exponential family distribution be denoted by $S(x|\beta,\lambda) = \exp(-\beta g(x;\lambda))$ and X_0, X_1, X_2 be independent random variables that have survival functions $S(x|\beta_0, \lambda)$, $S(x|\beta_1, \lambda)$ and $S(x|\beta_2, \lambda)$, respectively, where $x \geq 0$, $\lambda > 0$, $\beta_0 > 0$, $\beta_1 > 0$, and $\beta_2 > 0$. Define $T_1 = min\{X_0, X_1\}$ and $T_2 = min\{X_0, X_2\}$; then it can be shown that T_1 and T_2 have the following joint survival functions,

$$\begin{aligned} S_{T_1,T_2}(t_1, t_2) &= P(T_1 > t_1, T_2 > t_2) \\ &= P(X_1 > t_1, X_2 > t_2, X_0 > max\{t_1, t_2\}) \\ &= P(X_1 > t_1)P(X_2 > t_2)P(X_0 > max\{t_1, t_2\}) \\ &= \exp(-\beta_1 g(t_1; \lambda)) \exp(-\beta_2 g(t_2; \lambda)) \exp(-\beta_0 g(max\{t_1, t_2\}; \lambda)), \end{aligned} \tag{4}$$

which is called the joint MOB exponential family survival function with three parameters, λ, β_0, β_1, and β_2. Following the same procedure used by Shi and Wu [35], the following properties can be obtained accordingly:

Proposition 1: The joint distribution of T_1 and T_2 has the following two-parameter survival function,

$$S_{T_1,T_2}(t_1, t_2) = \begin{cases} S(t_1|\beta_0 + \beta_1, \lambda)S(t_2|\beta_2, \lambda) & t_1 > t_2 \\ S(t_1|\beta_1, \lambda)S(t_2|\beta_0 + \beta_2, \lambda) & t_2 > t_1 \\ S(t|\beta_0 + \beta_1 + \beta_2, \lambda) & t = t_1 = t_2. \end{cases} \tag{5}$$

Proposition 2: The joint PDF of T_1 and T_2 is given as the following two-parameter function,

$$f_{T_1,T_2}(t_1, t_2) = \begin{cases} f_1(t_1, t_2) = f(t_1|\beta_0 + \beta_1, \lambda)f(t_2|\beta_2, \lambda) & t_1 > t_2 \\ f_2(t_1, t_2) = f(t_1|\beta_1, \lambda)f(t_2|\beta_0 + \beta_2, \lambda) & t_2 > t_1 \\ f_0(t_1, t_2) = \frac{\beta_0}{\beta_0+\beta_1+\beta_2} f(t|\beta_0 + \beta_1 + \beta_2, \lambda) & t = t_1 = t_2. \end{cases} \tag{6}$$

Place n identical systems of two competing failure modes, which have latent lifetimes T_1 and T_2, under the progressive type II with censoring scheme, $\{R_1, R_2, \cdots, R_m\}$. The resulting observed type II progressively censored samples are presented as $(X_{1:m:n}, \delta_1, R_1)$, $(X_{2:m:n}, \delta_2, R_2)$, $(X_{3:m:n}, \delta_3, R_3)$,$\cdots$,$(X_{m-1:m:n}, \delta_{m-1}, R_{m-1})$, $(X_{m:m:n}, \delta_m, R_m)$, where $\sum_{i=1}^{m} R_i + m = n$ and the indicator $\delta_i = k$ is used to show the ith failure system due to the failure mode k, $k = 0$, 1, or 2. Let $I_k(\delta_i = k) = 1$ and $I_k(\delta_i \neq k) = 0$, where $k =$ 0, 1, or 2 and $i = 1, 2, 3, \cdots, m$. The random variable $n_0 = \sum_{i=1}^{m} I_0(\delta_i = 0)$ is the number of fail systems due to both failure modes, $n_1 = \sum_{i=1}^{m} I_1(\delta_i = 1)$ is the number of fail systems due to failure mode $k = 1$, and $n_2 = \sum_{i=1}^{m} I_2(\delta_i = 2)$ is the number of fail systems due to failure mode $k = 2$.

Let T be the failure time of the aforementioned competing risks model. It is easy to find the system survival function to be $S_T(t) = \exp(-(\beta_0 + \beta_1 + \beta_2)g(t; \lambda))$. Therefore, the p-th quantile lifetime, t_p, of the competing risks model can be obtained as $t_p = g^{-1}\left(\frac{-\ln(1-p)}{\beta_0+\beta_1+\beta_2}; \lambda\right)$, where $0 < p < 1$ and $g^{-1}(\cdot; \lambda)$ is the generalized inverse function of $g(t; \lambda)$.

3 Maximum Likelihood Estimation

Based on the progressively type II censored sample, $(X_{1:m:n}, \delta_1, R_1), (X_{2:m:n}, \delta_2, R_2), (X_{3:m:n}, \delta_3, R_3), \cdots, (X_{m-1:m:n}, \delta_{m-1}, R_{m-1}), (X_{m:m:n}, \delta_m, R_m)$ collected from the n systems mentioned above, the likelihood function can be presented as

$$L(\beta_0, \beta_1, \beta_2, \lambda) \propto \prod_{i=1}^{m} \left\{ (f_{T_1,T_2}(X_{i:m:n}, X_{i:m:n}))^{I_0(\delta_i)} \prod_{j=1}^{2} \right.$$
$$\left. \times \left[-\frac{\partial S_{T_1,T_2}(t_1, t_2)}{\partial t_j} |_{(X_{i:m:n}, X_{i:m:n})} \right]^{I_j(\delta_i)} (S_{T_1,T_2}(X_{i:m:n}, X_{i:m:n}))^{R_i} \right\}, \tag{7}$$

where

$$f_{T_1,T_2}(X_{i:m:n}, X_{i:m:n}) = \frac{\beta_0}{\beta_0 + \beta_1 + \beta_2} f(X_{i:m:n} | \beta_0 + \beta_1 + \beta_2, \lambda) \tag{8}$$
$$= \beta_0 g'(X_{i:m:n}; \lambda) \exp(-(\beta_0 + \beta_1 + \beta_2) g(X_{i:m:n}; \lambda))$$

$$-\frac{\partial S_{T_1,T_2}(t_1, t_2)}{\partial t_1} |(X_{i:m:n}, X_{i:m:n}) = f(X_{i:m:n} | \beta_1, \lambda) S(X_{i:m:n} | \beta_0 + \beta_2, \lambda) \tag{9}$$
$$= \beta_1 g'(X_{i:m:n}; \lambda) \exp(-(\beta_0 + \beta_1 + \beta_2) g(X_{i:m:n}; \lambda))$$

$$-\frac{\partial S_{T_1,T_2}(t_1, t_2)}{\partial t_2} |(X_{i:m:n}, X_{i:m:n}) = f(X_{i:m:n} | \beta_2, \lambda) S(X_{i:m:n} | \beta_0 + \beta_1, \lambda) \tag{10}$$
$$= \beta_2 g'(X_{i:m:n}; \lambda) \exp(-(\beta_0 + \beta_1 + \beta_2) g(X_{i:m:n}; \lambda))$$

$$S_{T_1,T_2}(X_{i:m:n}, X_{i:m:n}) = S(X_{i:m:n} | \beta_0 + \beta_1 + \beta_2, \lambda) \tag{11}$$
$$= \exp(-(\beta_0 + \beta_1 + \beta_2) g(X_{i:m:n}; \lambda)).$$

Therefore, the likelihood function can be represented as

$$L(\beta_0, \beta_1, \beta_2, \lambda) \propto \prod_{j=0}^{2} \beta_j^{n_j} \prod_{i=1}^{m} g'(X_{i:m:n}; \lambda) \exp$$
$$\times \left(-(\beta_0 + \beta_1 + \beta_2) \sum_{i=1}^{m} (R_i + 1) g(X_{i:m:n}; \lambda) \right), \tag{12}$$

and the log-likelihood function without constant term can be presented as

$$l(\beta_0, \beta_1, \beta_2, \lambda) = \sum_{j=0}^{2} n_j \ln(\beta_j) + \sum_{i=1}^{m} \ln(g'(X_{i:m:n}; \lambda)) - (\beta_0 + \beta_1 + \beta_2) \left(\sum_{i=1}^{m}(R_i + 1)g(X_{i:m:n}; \lambda)\right). \tag{13}$$

Taking the first-order partial derivative of $l(\beta_0, \beta_1, \beta_2, \lambda)$ with respective to $\beta_0, \beta_1, \beta_2$ and λ, respectively, the following results are obtained:

$$\frac{\partial l(\beta_0, \beta_1, \beta_2, \lambda)}{\partial \beta_0} = \frac{n_0}{\beta_0} - \left(\sum_{i=1}^{m}(R_i + 1)g(X_{i:m:n}; \lambda)\right), \tag{14}$$

$$\frac{\partial l(\beta_0, \beta_1, \beta_2, \lambda)}{\partial \beta_1} = \frac{n_1}{\beta_1} - \left(\sum_{i=1}^{m}(R_i + 1)g(X_{i:m:n}; \lambda)\right), \tag{15}$$

$$\frac{\partial l(\beta_0, \beta_1, \beta_2, \lambda)}{\partial \beta_2} = \frac{n_2}{\beta_2} - \left(\sum_{i=1}^{m}(R_i + 1)g(X_{i:m:n}; \lambda)\right), \tag{16}$$

$$\frac{\partial l(\beta_0, \beta_1, \beta_2, \lambda)}{\partial \lambda} = \sum_{i=1}^{m} \frac{g'_\lambda(X_{i:m:n}; \lambda)}{g'(X_{i:m:n}; \lambda)} - (\beta_0 + \beta_1 + \beta_2)\left(\sum_{i=1}^{m}(R_i + 1)g_\lambda(X_{i:m:n}; \lambda)\right), \tag{17}$$

where $g'_\lambda(x; \lambda) = \frac{\partial g'(x;\lambda)}{\partial \lambda}$. Setting $\frac{\partial l(\beta_0, \beta_1, \beta_2, \lambda)}{\partial \beta_j} = 0$, the MLE of β_j is given as

$$\hat{\beta}_j = \frac{n_j}{\left(\sum_{i=1}^{m}(R_i + 1)g(X_{i:m:n}; \lambda)\right)} \tag{18}$$

for $j = 0,1$, or 2, given $\lambda > 0$. Plugging $\hat{\beta}_j$ in the log-likelihood function, the profile log-likelihood function without constant term can be obtained as follows:

$$cl(\lambda) = \sum_{j=0}^{2} n_j \ln(n_j) - m \ln\left(\sum_{i=1}^{m}(R_i + 1)g(X_{i:m:n}; \lambda)\right) + \sum_{i=1}^{m} \ln(g'(X_{i:m:n}; \lambda)) - m. \tag{19}$$

The existence of MLE, $\hat{\lambda}$, depends upon some regular conditions of $g(x; \lambda)$ that make profile log-likelihood function have concave down and unimodal shape in terms of λ.

3.1 Special Family 1: Weibull Distribution

When $g(x,\lambda) = x^{\lambda}$, the two-parameter exponential life time distribution has Weibull distribution. The profile log-likelihood function of Eq. (19) can be represented as follows:

$$cl_w(\lambda) = \sum_{j=1}^{2} n_j \ln(n_j) - m \ln\left(\sum_{i=1}^{m}(R_i+1)X_{i:m:n}^{\lambda}\right) + m\ln(\lambda) + (\lambda-1)\left(\sum_{i=1}^{m}\ln(X_{i:m:n})\right) - m \tag{20}$$

and

$$\frac{dcl_w(\lambda)}{d\lambda} = \frac{m}{\lambda} + \sum_{i=1}^{m}\ln(X_{i:m:n}) - m\frac{\sum_{i=1}^{m}(R_i+1)X_{i:m:n}^{\lambda}\ln(X_{i:m:n})}{\sum_{i=1}^{m}(R_i+1)X_{i:m:n}^{\lambda}}. \tag{21}$$

The following propositions for Weibull distribution can be used to show the MLE $\hat{\lambda}$ of common shape parameter of Weibull distributions is uniquely defined:

Proposition 1: The profile log-likelihood function $cl_w(\lambda)$ is a concave function of λ.

Proposition 2: If $n_j > 0$ for $j = 0, 1, 2$, then MLEs of $\beta_j > 0$ for $j = 0, 1, 2$ and λ for Weibull distributions are uniquely defined.

3.2 Special Family 2: Burr XII Distribution

When $g(x,\lambda) = \ln(1+x^{\lambda})$, the two-parameter exponential life time distribution has Burr XII distribution that has inner shape parameter λ. The profile log-likelihood function of Eq. (19) can be represented as follows:

$$\begin{aligned} cl_B(\lambda) &= \sum_{j=1}^{2} n_j \ln(n_j) - m\ln\left(\sum_{i=1}^{m}(R_i+1)\ln\left(1+X_{i:m:n}^{\lambda}\right)\right) \\ &\quad + m\ln(\lambda) + (\lambda-1)\left(\sum_{i=1}^{m}\ln(X_{i:m:n})\right) - \sum_{i=1}^{m}\ln(1+X_{i:m:n}^{\lambda}) - m \\ &= \Psi(\lambda) - m\ln\left(\sum_{i=1}^{m}(R_i+1)\ln\left(1+X_{i:m:n}^{\lambda}\right)\right), \end{aligned} \tag{22}$$

where $\Psi(\lambda) = \sum_{j=1}^{2} n_j \ln(n_j) + \sum_{i=1}^{m} \ln(g'(X_{i:m:n}; \lambda) - m$. It is easy to show that $\Psi(\lambda)$ is a strictly concave function in $\lambda > 0$. Following the same argument by Wingo [36, 37] and Lio and Tsai [25],

Proposition 3: Given a positive value of $\beta_0 + \beta_1 + \beta_2$, the MLE, $\hat{\lambda}$, is always uniquely defined if and only if at least one observation is different from unity.

Proposition 4: Let $J \geq 2$ and $n_0 > 0, n_1 > 0, n_2 > 0$. Assume that $X_{i_1:m:n} \neq X_{i_2:m:n}$ for some $i_1 \neq i_2$ from $1 \leq i_1, i_2 \leq m$. Then MLEs of β_j for $j = 0, 1, 2$ and λ for Burr XII distributions are uniquely defined positive values.

Please note that $n_0 > 0$, $n_1 > 0$, and $n_2 > 0$ are sufficient conditions to ensure that MLEs $\hat{\beta}_j > 0$, $j = 0, 1, 2$. It is very often that $n_j = 0$, $j = 1, 2$, or 3 during the simulation study. Therefore, simulation study is only conducted to evaluate the performance of Bayesian estimators.

4 Bayesian Estimation

Let the model parameters given above be represented as $\Theta = (\theta_0, \theta_1, \theta_2, \theta_3) = (\beta_0, \beta_1, \beta_2, \lambda)$. Under the Bayesian framework, it is assumed that all unknown parameters, $\theta_l, l = 0, 1, 2, 3$, are independent and $\theta_l, l = 0, 1, 2$, have prior distributions with probability density functions, respectively, given as follows:

$$h_l(\theta_l; \alpha_l, \gamma_l) = \frac{1}{\Gamma(\alpha_l)\gamma_l^{\alpha_l}} \theta_l^{\alpha_l - 1} \exp\left\{-\frac{\theta_l}{\gamma_l}\right\}, \tag{23}$$

where $\alpha_l > 0$ and $\gamma_l > 0$ are hyper-parameters for $l = 0, 1, 2$. θ_3 has prior distribution with probability density function $h_3(\theta_3) \propto C$ where $C > 0$ is a constant. Combining (12), (23), and $h_3(\lambda)$, the joint posterior probability density function of Θ given a progressively type II censored data, $D = \{(X_{1:m:n}, \delta_1, R_1), (X_{2:m:n}, \delta_2, R_2), (X_{3:m:n}, \delta_3, R_3), \cdots, (X_{m-1:m:n}, \delta_{m-1}, R_{m-1}), (X_{m:m:n}, \delta_m, R_m)\}$, can be presented as

$$\Pi(\beta_0, \beta_1, \beta_2, \lambda | D) \propto \exp\left(-(\beta_0 + \beta_1 + \beta_2)\left(\sum_{i=1}^{m}(R_i + 1)g(X_{i:m:n}; \lambda)\right)\right)$$
$$\times \left(\prod_{j=0}^{2} \beta_j^{n_j} \prod_{i=1}^{m} g'(X_{i:m:n}; \lambda)\right)$$
$$\times\, h_0(\beta_0; \alpha_0, \gamma_0) h_1(\beta_1; \alpha_1, \gamma_1) h_2(\beta_2; \alpha_2, \gamma_2) h_3(\lambda). \tag{24}$$

Hence, the marginal posterior density functions of β_0, β_1, β_2, and λ given data D are, respectively, represented as

$$\Pi_0(\beta_0|D) = \int\int\int \Pi(\beta_0, \beta_1, \beta_2, \lambda|D) d\beta_1 d\beta_2 d\lambda, \tag{25}$$

$$\Pi_1(\beta_1|D) = \int\int\int \Pi(\beta_0, \beta_1, \beta_2, \lambda|D) d\beta_0 d\beta_2 d\lambda, \tag{26}$$

$$\Pi_2(\beta_2|D) = \int\int\int \Pi(\beta_0, \beta_1, \beta_2, \lambda|D) d\beta_0 d\beta_1 d\lambda, \tag{27}$$

and

$$\Pi_3(\lambda|D) = \int\int\int \Pi(\beta_0, \beta_1, \beta_2, \lambda|D) d\beta_0 d\beta_1 d\beta_2. \tag{28}$$

The joint marginal posterior density functions of any three parameters can be obtained as follows:

$$\Pi_{\beta_0,\beta_1,\beta_2}(\beta_0, \beta_1, \beta_2|D) = \int \Pi(\beta_0, \beta_1, \beta_2, \lambda|D) d\lambda, \tag{29}$$

$$\Pi_{\beta_0,\beta_1,\lambda}(\beta_0, \beta_1, \lambda|D) = \int \Pi(\beta_0, \beta_1, \beta_2, \lambda|D) d\beta_2, \tag{30}$$

$$\Pi_{\beta_0,\beta_2,\lambda}(\beta_0, \beta_2, \lambda|D) = \int \Pi(\beta_0, \beta_1, \beta_2, \lambda|D) d\beta_1, \tag{31}$$

and

$$\Pi_{\beta_1,\beta_2,\lambda}(\beta_1, \beta_2, \lambda|D) = \int \Pi(\beta_0, \beta_1, \beta_2, \lambda|D) d\beta_0. \tag{32}$$

Meanwhile, the full conditional posterior probability density function of β_0, given β_1,β_2, and λ, is

$$\Pi_0(\beta_0|\beta_1, \beta_2, \lambda, D) \propto \beta_0^{n_0+\alpha_0-1} \exp\left(-\beta_0\left(\frac{1}{\gamma_0} + \sum_{i=1}^{m}(R_i+1)g(X_{i:m:n}; \lambda)\right)\right), \tag{33}$$

the full conditional posterior probability density function of β_1, given β_0,β_2, and λ, is

$$\Pi_1(\beta_1|\beta_0, \beta_2, \lambda, D) \propto \beta_1^{n_1+\alpha_1-1} \exp\left(-\beta_1\left(\frac{1}{\gamma_1} + \sum_{i=1}^{m}(R_i+1)g(X_{i:m:n}; \lambda)\right)\right), \tag{34}$$

the full conditional posterior probability density function of β_2, given β_0,β_1, and λ, is

$$\Pi_2(\beta_2|\beta_0, \beta_1, \lambda, D) \propto \beta_2^{n_2+\alpha_2-1} \exp\left(-\beta_2\left(\frac{1}{\gamma_2}+\sum_{i=1}^{m}(R_i+1)g(X_{i:m:n};\lambda)\right)\right), \quad (35)$$

and the full conditional posterior probability density function of λ, given β_0,β_1, and β_2, is

$$\Pi_3(\lambda|\beta_0, \beta_1, \beta_2, D) \propto \exp\left(-(\beta_0+\beta_1+\beta_2)\left(\sum_{i=1}^{m}(R_i+1)g(X_{i:m:n};\lambda)\right)\right) \times \left(\prod_{i=1}^{m} g'(X_{i:m:n};\lambda)\right). \quad (36)$$

In this chapter, the loss functions considered are squared error, absolute error, and LINEX loss functions. The corresponding Bayesian estimators will be the posterior distribution mean and median under square error loss and absolute error loss functions, respectively. Under LINEX loss function, $L(\theta_l, \hat{\theta}_l) = \exp(\phi(\hat{\theta}_l - \theta_l)) - \phi(\hat{\theta}_l - \theta_l) - 1$, where $\hat{\theta}_l$ is the Bayesian estimator of θ_l and $\phi \neq 0$ is a given real number, and the Bayesian estimate is $\frac{-1}{\phi}\ln(E(\exp(-\phi\theta_l)|D))$ where $E(\cdot|D)$ is the posterior expectation. Among all the aforementioned posterior density functions for the parameters β_0, β_1, β_2, and λ, it can be noted that the respective posterior density functions of θ_l, $l = 0, 1, 2, 3$ are not in a closed function. Hence, in order to obtain the Bayes estimates, Markov-Chain Monte Carlo method through the application of Metropolis–Hastings (M–H) algorithm [18, 27] via the Gibbs scheme [17] is utilized to draw the samples of β_0, β_1, β_2, and λ, respectively, through (33), (34), (35), and (36).

4.1 A Markov-Chain Monte Carlo Process

Given $j = 0, 1, 2, 3$, the Markov chain $\theta_j^{(i)}$, $i = 1, 2, \cdots$, of the jth parameter, θ_j, can be constructed by applying the Metropolis–Hastings (M–H) algorithm stated as follows. Let $q_j(\theta_j^{(*)}|\theta_j^{(i)})$ be a proposed conditional transition probability density function for $\theta_j^{(*)}$, given $\theta_j^{(i)}$ for $j = 0, 1, 2, 3$. Given a current state value, $\theta_j^{(i)}$, of the parameter θ_j, $\theta_j^{(*)}$ is a candidate value for the parameter θ_j in the next state and generated by $q_j(\theta_j^{(*)}|\theta_j^{(i)})$. Then, $\theta_j^{(*)}$ is accepted as the value of the next state, $\theta_j^{(i+1)}$, with a probability of $\min\left\{1, \frac{\Pi_j(\theta_j^{(*)}|D)q_j(\theta_j^{(i)}|\theta_j^{(*)})}{\Pi_j(\theta_j^{(i)}|D)q_j(\theta_j^{(*)}|\theta_j^{(i)})}\right\}$. If $\theta_j^{(*)}$ is rejected as the value of the next state, then the next state $\theta_j^{(i+1)} = \theta_j^{(i)}$. The Markov chain for

$\{\beta_0^{(i)}, \beta_1^{(i)}, \beta_2^{(i)}, \lambda^{(i)}, i = 1, 2, 3, \cdots\} = \{\theta_0^{(i)}, \theta_1^{(i)}, \theta_2^{(i)}, \theta_3^{(i)}, i = 1, 2, 3, \cdots\}$ can be generated through the Markov-Chain Monte Carlo (MCMC) iterative process stated as follows:

Step 1: Set i=0

Step 2: Generate $\theta_0^{(*)}$ from $q_0(\theta_0^{(*)}|\theta_0^{(i)})$ and u_0 from uniform distribution over (0, 1) interval independently, and

$$\theta_0^{(i+1)} = \begin{cases} \theta_0^{(*)} \text{ if } u_0 \leq \min\left\{1, \frac{\Pi_0(\theta_0^{(*)}|\theta_1^{(i)},\theta_2^{(i)},\theta_3^{(i)},D)q_0(\theta_0^{(i)}|\theta_0^{(*)})}{\Pi_0(\theta_0^{(i)}|\theta_1^{(i)},\theta_2^{(i)},\theta_3^{(i)},D)q_0(\theta_0^{(*)}|\theta_0^{(i)})}\right\} \\ \theta_0^{(i)} \text{ otherwise.} \end{cases} \tag{37}$$

Step 3: Generate $\theta_1^{(*)}$ from $q_1(\theta_1^{(*)}|\theta_1^{(i)})$ and u_1 from uniform distribution over (0, 1) interval independently, and

$$\theta_1^{(i+1)} = \begin{cases} \theta_1^{(*)} \text{ if } u_1 \leq \min\left\{1, \frac{\Pi_1(\theta_1^{(*)}|\theta_0^{(i+1)},\theta_2^{(i)},\theta_3^{(i)},D)q_1(\theta_1^{(i)}|\theta_1^{(*)})}{\Pi_1(\theta_1^{(i)}|\theta_0^{(i+1)},\theta_2^{(i)},\theta_3^{(i)},D)q_1(\theta_1^{(*)}|\theta_1^{(i)})}\right\} \\ \theta_1^{(i)} \text{ otherwise.} \end{cases} \tag{38}$$

Step 4: Generate $\theta_2^{(*)}$ from $q_2(\theta_2^{(*)}|\theta_2^{(i)})$ and u_2 from uniform distribution over (0, 1) interval independently, and

$$\theta_2^{(i+1)} = \begin{cases} \theta_2^{(*)} \text{ if } u_2 \leq \min\left\{1, \frac{\Pi_2(\theta_2^{(*)}|\theta_0^{(i+1)},\theta_1^{(i+1)},\theta_3^{(i)},D)q_2(\theta_2^{(i)}|\theta_2^{(*)})}{\Pi_2(\theta_2^{(i)}|\theta_0^{(i+1)},\theta_1^{(i+1)},\theta_3^{(i)},D)q_2(\theta_2^{(*)}|\theta_2^{(i)})}\right\} \\ \theta_2^{(i)} \text{ otherwise.} \end{cases} \tag{39}$$

Step 5: Generate $\theta_3^{(*)}$ from $q_3(\theta_3^{(*)}|\theta_3^{(i)})$ and u_3 from uniform distribution over (0, 1) interval independently, and

$$\theta_3^{(i+1)} = \begin{cases} \theta_3^{(*)} \text{ if } u_3 \leq \min\left\{1, \frac{\Pi_3(\theta_3^{(*)}|\theta_0^{(i+1)},\theta_1^{(i+1)},\theta_2^{(i+1)},D)q_3(\theta_3^{(i)}|\theta_3^{(*)})}{\Pi_3(\theta_3^{(i)}|\theta_0^{(i+1)},\theta_1^{(i+1)},\theta_2^{(i+1)},D)q_3(\theta_3^{(*)}|\theta_3^{(i)})}\right\} \\ \theta_3^{(i)} \text{ otherwise.} \end{cases} \tag{40}$$

Step 6: Set $i = i + 1$ go to Step 2.

Starting with initial values, $\theta_0^{(0)}$,$\theta_1^{(0)}$ $\theta_2^{(0)}$, and $\theta_3^{(0)}$, the above iterative process is running through a huge number of periods (says N). For $j = 0, 1, 2, 3$, the empirical distributions of θ_j could be described by the realizations of θ_j after a burn-in period, N_b. The Bayes estimators of θ_j can be approximated based on the values of $\left\{\theta_j^{(i)}|i = N_b, \ldots, N\right\}$, respectively. For instance, if the squared loss function is used, then the Bayes estimates of θ_j are the means of $\left\{\theta_j^{(i)}|i = N_b, \ldots, N\right\}$; if the absolute value of difference loss function is used, then the Bayes estimates of θ_j are the medians of the empirical distributions of $\left\{\theta_j^{(i)} | i = N_b, \ldots, N\right\}$; and if LINEX loss function is used, then the Bayes estimates of θ_j can be evaluated by

$$\hat{\theta}_{l,\phi} = \frac{-1}{\phi} \ln \left(\frac{1}{N - N_b} \sum_{k=N_b+1}^{N} \exp(-\phi \theta_l^{(k)}) \right).$$

In order to find the Bayesian estimation of a function, $\eta(\Theta)$, of Θ, the Markov chain $\eta^{(i)}(\Theta), i = 1, 2, 3, \cdots$ can be approximately obtained by plugging in method using the Markov chain $\Theta^{(i)}, i = 1, 2, \cdots$. The posterior distribution of $\eta(\Theta)$ can be approximated by using the empirical distribution based on the Markov chain $\eta^{(i)}(\Theta), i = 1, 2, 3, \cdots$. Then the Bayesian estimate can be derived for $\eta(\Theta)$, accordingly.

It should be mentioned that $\Pi_0(\theta_0|\theta_1, \theta_2, \theta_3, D)$, $\Pi_1(\theta_1|\theta_0, \theta_2, \theta_3, D)$, $\Pi_2(\theta_2|\theta_0, \theta_1, \theta_3, D)$, and $\Pi_3(\theta_3|\theta_0, \theta_1, \theta_2, D)$ can be replaced by $\Pi(\theta_0, \theta_1, \theta_2, \theta_3|D)$ during the implementation of Metropolis–Hastings algorithm, and when the MCMC process is implemented based on non-informative priors (i.e., $h_l(\theta_l) \propto C$ for $l = 0, 1, 2, 3$ where C is a constant), the MCMC process will approach to the maximum likelihood estimates for the parameters μ_1 and μ_2 and ρ, respectively (see, for example, Chib and Greenberg [9]). Moreover, the full conditional posteriors for $\beta_l, l = 0, 1, 2$ are gamma distribution with shape parameter $n_l + \alpha_l$ and rate parameter $\frac{1}{\gamma_l} + \sum_i^m (R_i + 1) g(X_{i:m:n}; \lambda)$ that is only dependent on given λ. Therefore, the MCMC jumps, Steps 2, 3 and 4 can be replaced by taking sample from the corresponding gamma distribution, instead. Step 5 can be modified as follows,

Step 5*: Let $\theta_3^{old} = \theta_3^{(i)}$.

Step 5.1: Generate θ_3^* from $q_3(\theta_3^*|\theta_3^{old})$ and u_3 from uniform distribution over (0,1) interval independently, and

$$\theta_3^{(i+1)} = \begin{cases} \theta_3^{(*)} & \text{if } u_3 \leq \min\left\{1, \frac{\Pi_3(\theta_3^{(*)}|\theta_0^{(i+1)}, \theta_1^{(i+1)}, \theta_2^{(i+1)}, D) q_3(\theta_3^{(old)}|\theta_3^{(*)})}{\Pi_3(\theta_3^{(old)}|\theta_0^{(i+1)}, \theta_1^{(i+1)}, \theta_2^{(i+1)}, D) q_3(\theta_3^{(*)}|\theta_3^{(old)})}\right\} \\ \theta_3^{(old)} & \text{otherwise.} \end{cases} \tag{41}$$

Step 5.2: Let $\theta_3^{old} = \theta_3^{(i+1)}$. Repeat Step 5.1 and Step 5.2 for some more times.

5 Simulation Studies

A simulation study is conducted to investigate the performance of the proposed Bayesian estimates of the competing risks model parameters and system lifetime utilizing square error, absolute error, and LINEX loss functions based on the progressively type II censored data that includes failure times and the associated causes. The simulation inputs, which include sample sizes $n = 30$ and 50, progressive censoring $R_i, i = 1, 2, 3, \cdots, m$, and population parameters, β_0, β_1, β_2, and λ, are listed in Tables 1, 2, 3, 4, 5, 6, 7, 8, 9, 10, 11, 12, 13, 14, 15, 16, 17, and 18. For $\beta_l, l = 0, 1, 2$, two prior distributions that include non-informative and light informative gamma priors with hyper-parameters $\alpha_0 = 2$, $\gamma_0 = 0.1$; $\alpha_1 = 6$, $\gamma_1 = 0.2$; $\alpha_2 = 10$, $\gamma_2 = 0.1$ are applied. For λ, only simulation inputs, the simulation was conducted by 10,000 iterations. Each iteration generates Markov chain of size 50,000 for each estimator, and Bayesian estimate was calculated by using burn-in at 40,000. Parts of simulation results have been displayed in Tables 1, 2, 3, 4, 5, 6, 7, 8, 9, 10, 11, 12, 13, 14, 15, 16, 17, and 18. that show the general behaviors from the simulation study. that show the general behaviors from the simulation study.

Tables 1, 2, and 3 show the simulation results for the competing risks model of two independent failure modes that have the distributed latent lifetimes, and Tables 4, 5, and 6 display the simulation results for dependent two failure modes that have the Weibull distributed latent lifetimes. These six tables use the same parameters $\beta_l, l = 1, 2$ and λ and dependent factor with $\beta_0 = 0.2$ for Tables 4, 5, and 6. In viewing these six tables, it can be noted that the Bayesian estimates of distribution parameters for dependent system are a little bit more accurate than those for independent system. But there are no much difference between Bayesian estimates of quantile lifetime estimates for both systems. Meanwhile Tables 1, 2, 3, 4, 5, 6, 7, 8, and 9 show that the Bayesian estimates are getting more accurate when the dependent factor β_0 increases. Tables 10, 11, and 12 have the simulation results by using non-informative priors. Comparing the simulation results from Tables 4, 5, and 6 and the simulation results from Tables 10, 11, and 12, it can be seen that the informative prior does improve the accuracy of Bayesian estimates. Tables 13, 14, 15, 16, 17, and 18 display the simulation results for the Burr XII distributed latent failure time system. Again, it can be seen that when dependent factor β_0 increases, the accuracy of Bayesian estimate is improved.

6 An Illustrative Example

The data set about the effect of laser treatment to delay the onset of blindness from 71 patients under the Diabetic Retinopathy Study conducted by the National Eye Institute will be used to illustrate the proposed Bayesian estimation procedure. At the beginning, one eye from the ith patient for $i = 1, 2, \cdots, 71$ was randomly selected for giving the laser treatment and the other eye without giving the laser treatment. Then the minimum time, X_i, in terms of day to blindness and the cause index $\delta_i = 1, 2, 0$ for specifying treated, untreated, or both eyes was recorded. More detail description of the complete data set can be obtained from the report by Csorgo and Welsh [13]. Feizjavadian and Hashemi [16] investigated the maximum likelihood estimates and approximated maximum likelihood estimates of the competing risks model with two dependent causes whose latent times have

Table 1 Computed MSEs and biases (in parentheses) of the Bayes estimators with informative priors based on simulation for two independent Weibull distributions

			$(\lambda, \beta_1, \beta_2) = (0.6, 1.2, 1.0)$			$(\lambda, \beta_1, \beta_2) = (0.6, 1.2, 1.0)$		
	m	Scheme	Squared error loss			Absolute error loss		
1	15	(0,...,0,15)	0.0207(0.0698)	0.1187(0.1310)	0.2109(0.3309)	0.0201(0.0658)	0.1058(0.0872)	0.1806(0.2871)
2		(15,0,...,0)	0.0186(0.0608)	0.0780(0.0623)	0.1429(0.2623)	0.0175(0.0538)	0.0725(0.0306)	0.1247(0.2305)
3		(3,0,0,...,3,0,0)	0.0182(0.0639)	0.0961(0.0959)	0.1744(0.2960)	0.0175(0.0593)	0.0871(0.0589)	0.1507(0.2589)
4	20	(0,...,0,30)	0.0149(0.0597)	0.1512(0.1579)	0.2544(0.3579)	0.0147(0.0575)	0.1358(0.1155)	0.2221(0.3156)
5		(30,0,...,0)	0.0132(0.0488)	0.0779(0.0617)	0.1426(0.2617)	0.0125(0.0436)	0.0730(0.0349)	0.1269(0.2349)
6		(3,0,3,0,...,3,0)	0.0130(0.0537)	0.1131(0.1176)	0.2000(0.3175)	0.0126(0.0508)	0.1027(0.0824)	0.1756(0.2824)
7	30	(0,...,0,20)	0.0154(0.0657)	0.1346(0.1479)	0.2338(0.3479)	0.0150(0.0628)	0.1226(0.1170)	0.2094(0.3169)
8		(20,0,...,0)	0.0097(0.0409)	0.0655(0.0530)	0.1268(0.2531)	0.0093(0.0376)	0.0622(0.0328)	0.1154(0.2329)
9		(2,0,0,...,2,0,0)	0.0114(0.0513)	0.0939(0.0933)	0.1712(0.2932)	0.0111(0.0487)	0.0873(0.0689)	0.1549(0.2689)

Table 2 Estimated MSEs and biases (in parentheses) of the Bayes estimators with informative priors based on simulation study for Weibull distributions

	m	Scheme	$(\lambda, \beta_1, \beta_2) = (0.6, 1.2, 1.0)$ LINEX with $\phi = 0.5$			$(\lambda, \beta_1, \beta_2) = (0.6, 1.2, 1.0)$ LINEX with $\phi = -0.5$		
1	15	(0,. . . ,0,15)	0.0200(0.0665)	0.1016(0.0926)	0.1785(0.2925)	0.0214(0.0732)	0.1415(0.1732)	0.2505(0.3731)
2		(15,0,. . . ,0)	0.0179(0.0574)	0.0697(0.0331)	0.1229(0.2331)	0.0194(0.0642)	0.0893(0.0936)	0.1667(0.2936)
3		(3,0,0,. . . ,3,0,0)	0.0176(0.0608)	0.0838(0.0626)	0.1488(0.2626)	0.0189(0.0670)	0.1125(0.1321)	0.2054(0.3321)
4	20	(0,. . . ,0,30)	0.0145(0.0575)	0.1310(0.1209)	0.2193(0.3208)	0.0153(0.0620)	0.1773(0.1986)	0.2967(0.3986)
5		(30,0,. . . ,0)	0.0127(0.0464)	0.0706(0.0370)	0.1254(0.2370)	0.0136(0.0513)	0.0873(0.0880)	0.1624(0.2880)
6		(3,0,3,0,. . . ,3,0)	0.0126(0.0516)	0.0992(0.0862)	0.1737(0.2862)	0.0133(0.0559)	0.1308(0.1514)	0.2314(0.3514)
7	30	(0,. . . ,0,20)	0.0150(0.0636)	0.1197(0.1209)	0.2081(0.3209)	0.0157(0.0678)	0.1527(0.1769)	0.2635(0.3768)
8		(20,0,. . . ,0)	0.0094(0.0391)	0.0607(0.0345)	0.1145(0.2346)	0.0099(0.0427)	0.0714(0.0724)	0.1404(0.2725)
9		(2,0,0,. . . ,2,0,0)	0.0111(0.0496)	0.0853(0.0714)	0.1538(0.2713)	0.0116(0.0531)	0.1044(0.1164)	0.1909(0.3163)

Table 3 Estimated MSEs and biases (in parentheses) of the Bayes estimators for 0.1th lifetime, median lifetime, and 0.9th lifetime with informative priors based on simulation study for Weibull distributions with $(\lambda, \beta_1, \beta_2) = (0.6, 1.2, 1.0)$

	m	Scheme	$q_{0.1}, q_{0.5}, q_{0.9}$ Absolute value error			$q_{0.1}, q_{0.5}, q_{0.9}$ LINEX with $\phi = 0.5$		
1	15	(0,...,0,15)	6.86×10^{-5}(0.0048)	0.0029(0.0038)	0.4152(−0.0827)	8.44×10^{-5}(0.0047)	0.0035(0.0107)	0.2640(−0.0311)
2		(15,0,...,0)	9.20×10^{-5}(0.0059)	0.0043(0.0082)	0.1422(−0.0909)	10.01×10^{-5}(0.0058)	0.0046(0.0152)	0.1427(−0.0481)
3		(3,0,0,...,3,0,0)	$6, 87 \times 10^{-5}$(0.0049)	0.0032(0.0051)	0.1969(−0.0965)	8.81×10^{-5}(0.0049)	0.0035(0.0117)	0.1816(−0.0442)
4	20	(0,...,0,30)	3.09×10^{-5}(0.0030)	0.0027(−0.0011)	0.5880(−0.0670)	3.65×10^{-5}(0.0030)	0.0034(0.0060)	0.3533(−0.0282)
5		(30,0,...,0)	5.07×10^{-5}(0.0041)	0.0033(0.0030)	0.1387(−0.0940)	6.83×10^{-5}(0.0041)	0.0035(0.0089)	0.1394(−0.0575)
6		(3,0,3,0,...,3,0)	3.17×10^{-5}(0.0030)	0.0023(−0.0014)	0.2298(−0.1032)	3.88×10^{-5}(0.0030)	0.0026(0.0045)	0.2079(−0.0547)
7	30	(0,...,0,20)	3.30×10^{-5}(0.0033)	0.0019(−0.0019)	0.2330(−0.1249)	3.90×10^{-5}(0.0032)	0.0020(0.0020)	0.2127(−0.0845)
8		(20,0,...,0)	3.31×10^{-5}(0.0030)	0.0025(−0.0010)	0.1118(−0.1066)	4.23×10^{-5}(0.0030)	0.0026(0.0033)	0.1113(−0.0784)
9		(2,0,0,...,2,0,0)	2.93×10^{-5}(0.0029)	0.0021(−0.0013)	0.1590(−0.1142)	3.56×10^{-5}(0.0029)	0.0022(0.0027)	0.1548(−0.0787)

Table 4 Estimated MSEs and biases (in parentheses) of the Bayes estimators with informative priors based on simulation study for Weibull distributions

	m	Scheme	$(\lambda, \beta_0, \beta_1, \beta_2) = (0.6, 0.2, 1.2, 1.0)$ Squared error loss				$(\lambda, \beta_0, \beta_1, \beta_2) = (0.6, 0.2, 1.2, 1.0)$ Absolute error loss			
1	15	(0,...,0,15)	0.017(0.063)	0.005(0.010)	0.112(0.116)	0.198(0.316)	0.017(0.059)	0.005(−0.012)	0.100(0.071)	0.169(0.271)
2		(15,0,...,0)	0.018(0.059)	0.005(0.005)	0.077(0.057)	0.140(0.257)	0.017(0.052)	0.005(−0.016)	0.071(0.024)	0.121(0.224)
3		(3,0,0,...,3,0,0)	0.016(0.059)	0.005(0.009)	0.094(0.091)	0.171(0.291)	0.016(0.054)	0.005(−0.012)	0.086(0.053)	0.147(0.253)
4	20	(0,...,0,30)	0.012(0.052)	0.006(0.013)	0.135(0.140)	0.231(0.340)	0.012(0.050)	0.005(−0.008)	0.122(0.097)	0.200(0.297)
5		(30,0,...,0)	0.012(0.047)	0.005(0.005)	0.077(0.058)	0.140(0.258)	0.012(0.042)	0.005(−0.014)	0.072(0.029)	0.124(0.229)
6		(3,0,3,0,...,3,0)	0.011(0.048)	0.005(0.009)	0.111(0.109)	0.195(0.309)	0.011(0.045)	0.005(−0.010)	0.101(0.072)	0.170(0.272)
7	30	(0,...,0,20)	0.014(0.060)	0.006(0.014)	0.128(0.139)	0.223(0.339)	0.013(0.058)	0.006(−0.003)	0.116(0.107)	0.199(0.307)
8		(20,0,...,0)	0.010(0.042)	0.005(0.005)	0.069(0.055)	0.131(0.255)	0.009(0.039)	0.005(−0.010)	0.065(0.034)	0.118(0.233)
9		(2,0,0,...,2,0,0)	0.010(0.047)	0.006(0.010)	0.093(0.089)	0.169(0.289)	0.010(0.044)	0.006(−0.006)	0.087(0.063)	0.152(0.263)

Table 5 Estimated MSEs and biases (in parentheses) of the Bayes estimators with informative priors based on simulation study for Weibull distributions

	m	Scheme	$(\lambda, \beta_0, \beta_1, \beta_2) = (0.6, 0.2, 1.2, 1.0)$ LINEX with $\phi = 0.5$				$(\lambda, \beta_0, \beta_1, \beta_2) = (0.6, 0.2, 1.2, 1.0)$ LINEX with $\phi = -0.5$			
1	15	(0,…,0,15)	0.017(0.060)	0.005(0.007)	0.096(0.077)	0.167(0.277)	0.018(0.066)	0.005(0.014)	0.133(0.158)	0.236(0.358)
2		(15,0,…,0)	0.017(0.056)	0.005(0.002)	0.068(0.027)	0.119(0.227)	0.019(0.062)	0.005(0.008)	0.088(0.090)	0.164(0.290)
3		(3,0,0,…,3,0,0)	0.016(0.056)	0.005(0.006)	0.082(0.057)	0.145(0.257)	0.017(0.061)	0.005(0.013)	0.111(0.129)	0.202(0.329)
4	20	(0,…,0,30)	0.012(0.050)	0.005(0.009)	0.117(0.103)	0.198(0.303)	0.012(0.054)	0.006(0.016)	0.158(0.181)	0.271(0.381)
5		(30,0,…,0)	0.012(0.045)	0.005(0.002)	0.070(0.032)	0.122(0.231)	0.013(0.049)	0.005(0.008)	0.086(0.085)	0.160(0.285)
6		(3,0,3,0,…,3,0)	0.011(0.046)	0.005(0.006)	0.098(0.077)	0.168(0.277)	0.012(0.050)	0.006(0.013)	0.128(0.144)	0.226(0.344)
7	30	(0,…,0,20)	0.013(0.058)	0.006(0.012)	0.113(0.111)	0.198(0.311)	0.014(0.062)	0.006(0.017)	0.145(0.169)	0.253(0.369)
8		(20,0,…,0)	0.010(0.041)	0.005(0.003)	0.063(0.035)	0.118(0.235)	0.010(0.044)	0.006(0.008)	0.075(0.076)	0.146(0.276)
9		(2,0,0,…,2,0,0)	0.010(0.045)	0.006(0.008)	0.084(0.066)	0.151(0.266)	0.011(0.048)	0.006(0.013)	0.104(0.114)	0.189(0.313)

Table 6 Estimated MSEs and biases (in parentheses) of the Bayes estimators for 0.1th lifetime, median lifetime, and 0.9th lifetime with informative priors based on simulation study for Weibull distributions with $(\lambda, \beta_0, \beta_1, \beta_2) = (0.6, 0.2, 1.2, 1.0)$

	m	Scheme	$q_{0.1}, q_{0.5}, q_{0.9}$ Square error loss			$q_{0.1}, q_{0.5}, q_{0.9}$ LINEX with $\phi = 0.5$		
1	15	(0,...,0,15)	6.25×10^{-5}(0.0040)	0.0025(0.0109)	1.3253(0.0985)	6.22×10^{-5}(0.0040)	0.0024(0.0103)	0.1544(−0.0165)
2		(15,0,...,0)	9.98×10^{-5}(0.0052)	0.0035(0.0160)	0.1208(0.0074)	9.92×10^{-5}(0.0052)	0.0034(0.0152)	0.0920(−0.0289)
3		(3,0,0,...,3,0,0)	6.71×10^{-5}(0.0042)	0.0027(0.0113)	0.1923(0.0251)	6.68×10^{-5}(0.0042)	0.0026(0.0107)	0.1140(−0.0302)
4	20	(0,...,0,30)	2.56×10^{-5}(0.0025)	0.0019(0.0049)	0.5771(0.0723)	2.55×10^{-5}(0.0024)	0.0018(0.0044)	0.1811(−0.0267)
5		(30,0,...,0)	5.41×10^{-5}(0.0037)	0.0027(0.0102)	0.1122(−0.0107)	5.38×10^{-5}(0.0037)	0.0026(0.0096)	0.0913(−0.0387)
6		(3,0,3,0,...,3,0)	3.04×10^{-5}(0.0026)	0.0020(0.0057)	0.3469(0.0296)	3.03×10^{-5}(0.0026)	0.0019(0.0052)	0.1442(−0.0308)
7	30	(0,...,0,20)	3.02×10^{-5}(0.0028)	0.0014(0.0031)	0.1814(−0.0264)	3.01×10^{-5}(0.0028)	0.0014(0.0028)	0.1275(−0.0643)
8		(20,0,...,0)	3.44×10^{-5}(0.0028)	0.0019(0.0055)	0.0861(−0.0389)	3.42×10^{-5}(0.0028)	0.0018(0.0051)	0.0770(−0.0569)
9		(2,0,0,...,2,0,0)	2.62×10^{-5}(0.0024)	0.0015(0.0032)	0.1245(−0.0302)	2.62×10^{-5}(0.0024)	0.0015(0.0029)	0.0999(−0.0564)

Table 7 Estimated MSEs and biases (in parentheses) of the Bayes estimators with informative priors based on simulation study for Weibull distribution

	m	Scheme	$(\lambda, \beta_0, \beta_1, \beta_2) = (0.6, 0.4, 1.2, 1.0)$ Square error loss				$(\lambda, \beta_0, \beta_1, \beta_2) = (0.6, 0.4, 1.2, 1.0)$ Absolute value error loss			
1	15	(0,...,0,15)	0.010(0.009)	0.025(−0.128)	0.056(0.025)	0.018(−0.009)	0.011(0.023)	0.032(−0.154)	0.057(−0.033)	0.020(−0.040)
2		(15,0,...,0)	0.012(0.031)	0.024(−0.124)	0.066(0.037)	0.023(0.014)	0.013(0.034)	0.030(−0.145)	0.062(0.001)	0.023(−0.009)
3		(3,0,0,...,3,0,0)	0.009(0.025)	0.024(−0.125)	0.060(0.034)	0.020(0.007)	0.011(0.035)	0.030(−0.148)	0.057(−0.010)	0.020(−0.020)
4	20	(0,...,0,30)	0.008(−0.031)	0.024(−0.127)	0.052(−0.031)	0.021(−0.047)	0.010(−0.015)	0.032(−0.155)	0.064(−0.101)	0.026(−0.079)
5		(30,0,...,0)	0.010(0.023)	0.021(−0.109)	0.066(0.034)	0.026(0.013)	0.010(0.027)	0.026(−0.129)	0.063(0.004)	0.025(−0.007)
6		(3,0,3,0,...,3,0)	0.008(0.003)	0.022(−0.115)	0.057(0.010)	0.020(−0.013)	0.009(0.018)	0.028(−0.138)	0.058(−0.035)	0.022(−0.038)
7	30	(0,...,0,20)	0.009(0.011)	0.017(−0.089)	0.058(0.044)	0.023(0.007)	0.011(0.033)	0.021(−0.109)	0.057(0.008)	0.023(−0.015)
8		(20,0,...,0)	0.014(0.025)	0.018(−0.086)	0.066(0.032)	0.030(0.017)	0.014(0.030)	0.021(−0.102)	0.064(0.009)	0.029(0.001)
9		(2,0,0,...,2,0,0)	0.008(0.027)	0.017(−0.087)	0.062(0.051)	0.026(0.023)	0.009(0.041)	0.021(−0.105)	0.060(0.024)	0.025(0.004)

Table 8 Estimated MSEs and biases (in parentheses) of the Bayes estimators with non-informative prior distributions based on Monte Carlo simulation for Weibull distributions

	m	Scheme	$(\lambda, \beta_0, \beta_1, \beta_2) = (0.6, 0.4, 1.2, 1.0)$ LINEX with $\phi = 0.5$				$(\lambda, \beta_0, \beta_1, \beta_2) = (0.6, 0.4, 1.2, 1.0)$ LINEX with $\phi = -0.5$			
4	15	(0,. . .,0,15)	0.010(−0.001)	0.026(−0.133)	0.050(−0.031)	0.018(−0.034)	0.009(0.019)	0.024(−0.123)	0.073(0.088)	0.020(0.017)
5		(15,0,. . .,0)	0.012(0.027)	0.025(−0.128)	0.059(0.004)	0.022(−0.004)	0.012(0.034)	0.023(−0.119)	0.077(0.073)	0.026(0.032)
6		(3,0,0,. . .,3,0,0)	0.010(0.019)	0.025(−0.129)	0.052(−0.008)	0.019(−0.014)	0.009(0.032)	0.023(−0.119)	0.073(0.081)	0.022(0.028)
7	20	(0,. . .,0,30)	0.010(−0.043)	0.025(−0.132)	0.054(−0.102)	0.023(−0.079)	0.007(−0.019)	0.023(−0.121)	0.065(0.049)	0.021(−0.013)
8		(30,0,. . .,0)	0.010(0.020)	0.022(−0.113)	0.060(0.006)	0.024(−0.002)	0.010(0.025)	0.021(−0.105)	0.075(0.064)	0.028(0.029)
9		(3,0,3,0,. . .,3,0)	0.008(−0.005)	0.023(−0.119)	0.051(−0.041)	0.020(−0.037)	0.007(0.010)	0.021(−0.109)	0.070(0.065)	0.022(0.012)
10	30	(0,. . .,0,20)	0.009(0.004)	0.018(−0.093)	0.051(0.001)	0.022(−0.015)	0.008(0.018)	0.017(−0.084)	0.071(0.092)	0.025(0.031)
11		(20,0,. . .,0)	0.014(0.024)	0.018(−0.089)	0.061(0.011)	0.028(0.004)	0.014(0.026)	0.017(−0.082)	0.072(0.054)	0.032(0.030)
12		(2,0,0,. . .,2,0,0)	0.009(0.023)	0.018(−0.091)	0.055(0.021)	0.024(0.006)	0.008(0.031)	0.017(−0.082)	0.073(0.083)	0.028(0.040)

Table 9 Estimated MSEs and biases (in parentheses) of the Bayes estimators for 0.1th lifetime, median lifetime, and 0.9th lifetime with informative prior distributions based on simulation study for Weibull distributions with $(\lambda, \beta_0, \beta_1, \beta_2) = (0.6, 0.4, 1.2, 1.0)$

	m	Scheme	$q_{0.1}, q_{0.5}, q_{0.9}$ Absolute value loss			$q_{0.1}, q_{0.5}, q_{0.9}$ LINEX with $\phi = 0.5$		
1	15	(0,. . . ,0,15)	4.00×10^{-5}(0.0046)	0.0018(0.0199)	0.0370(0.1157)	4.53×10^{-5}(0.0046)	0.0019(0.0223)	0.1930(0.3723)
2		(15,0,. . . ,0)	5.99×10^{-5}(0.0046)	0.0025(0.0229)	0.0610(0.1030)	6.57×10^{-5}(0.0046)	0.0027(0.0282)	0.0706(0.1569)
3		(3,0,0,. . . ,3,0,0)	4.08×10^{-5}(0.0047)	0.0020(0.0221)	0.0379(0.0968)	4.71×10^{-5}(0.0047)	0.0021(0.0258)	0.0971(0.2427)
4	20	(0,. . . ,0,30)	2.02×10^{-5}(0.0028)	0.0011(0.0188)	0.0851(0.1971)	2.00×10^{-5}(0.0028)	0.0015(0.0310)	0.4096(0.5755)
5		(30,0,. . . ,0)	4.12×10^{-5}(0.0034)	0.0020(0.0187)	0.0759(0.0992)	4.40×10^{-5}(0.0034)	0.0022(0.0232)	0.0801(0.1443)
6		(3,0,3,0,. . . ,3,0)	2.43×10^{-5}(0.0034)	0.0013(0.0185)	0.0398(0.1109)	2.60×10^{-5}(0.0034)	0.0014(0.0225)	0.1886(0.3594)
7	30	(0,. . . ,0,20)	2.51×10^{-5}(0.0032)	0.0012(0.0154)	0.0313(0.0692)	2.41×10^{-5}(0.0032)	0.0013(0.0158)	0.1529(0.2934)
8		(20,0,. . . ,0)	5.21×10^{-5}(0.0033)	0.0021(0.0171)	0.0849(0.0956)	5.42×10^{-5}(0.0033)	0.0023(0.0205)	0.0876(0.1249)
9		(2,0,0,. . . ,2,0,0)	2.77×10^{-5}(0.0033)	0.0014(0.0176)	0.0356(0.0555)	2.85×10^{-5}(0.0033)	0.0015(0.0195)	0.0697(0.1644)

Table 10 Estimated MSEs and biases (in parentheses) of the Bayes estimators with non-informative prior distributions based on simulation study for Weibull distributions

	m	Scheme	$(\lambda, \beta_0, \beta_1, \beta_2) = (0.6, 0.2, 1.2, 1.0)$ Square error loss				$(\lambda, \beta_0, \beta_1, \beta_2) = (0.6, 0.2, 1.2, 1.0)$ Absolute value error loss			
4	15	(0,...,0,15)	0.036(0.138)	0.012(0.023)	0.395(0.495)	0.634(0.695)	0.035(0.135)	0.012(−0.009)	0.334(0.429)	0.546(0.629)
5		(15,0,...,0)	0.026(0.097)	0.012(0.024)	0.410(0.506)	0.652(0.706)	0.025(0.091)	0.011(−0.009)	0.348(0.440)	0.563(0.640)
6		(3,0,0,...,3,0,0)	0.031(0.122)	0.012(0.026)	0.406(0.506)	0.648(0.706)	0.030(0.118)	0.011(−0.006)	0.343(0.440)	0.559(0.640)
7	20	(0,...,0,30)	0.049(0.193)	0.020(0.067)	1.197(0.998)	1.636(1.198)	0.049(0.191)	0.016(0.035)	1.069(0.931)	1.481(1.131)
8		(30,0,...,0)	0.033(0.136)	0.020(0.066)	1.199(0.999)	1.629(1.199)	0.032(0.131)	0.016(0.034)	1.071(0.933)	1.484(1.133)
9		(3,0,3,0,...,3,0)	0.045(0.182)	0.020(0.067)	1.188(0.995)	1.626(1.198)	0.045(0.179)	0.016(0.035)	1.060(0.929)	1.472(1.129)
10	30	(0,...,0,20)	0.152(0.366)	0.045(0.150)	4.296(2.000)	5.137(2.200)	0.151(0.365)	0.037(0.118)	4.035(1.934)	4.849(2.134)
11		(20,0,...,0)	0.060(0.206)	0.045(0.149)	4.301(2.001)	5.142(2.201)	0.059(0.204)	0.036(0.116)	4.040(1.934)	4.853(2.134)
12		(2,0,0,...,2,0,0)	0.100(0.292)	0.046(0.152)	4.283(1.995)	5.121(2.195)	0.099(0.290)	0.037(0.120)	4.022(1.929)	4.834(2.129)

Table 11 Estimated MSEs and biases (in parentheses) of the Bayes estimators with non-informative priors based on simulation study for Weibull distributions

	m	Scheme	$(\lambda, \beta_0, \beta_1, \beta_2) = (0.6, 0.2, 1.2, 1.0, 0.6)$ LINEX with $\phi = 0.5$				$(\lambda, \beta_0, \beta_1, \beta_2) = (0.6, 0.2, 1.2, 1.0)$ LINEX with $\phi = -0.5$			
4	15	(0,...,0,15)	0.036(0.136)	0.011(0.018)	0.309(0.416)	0.516(0.616)	0.037(0.141)	0.013(0.029)	0.510(0.586)	0.785(0.786)
5		(15,0,...,0)	0.025(0.094)	0.011(0.018)	0.322(0.426)	0.532(0.626)	0.027(0.100)	0.013(0.029)	0.528(0.597)	0.807(0.797)
6		(3,0,0,...,3,0,0)	0.030(0.119)	0.011(0.020)	0.318(0.426)	0.528(0.626)	0.032(0.124)	0.013(0.032)	0.523(0.597)	0.802(0.797)
7	20	(0,...,0,30)	0.049(0.192)	0.018(0.060)	0.984(0.895)	1.382(1.095)	0.050(0.195)	0.021(0.074)	1.468(1.115)	1.954(1.316)
8		(30,0,...,0)	0.033(0.133)	0.018(0.060)	0.985(0.896)	1.384(1.096)	0.034(0.138)	0.021(0.073)	1.471(1.117)	1.958(1.317)
9		(3,0,3,0,...,3,0)	0.045(0.180)	0.018(0.061)	0.975(0.892)	1.373(1.093)	0.046(0.184)	0.021(0.074)	1.457(1.113)	1.943(1.313)
10	30	(0,...,0,20)	0.151(0.364)	0.042(0.142)	3.692(1.850)	4.472(2.050)	0.154(0.368)	0.049(0.159)	5.045(2.172)	5.954(2.372)
11		(20,0,...,0)	0.059(0.204)	0.041(0.140)	3.696(1.851)	4.476(2.051)	0.060(0.208)	0.049(0.158)	5.050(2.172)	5.959(2.372)
12		(2,0,0,...,2,0,0)	0.099(0.290)	0.043(0.144)	3.680(1.846)	4.458(2.046)	0.101(0.293)	0.050(0.161)	5.029(2.167)	5.936(2.367)

Table 12 Estimated MSEs and biases (in parentheses) of the Bayes estimators for 0.1th lifetime, median lifetime, and 0.9th lifetime with non-informative prior distributions based on simulation study for Weibull distributions with $(\lambda, \beta_0, \beta_1, \beta_2) = (0.6, 0.2, 1.2, 1.0)$

	m	Scheme	$q_{0.1}, q_{0.5}, q_{0.9}$ Absolute value loss			$q_{0.1}, q_{0.5}, q_{0.9}$ LINEX with $\phi = 0.5$		
1	15	(0,...,0,15)	7.50×10^{-5}(0.0061)	0.0018(−0.0105)	0.1931(−0.3154)	9.81×10^{-5}(0.0061)	0.0020(−0.0023)	0.1549(−0.2878)
2		(15,0,...,0)	5.71×10^{-5}(0.0044)	0.0028(−0.0234)	0.1845(−0.3454)	8.18×10^{-5}(0.0044)	0.0028(−0.0147)	0.1667(−0.3158)
3		(3,0,0,...,3,0,0)	6.08×10^{-5}(0.0051)	0.0020(−0.0168)	0.1735(−0.3353)	8.22×10^{-5}(0.0051)	0.0020(−0.0086)	0.1534(−0.3061)
4	20	(0,...,0,30)	4.48×10^{-5}(0.0049)	0.0017(−0.0306)	0.2546(−0.4913)	5.49×10^{-5}(0.0049)	0.0015(−0.0262)	0.2411(−0.4752)
5		(30,0,...,0)	3.55×10^{-5}(0.0028)	0.0032(−0.0455)	0.2880(−0.5197)	4.65×10^{-5}(0.0028)	0.0028(−0.0405)	0.2731(−0.5035)
6		(3,0,3,0,...,3,0)	4.17×10^{-5}(0.0045)	0.0019(−0.0335)	0.2610(−0.4965)	5.23×10^{-5}(0.0045)	0.0017(−0.029)	0.2472(−0.4805)
7	30	(0,...,0,20)	1.47×10^{-4}(0.0100)	0.0015(−0.0286)	0.3575(−0.5953)	1.64×10^{-4}(0.0100)	0.0014(−0.0265)	0.3514(−0.5900)
8		(20,0,...,0)	3.29×10^{-5}(0.0022)	0.0047(−0.0633)	0.4408(−0.6602)	3.84×10^{-5}(0.0022)	0.0045(−0.0609)	0.4328(−0.6541)
9		(2,0,0,...,2,0,0)	6.23×10^{-5}(0.0057)	0.0027(−0.0453)	0.3922(−0.6235)	7.19×10^{-5}(0.0057)	0.0025(−0.043)	0.3853(−0.6177)

Table 13 Estimated MSEs and biases (in parentheses) of the Bayes estimators with informative priors based on simulation study for Burr XII distributions

	m	Scheme	$(\lambda, \beta_0, \beta_1, \beta_2) = (0.6, 0.2, 1.2, 1.0)$ Squared error loss				$(\lambda, \beta_0, \beta_1, \beta_2) = (0.6, 0.2, 1.2, 1.0)$ Absolute error loss			
1	15	(0,...,0,15)	0.019(0.063)	0.005(0.009)	0.097(0.097)	0.176(0.297)	0.018(0.059)	0.005(−0.013)	0.088(0.056)	0.150(0.256)
2		(15,0,...,0)	0.016(0.051)	0.005(0.002)	0.071(0.045)	0.129(0.245)	0.015(0.044)	0.005(−0.018)	0.067(0.013)	0.112(0.213)
3		(3,0,0,...,3,0,0)	0.016(0.055)	0.005(0.006)	0.085(0.071)	0.153(0.271)	0.015(0.050)	0.005(−0.016)	0.078(0.036)	0.132(0.236)
4	20	(0,...,0,30)	0.013(0.056)	0.006(0.013)	0.126(0.137)	0.221(0.337)	0.013(0.053)	0.005(−0.007)	0.113(0.097)	0.192(0.297)
5		(30,0,...,0)	0.011(0.038)	0.005(0.004)	0.067(0.041)	0.124(0.241)	0.010(0.033)	0.005(−0.014)	0.064(0.014)	0.110(0.214)
6		(3,0,3,0,...,3,0)	0.011(0.047)	0.005(0.008)	0.094(0.088)	0.169(0.288)	0.011(0.044)	0.005(−0.012)	0.086(0.055)	0.148(0.255)
7	30	(0,...,0,20)	0.012(0.054)	0.006(0.010)	0.101(0.102)	0.182(0.302)	0.012(0.051)	0.005(−0.006)	0.093(0.075)	0.163(0.275)
8		(20,0,...,0)	0.008(0.032)	0.005(0.004)	0.057(0.032)	0.110(0.232)	0.008(0.029)	0.005(−0.011)	0.055(0.012)	0.100(0.212)
9		(2,0,0,...,2,0,0)	0.009(0.041)	0.005(0.006)	0.076(0.069)	0.143(0.269)	0.009(0.039)	0.005(−0.010)	0.071(0.046)	0.130(0.246)

Table 14 Estimated MSEs and biases (in parentheses) of the Bayes estimators with informative priors based on simulation study for Burr XII distributions

	m	Scheme	$(\lambda, \beta_0, \beta_1, \beta_2, \lambda) = (0.6, 0.2, 1.2, 1.0)$ LINEX with $\phi = 0.5$				$(\lambda, \beta_0, \beta_1, \beta_2, \lambda) = (0.6, 0.2, 1.2, 1.0)$ LINEX with $\phi = -0.5$			
1	15	(0,...,0,15)	0.018(0.060)	0.005(0.006)	0.085(0.061)	0.149(0.261)	0.019(0.067)	0.005(0.013)	0.115(0.136)	0.209(0.336)
2		(15,0,...,0)	0.015(0.048)	0.005(−0.001)	0.064(0.016)	0.111(0.216)	0.017(0.054)	0.005(0.006)	0.080(0.076)	0.151(0.276)
3		(3,0,0,...,3,0,0)	0.015(0.052)	0.005(0.002)	0.075(0.039)	0.131(0.239)	0.017(0.058)	0.005(0.009)	0.098(0.106)	0.180(0.306)
4	20	(0,...,0,30)	0.013(0.054)	0.005(0.010)	0.109(0.102)	0.190(0.302)	0.013(0.058)	0.006(0.016)	0.147(0.176)	0.258(0.376)
5		(30,0,...,0)	0.011(0.036)	0.005(0.001)	0.062(0.016)	0.109(0.216)	0.011(0.041)	0.005(0.007)	0.075(0.067)	0.141(0.267)
6		(3,0,3,0,...,3,0)	0.011(0.045)	0.005(0.005)	0.083(0.059)	0.147(0.259)	0.012(0.049)	0.006(0.011)	0.108(0.120)	0.196(0.320)
7	30	(0,...,0,20)	0.012(0.053)	0.005(0.008)	0.091(0.078)	0.162(0.278)	0.013(0.056)	0.006(0.013)	0.114(0.128)	0.205(0.328)
8		(20,0,...,0)	0.008(0.031)	0.005(0.002)	0.053(0.014)	0.099(0.214)	0.009(0.0340)	0.005(0.006)	0.061(0.052)	0.122(0.252)
9		(2,0,0,...,2,0,0)	0.009(0.040)	0.005(0.003)	0.070(0.048)	0.129(0.248)	0.009(0.043)	0.005(0.008)	0.084(0.090)	0.160(0.290)

Table 15 Estimated MSEs and biases (in parentheses) of the Bayes estimators for 0.1th lifetime, median lifetime, and 0.9th lifetime with informative priors based on simulation study for Burr XII distributions with $(\lambda, \beta_0, \beta_1, \beta_2) = (0.6, 0.2, 1.2, 1.0)$

			$q_{0.1}, q_{0.5}, q_{0.9}$			$q_{0.1}, q_{0.5}, q_{0.9}$		
	m	Scheme	Square error loss			LINEX with $\phi = 0.5$		
1	15	(0,...,0,15)	$6.40 \times 10^{-5}(0.0046)$	0.0025(0.0066)	0.1258(−0.0738)	$8.04 \times 10^{-5}(0.0046)$	0.0027(0.0117)	0.1270(−0.0225)
2		(15,0,...,0)	$6.90 \times 10^{-5}(0.0051)$	0.0035(0.0081)	0.0854(−0.0643)	$9.91 \times 10^{-5}(0.0051)$	0.0037(0.0149)	0.0879(−0.0321)
3		(3,0,0,...,3,0,0)	$5.71 \times 10^{-5}(0.0044)$	0.0027(0.0063)	0.1006(−0.0702)	$7.51 \times 10^{-5}(0.0044)$	0.0029(0.0119)	0.1044(−0.0276)
4	20	(0,...,0,30)	$2.70 \times 10^{-5}(0.0028)$	0.0016(−0.0008)	0.1439(−0.0959)	$3.24 \times 10^{-5}(0.0028)$	0.0017(0.0038)	0.1422(−0.0479)
5		(30,0,...,0)	$4.01 \times 10^{-5}(0.0035)$	0.0028(0.0032)	0.0828(−0.0687)	$5.59 \times 10^{-5}(0.0035)$	0.0029(0.0089)	0.0842(−0.0412)
6		(3,0,3,0,...,3,0)	$2.74 \times 10^{-5}(0.0028)$	0.0018(0.0009)	0.1061(−0.0814)	$3.43 \times 10^{-5}(0.0028)$	0.0019(0.0055)	0.1092(0.1092)
7	30	(0,...,0,20)	$2.71 \times 10^{-5}(0.0029)$	0.0015(0.0010)	0.0988(−0.0953)	$3.30 \times 10^{-5}(0.0029)$	0.0016(0.0041)	0.1003(−0.0626)
8		(20,0,...,0)	$2.80 \times 10^{-5}(0.0027)$	0.0022(0.0006)	0.0712(−0.0741)	$3.67 \times 10^{-5}(0.0027)$	0.0022(0.0048)	0.0715(−0.0534)
9		(2,0,0,...,2,0,0)	$2.28 \times 10^{-5}(0.0025)$	0.0017(−0.0005)	0.0811(−0.090)	$2.83 \times 10^{-5}(0.0024)$	0.0017(0.0030)	0.0818(−0.0631)

Table 16 Estimated MSEs and biases (in parentheses) of the Bayes estimators with informative priors based on simulation study for Burr XII distributions

	m	Scheme	$(\lambda, \beta_0, \beta_1, \beta_2) = (0.6, 0.4, 1.2, 1.0)$ Squared error loss				$(\lambda, \beta_0, \beta_1, \beta_2) = (0.6, 0.4, 1.2, 1.0)$ Absolute error loss			
1	15	(0,. . .,0,15)	0.014(0.042)	0.023(−0.119)	0.089(0.075)	0.159(0.275)	0.014(0.038)	0.029(−0.143)	0.081(0.034)	0.135(0.233)
2		(15,0,. . .,0)	0.015(0.044)	0.024(−0.122)	0.070(0.042)	0.127(0.241)	0.014(0.038)	0.029(−0.143)	0.067(0.008)	0.110(0.208)
3		(3,0,0,. . .,3,0,0)	0.013(0.040)	0.023(−0.119)	0.078(0.054)	0.139(0.254)	0.013(0.035)	0.028(−0.141)	0.073(0.017)	0.120(0.217)
4	20	(0,. . .,0,30)	0.010(0.033)	0.020(−0.104)	0.106(0.088)	0.182(0.288)	0.010(0.031)	0.025(−0.125)	0.098(0.048)	0.157(0.248)
5		(30,0,. . .,0)	0.010(0.034)	0.021(−0.108)	0.067(0.033)	0.121(0.233)	0.010(0.028)	0.025(−0.127)	0.065(0.005)	0.107(0.205)
6		(3,0,3,0,. . .,3,0)	0.009(0.031)	0.021(−0.105)	0.088(0.070)	0.156(0.270)	0.009(0.029)	0.025(−0.125)	0.082(0.036)	0.136(0.236)
7	30	(0,. . .,0,20)	0.010(0.037)	0.017(−0.081)	0.093(0.080)	0.165(0.280)	0.010(0.035)	0.019(−0.098)	0.086(0.051)	0.147(0.251)
8		(20,0,. . .,0)	0.008(0.029)	0.017(−0.087)	0.061(0.029)	0.112(0.229)	0.008(0.026)	0.020(−0.102)	0.059(0.008)	0.102(0.208)
9		(2,0,0,. . .,2,0,0)	0.008(0.030)	0.017(−0.084)	0.074(0.052)	0.135(0.252)	0.008(0.028)	0.020(−0.100)	0.070(0.027)	0.121(0.228)

Table 17 Estimated MSEs and biases (in parentheses) of the Bayes estimators with informative priors based on simulation study for Burr XII distributions

	m	Scheme	$(\lambda, \beta_0, \beta_1, \beta_2, \lambda) = (0.6, 0.4, 1.2, 1.0)$ LINEX with $\phi = 0.5$				$(\lambda, \beta_0, \beta_1, \beta_2, \lambda) = (0.6, 0.4, 1.2, 1.0)$ LINEX with $\phi = -0.5$			
1	15	(0,…,0,15)	0.014(0.039)	0.024(−0.124)	0.078(0.039)	0.134(0.239)	0.015(0.045)	0.022(−0.114)	0.104(0.115)	0.190(0.315)
2		(15,0,…,0)	0.014(0.041)	0.024(−0.126)	0.064(0.011)	0.108(0.211)	0.015(0.048)	0.023(−0.117)	0.080(0.074)	0.149(0.274)
3		(3,0,0,…,3,0,0)	0.013(0.037)	0.024(−0.124)	0.069(0.022)	0.118(0.222)	0.014(0.042)	0.022(−0.115)	0.090(0.090)	0.165(0.290)
4	20	(0,…,0,30)	0.010(0.031)	0.021(−0.108)	0.094(0.054)	0.156(0.254)	0.010(0.035)	0.019(−0.099)	0.123(0.125)	0.213(0.325)
5		(30,0,…,0)	0.010(0.031)	0.022(−0.112)	0.062(0.008)	0.105(0.208)	0.011(0.036)	0.021(−0.104)	0.075(0.060)	0.139(0.260)
6		(3,0,3,0,…,3,0)	0.009(0.030)	0.021(−0.110)	0.079(0.040)	0.135(0.240)	0.009(0.033)	0.020(−0.101)	0.101(0.103)	0.182(0.303)
7	30	(0,…,0,20)	0.010(0.036)	0.017(−0.085)	0.084(0.055)	0.146(0.255)	0.010(0.039)	0.016(−0.077)	0.104(0.106)	0.186(0.306)
8		(20,0,…,0)	0.008(0.028)	0.018(−0.090)	0.057(0.010)	0.101(0.210)	0.008(0.031)	0.017(−0.083)	0.065(0.050)	0.125(0.250)
9		(2,0,0,…,2,0,0)	0.008(0.029)	0.018(−0.088)	0.068(0.030)	0.120(0.230)	0.008(0.032)	0.017(−0.080)	0.081(0.074)	0.151(0.274)

Table 18 Estimated MSEs and biases (in parentheses) of the Bayes estimators for 0.1th lifetime, median lifetime, and 0.9th lifetime with informative priors based on simulation study for Burr XII distributions with $(\lambda, \beta_0, \beta_1, \beta_2) = (0.6, 0.4, 1.2, 1.0)$

	m	Scheme	$q_{0.1}, q_{0.5}, q_{0.9}$ Square error loss			$q_{0.1}, q_{0.5}, q_{0.9}$ LINEX with $\phi = 0.5$		
1	15	(0,...,0,15)	4.06×10^{-5}(0.0036)	0.0021(0.0111)	0.1060(0.0169)	5.24×10^{-5}(0.0036)	0.0023(0.0162)	0.1184(0.0696)
2		(15,0,...,0)	6.06×10^{-5}(0.0049)	0.0033(0.0156)	0.0695(0.0124)	8.74×10^{-5}(0.0049)	0.0036(0.0221)	0.0768(0.0451)
3		(3,0,0,...,3,0,0)	4.46×10^{-5}(0.0039)	0.0025(0.0125)	0.0845(0.0153)	5.94×10^{-5}(0.0039)	0.0027(0.0180)	0.0954(0.0954)
4	20	(0,...,0,30)	1.93×10^{-5}(0.0023)	0.0014(0.0067)	0.1277(0.0130)	2.35×10^{-5}(0.0023)	0.0017(0.0113)	0.1359(0.0632)
5		(30,0,...,0)	3.44×10^{-5}(0.0035)	0.0025(0.0113)	0.0663(0.0075)	4.86×10^{-5}(0.0035)	0.0027(0.0168)	0.0720(0.0355)
6		(3,0,3,0,...,3,0)	1.92×10^{-5}(0.0024)	0.0015(0.0067)	0.0997(0.00214)	2.44×10^{-5}(0.0024)	0.0017(0.0112)	0.1013(0.0435)
7	30	(0,...,0,20)	1.94×10^{-5}(0.0023)	0.0013(0.0053)	0.0761(−0.0197)	2.38×10^{-5}(0.0023)	0.0014(0.0083)	0.0831(0.0138)
8		(20,0,...,0)	2.39×10^{-5}(0.0027)	0.0019(0.0076)	0.0561(−0.0098)	3.16×10^{-5}(0.0027)	0.0020(0.0116)	0.0592(0.0109)
9		(2,0,0,...,2,0,0)	1.80×10^{-5}(0.0022)	0.0014(0.0052)	0.0640(−0.0147)	2.24×10^{-5}(0.0022)	0.0015(0.0086)	0.0690(0.0130)

the MOB Weibull distribution by using type II progressive hybrid censored samples generated from the complete data set with time transformed to in terms of year. They reported the obtained estimations of the parameters were closed to the maximum likelihood estimates by using the complete data set. For easy reference, the complete data set reported by Csorgo and Welsh [13] is also reported in Table 19. In this section, Bayesian estimates for the competing risks model with two dependent causes whose latent times have the MOB Weibull distribution are studied based on progressive type II censored sample generated from the complete data reported in Table 19. Following the same suggestion by Feizjavadian and Hashemi [16], we also converted times in terms of day to be times in terms of year.

Table 20 displays a progressively type II censored sample that was generated from Table 19 with censoring scheme (2, 0, 0, 2, 0, 0, 2, 0, 0, 2, 0, 0, 2, 0, 0, 2, 0, 0, 2, 0, 0, 2, 0, 0, 2, 0, 0, 2, 0, 0, 20) and $m = 31$. Gamma prior, $h_0(\beta_0; 2.0, 0.1)$, Gamma prior, $h_1(\beta_1; 6, 0.2)$, Gamma prior, $h_2(\beta_2; 10, 0.1)$, and non-informative prior, $h_3(\lambda)$, are used. During the implementation of MCMC process, the Markov chain, $\theta_j^{(i+1)}$ is generated from Gamma distribution with shape parameter $n_j + \alpha_j$ and rate parameter $\frac{1}{\gamma_j} + \sum_{i=1}^{m}(R_i + 1)X_{i:m:n}^{\lambda^{(i)}}$ for $j = 0, 1, 2$. Meanwhile, Step 5 was replaced by Step 5* for 150 times to ensure the Markov chain of $\theta_3^{(i)}$, $i = 1, 2, 3, \cdots$ after burn-in reach stable and independent. Figure 1 displays time series plots, histogram, and ACF plots (from left column to right column) for the Markov chains of λ, β_0, β_1, and β_2 (from top row to bottom row) after burn-in, respectively. Figure 2 displays time series plots, histogram and ACF plots (from left column to right column) for the Markov chains of ten-percentile lifetime, median lifetime, and ninety-percentile lifetime (from top row to bottom row) after burn-in, respectively. It should be mentioned that all plots produced by R and histograms were using option freq=FALSE. Using square error loss function, the Bayesian estimates of λ, β_0, β_1, β_2, and three lifetimes are given in Table 21.

7 Conclusion

This chapter has provided a brief review of competing risks research work and presented a competing risks model with two latent failures that have MOB exponential family distribution. The MOB exponential family distribution covers Burr XII, Gompertz and Weibull distributions as special cases. Bayesian estimation via Markov-Chain and Monte Carlo process has been focused to estimate the model parameters of competing risks model when both competing causes have Burr XII and Weibull distributed failure times. The current simulation study is based on progressive type II censored sample. The extension to some other hybrid progressive censoring schemes should not be difficult. Furthermore, some potential work to find general conditions for MOB family distribution for the uniqueness of maximum likelihood estimation and the linkage with copula bivariate distribution would be interesting.

Table 19 Minimum time in day to blindness and associated causes for 71 patients under diabetic retinopathy study

i	X	δ	i	X	δ	i	X	δ	i	X	δ	i	X	δ	i	X	δ	i	X	δ	i	X	δ	i	X	δ	i	X	δ	i	X	δ	i	X	δ
1	266	1	2	91	2	3	154	2	4	285	0	5	583	1	6	547	2	7	79	1	8	622	0	9	707	2	10	469	2	11	93	1	12	1313	2
13	805	1	14	344	1	15	790	2	16	125	2	17	777	2	18	306	1	19	415	1	20	307	2	21	637	2	22	577	2	23	178	1	24	517	2
25	272	0	26	1137	0	27	1484	1	28	315	1	29	287	2	30	1252	1	31	717	2	32	642	1	33	141	2	34	407	1	35	356	1	36	1653	0
37	427	2	38	699	1	39	36	2	40	667	1	41	588	2	42	471	0	43	126	1	44	350	2	45	350	1	46	663	0	47	567	2	48	966	0
49	203	0	50	84	1	51	392	1	52	1140	2	53	901	1	54	1247	0	55	448	2	56	904	2	57	276	1	58	520	1	59	485	2	60	248	2
61	503	1	62	423	2	63	285	2	64	315	2	65	727	2	66	210	2	67	409	2	68	584	1	69	355	1	70	1302	1	71	227	2			

Table 20 Progressively type II censored sample with 31 observations obtained from Table 19

X	δ	X	δ	X	δ	X	δ	X	δ	X	δ	X	δ	X	δ	X	δ	X	δ	X	δ	X	δ	X	δ	X	δ	X	δ	X	δ
36	2	79	1	84	1	91	2	93	1	125	2	126	1	141	2	154	2	178	1	203	0	210	2	227	2	248	2	266	1	272	0
276	1	285	0	285	2	315	2	344	1	350	2	356	1	407	1	409	2	423	2	427	2	448	2	471	0	485	2	503	1		

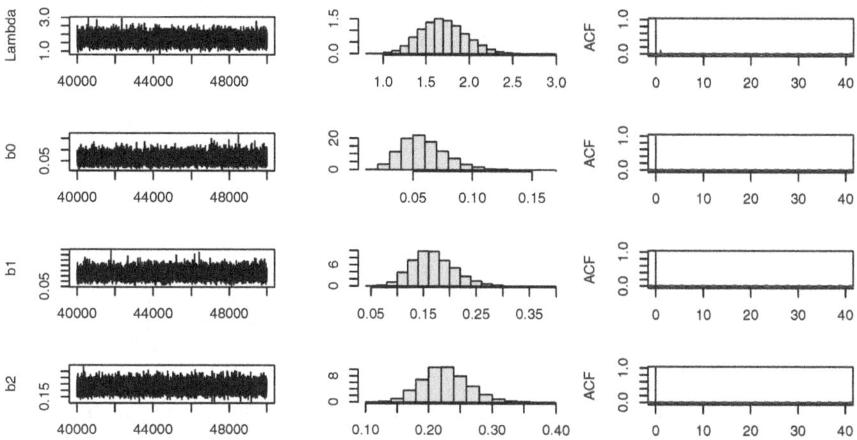

Fig. 1 Time series plots (left column), histogram (middle column), and ACF plots (right column)

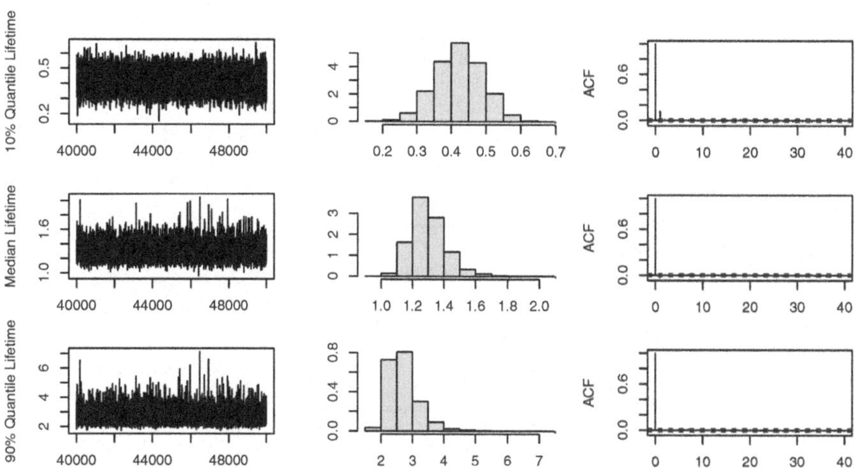

Fig. 2 Time series plots (left column), histogram (middle column), and ACF plots (right column)

Table 21 Bayesian estimates using square

Parameter	λ	β_0	β_1	β_2	$t_{0.1}$	$t_{0.5}$	$t_{0.9}$
Estimate	1.7031	0.0589	0.1685	0.2266	154.18	474.17	986.99

Appendix

Proof of Proposition 1

Let $h(\lambda) = \sum_{i=1}^{m}(R_i + 1)X_{i:m:n}^{\lambda}$. Then the first derivative, $h'(\lambda)$, and the second derivative, $h''(\lambda)$ of $h_w(\lambda)$, with respective to λ are, respectively, obtained as

$$h'(\lambda) = \sum_{i=1}^{m} (R_i + 1) X_{i:m:n}^{\lambda} \ln(X_{i:m:n})$$

$$h''(\lambda) = \sum_{i=1}^{m} (R_i + 1) X_{i:m:n}^{\lambda} (\ln(X_{i:m:n}))^2.$$

Let

$$h''(\lambda)h(\lambda) - (h'(\lambda))^2 = \left(\sum_{i=1}^{m} a_i^2\right)\left(\sum_{i=1}^{m} b_i^2\right) - \left(\sum_{i=1}^{m} a_i b_i\right)^2,$$

where $a_i = (R_i + 1)^{1/2} X_{i:m:n}^{\lambda/2} \ln(X_{i:m:n})$, $b_i = (R_i + 1)^{1/2} X_{i:m:n}^{\lambda/2}$. By Cauchy–Schwarz inequality, $(\sum_{i=1}^{m} a_i^2)(\sum_{i=1}^{m} b_i^2) - (\sum_{i=1}^{m} a_i b_i)^2 \geq 0$.

Therefore, $h''(\lambda)h_w(\lambda) - (h'(\lambda))^2 \geq 0$. Hence,

$$\frac{d^2 cl_w(\lambda)}{d\lambda d\lambda} = -\frac{m}{\lambda^2} - m\frac{h''(\lambda)h(\lambda) - (h'(\lambda))^2}{(h(\lambda))^2} \leq 0,$$

which implies $cl_w(\lambda)$ is a concave function. Proposition 1 is proved.

Proof of Proposition 2

Consider the following equation,

$$\frac{1}{\lambda} = \frac{\sum_{i=1}^{m}(R_i + 1) X_{i:m:n}^{\lambda} \ln(X_{i:m:n})}{\sum_{i=1}^{m}(R_i + 1) X_{i:m:n}^{\lambda}} - \frac{\sum_{i=1}^{m} \ln(X_{i:m:n})}{m}.$$

Let $\xi(\lambda) = \frac{1}{\lambda}$. $\xi(\lambda)$ is the decreasing function, and $\xi(\lambda) \to \infty$ as $\lambda \to 0^+$ and $\xi(\lambda) \to 0$ as $\lambda \to \infty$. Let

$$\zeta(\lambda) = \frac{\sum_{i=1}^{m}(R_i + 1) X_{i:m:n}^{\lambda} \ln(X_{i:m:n})}{\sum_{i=1}^{m}(R_i + 1) X_{i:m:n}^{\lambda}} - \frac{1}{m}\sum_{i=1}^{m} \ln(X_{i:m:n}).$$

Follow the same proof of Proposition 1, it can be proved that $\zeta'(\lambda) > 0$. Hence, $\zeta(\lambda)$ is an increasing function. Moreover, $\zeta(\lambda) \to \varpi$ as $\lambda \to 0^+$ where $\varpi = \frac{1}{n}(\sum_{i=1}^{m}(R_i + 1)\ln(X_{i:m:n})) - \frac{1}{m}\sum_{i=1}^{m} \ln(X_{i:m:n})$ and $\zeta(\lambda) \to (\ln(m) - \frac{1}{m}\sum_{i=1}^{m} \ln(X_{i:m:n})) > 0$ as $\lambda \to \infty$.

Proof of Proposition 3

Let $\phi(\lambda) = \frac{\partial l(\beta_0, \beta_1, \beta_2, \lambda)}{\partial \lambda}$. It can be noticed that

$$\begin{aligned}\phi(\lambda) &= \frac{m}{\lambda} + \sum_{i=1}^{m} \ln(X_{i:m:n}) - \sum_{i=1}^{m} \frac{X_{i:m:n}^{\lambda} \ln(X_{i:m:n})}{1 + X_{i:m:n}^{\lambda}} \\ &\quad - (\beta_0 + \beta_1 + \beta_2) \left(\sum_{i=1}^{m} (R_i + 1) \frac{X_{i:m:n}^{\lambda} \ln(X_{i:m:n})}{1 + X_{i:m:n}^{\lambda}} \right).\end{aligned}$$

It is trivial that $\phi(\lambda) = \infty$ as $\lambda \to 0^+$. Next, define the following index sets:

$M = \{i | i = 1, 2, \cdots, m, X_{i:m:n} < 1.0\}$, $P = \{i | i = 1, 2, \cdots, m, X_{i:m:n} > 1.0\}$. By basic calculation, the following results are obtained:

$$\sum_{i=1}^{m} \frac{X_{i:m:n}^{\lambda} \ln(X_{i:m:n})}{1 + X_{i:m:n}^{\lambda}} \to \sum_{i \in P} \ln(X_{i:m:n}), \text{ as } \lambda \to \infty.$$

Therefore, for any given $\beta_j > 0$, $j = 0, 1, 2$, the following can be proved

$$\phi(\infty) = \sum_{i \in M} \ln(X_{i:m:n}) - (\beta_0 + \beta_1 + \beta_2) \left(\sum_{i \in P} (R_i + 1) \ln(X_{i:m:n}) \right).$$

Since at least one of the index sets M and P is nonempty, it can be seen that $\phi(\infty) < 0$. Therefore, there exists at least one real solution of $\phi(\lambda) = 0$ on the positive real line. Furthermore, $\frac{\partial \phi(\lambda)}{\partial \lambda} < 0$ implies that $\phi(\lambda)$ is monotone decreasing in λ for $\lambda > 0$. Proposition 3 is proven.

Proof of Proposition 4

When β_j, $j = 0, 1, 2$, and common λ are unknown, the MLE of λ can be obtained by maximizing the profile log-likelihood function $cl_B(\lambda)$. Let

$$\xi(\lambda) = \frac{\partial cl_B(\lambda | \lambda_0, \lambda_1, \lambda_2)}{\partial \lambda};$$

then

$$\xi(\lambda) = \frac{m}{\lambda} + \sum_{i=1}^{m} \ln(X_{i:m:n}) - \sum_{i=1}^{m} \frac{X_{i:m:n}^{\lambda} \ln(X_{i:m:n})}{1 + X_{i:m:n}^{\lambda}}$$

$$- m \frac{\sum_{i=1}^{m} (R_i + 1) \frac{X_{i:m:n}^{\lambda} \ln(X_{i:m:n})}{1+X_{i:m:n}^{\lambda}}}{\sum_{i=1}^{m} (R_i + 1) \ln(1 + X_{i:m:n}^{\lambda})}.$$

By utilizing the same argument as Wingo [36] and Lio and Tsai [25], $\xi(\lambda) = 0$ has a unique solution on the positive real line. Proposition 4 is proven.

References

1. Ashour, S.K., Nassar, M.: Inference for Weibull distribution under adaptive type-I progressive hybrid censored competing risks data. Commun. Stat. Theory Methods **46**, 4756–4773 (2017)
2. Balakrishnan, N., Aggarwala, R.: Progressive Censoring: Theory, Methods, and Applications. Birkhauser, Boston (2000)
3. Balakrishnan, N., Cramer, E.: The Art of Progressive Censoring. Birkhauser, Boston (2014)
4. Balakrishnan, N., Han, D.: Exact inference for a simple step-stress model with competing risks for failure from exponential distribution under type-II censoring. J. Stat. Plan. Infer. **138**, 4172–4186 (2008)
5. Balakrishnan, N., Kundu, D.: Hybrid censoring: models, inferential results and applications. Comput. Stat. Data Anal. **57**, 166–209 (2013)
6. Bunea, C., Mazzuchi, T.A.: Competing failure modes in accelerated life testing. J. Stat. Plan. Infer. **136**, 1608–1620 (2006)
7. Cai, J., Shi, Y., Liu, B.: Analysis of incomplete data in the presence of dependent competing risks from Marshall-Olkin bivariate Weibull distribution under progressive hybrid censoring. Commun. Stat. Theory Methods **46**, 6497–6511 (2017)
8. Chen, D.G., Lio, Y.L.: Parameter estimations for generalized exponential distribution under progressive type-I interval censoring. Comput. Stat. Data Anal. **54**, 1581–1591 (2010)
9. Chib, S., Greenberg, E.: Understanding the Metropolis-Hastings algorithm. American Statistician 49, 327–335 (1995)
10. Childs, A., Chandrasekar, B., Balakrishnan, N., Kundu, D.: Exact likelihood inference based on Type-I and Type-II hybrid censored samples from the exponential distribution. Ann. Inst. Stat. Math. **55**, 319–330 (2003)
11. Childs, A., Chandrasekar, B., Balakrishnan, N.: Exact likelihood inference for an exponential parameter under progressive hybrid censoring schemes. In: Statistical Models and Methods for Biomedical and Technical Systems, pp. 319–330. Springer, Boston (2008)
12. Cramer, E., Schmiedt, A.B.: Progressively type-II censored competing risks data from Lomax distributions. Comput. Stat. Data Anal. **55**, 1285–1303 (2011)
13. Csorgo, S., Welsh, A.H.: Testing for exponential and Marshall-Olkin distribution. J. Stat. Plan. Infer. **23**, 287–300 (1989)
14. Epstein, B.: Truncated life tests in the exponential case. Ann. Math. Stat. **25**, 55–564 (1954)
15. Escarela, G., Carriere, J.: Fitting competing risks with an assumed copula. Stat. Methods Med. Res. **12**, 333–349 (2003)
16. Feizjavadian, S.H., Hashemi, R.: Analysis of dependent competing risks in the presence of progressive hybrid censoring using Marshall-Olkin bivariate Weibull distribution. Comput. Stat. Data Anal. **82**, 19–34 (2015)
17. Geman, S., Geman, D.: Stochastic relaxation, Gibbs distributions and the Bayesian restoration of images. IEEE Trans. Pattern Anal. Mach. Intell. **6**, 721–741 (1984)
18. Hastings, W.K.: Monte Carlo sampling methods using Markov chains and their applications. Biometrika **57**, 97–109 (1970)
19. Kundu, D., Basu, S.: Analysis of incomplete data in presence of competing risks. J. Stat. Plan. Infer. **87**, 221–239 (2000)

20. Kundu, D., Howlader, H.: Bayesian Inference and prediction of the inverse Weibull distribution for type-II censored data. Comput. Stat. Data Anal. **54**, 1547–1558 (2010)
21. Kundu, D., Joarder, A.: Analysis of type-II progressively hybrid censored data. Comput. Stat. Data Anal. **50**, 2509–2528 (2006)
22. Kundu, D., Kannan, N., Balakrishnan, N.: Analysis of progressively censored competing risks data. In: Rao, C.R., Balakrishnana, N. (eds.) Handbook of Statistics on Survival Analysis, vol. 23, pp. 331–348. Elsevier Publications, Amsterdam (2004)
23. Lin, C.T., Huang, Y.L.: On progressive hybrid censored exponential distribution. J. Stat. Comput. Simul. **82**, 689–709 (2012)
24. Lin, Y.-J., Lio, Y.L.: Bayesian inference under progressive type-I interval censoring. J. Appl. Stat. **39**, 1811–1824 (2012)
25. Lio, Y.L., Tsai, T.-R.: Estimation of $\delta = P(X < Y)$ for Burr XII distribution based on the progressively first failure-censored samples. J. Appl. Stat. **39**, 309–322 (2012)
26. Marshall, A.W., Olkin, I.: A multivariate exponential distribution. J. Am. Stat. Assoc. **62**(317), 30–44 (1967)
27. Metropolis, N., Rosenbluth, A.W., Rosenbluth, M.N., Teller, A.H., Teller, E.: Equations of state calculations by fast computing machines. J. Chem. Phys. **21**, 1087–1091 (1953)
28. Miyakawa, M.: Analysis of incomplete data in competing risks model. IEEE Trans. Reliab. **33**, 293–296 (1984)
29. Ng, H.K.T., Kundu, D., Chan, P.S.: Statistical analysis of exponential lifetimes under an adaptive Type-II progressively censoring scheme. Nav. Res. Logist. **56**, 687–698 (2009)
30. Pareek, B., Kundu, D., Kumar, S.: On progressively censored competing risks data for Weibull distributions. Comput. Stat. Data Anal. **53**, 4083–4094 (2009)
31. Park, C., Kulasekera, K.B.: Parametric inference of incomplete data with competing risks among several groups. IEEE Trans. Reliab. **53**, 11–21 (2004)
32. Qin, X., Gui, W.: Statistical inference of Burr-XII distribution under progressive type-II censored competing risks data with binomial removals. J. Comput. Appl. Math. **378**, 112922 (2020)
33. Sarhan, A.M.: Analysis of incomplete censored data in competing risks models with generalized exponential distributions. IEEE Trans. Reliab. **56**, 132–138 (2007)
34. Shih, J.-H., Emura, T.: Likelihood-based inference for bivariate latent failure time models with competing risks under the generalized FGM copula. Comput. Stat. **33**, 1293–1323 (2018)
35. Shi, Y., Wu, M.: Statistical analysis of dependent competing risks model from Gompertz distribution under progressively hybrid censoring. SpringerPlus. **5**, 1745 (2016)
36. Wingo, D.R.: Maximum likelihood methods for fitting the Burr type XII distribution to life test data. Biomet. J. **25**, 77–84 (1983)
37. Wingo, D.R.: Maximum likelihood methods for fitting the Burr type XII distribution to multiply (progressively) censored life data. Metrika **40**, 203–210 (1993)
38. Xu, A., Tang, Y.: Objective Bayesian analysis of accelerated competing failure models under type-I censoring. Comput. Stat. Data Anal. **55**, 2830–2839 (2011)
39. Zheng, M., Klein, J.P.: A self-consistent estimator of marginal survival functions based on dependent competing risk data and an assumed copula. Commun. Stat. Theory Methods. **23**, 2299–2311 (1994)
40. Zheng, M., Klein, J.P.: Estimates of marginal survival for dependent competing risks based on an assumed copula. Biometrika **82**, 127–138 (1995)

Part II
Stochastic Processes in Reliability Analysis

Bayesian Computations for Reliability Analysis in Dynamic Environments

Atilla Ay and Refik Soyer

Abstract In this chapter, we consider systems operating under a dynamic environment that causes changes in the failure characteristics of the system. We discuss different modeling strategies to describe the evolution of the dynamic environment and develop Bayesian analysis of the models using Markov Chain Monte Carlo methods and data augmentation techniques. We present illustrations from repairable systems using data from software testing, railroad track maintenance, and power outages.

1 Introduction and Overview

Stochastic processes play an important role in reliability analysis of systems that operate under dynamic environments. As noted by Singpurwalla [27], the physics of failure is affected by the dynamic environment and the changes in failure behavior of the system can be described by stochastic processes. According to [29], the first use of stochastic processes in reliability analysis dates back to [15], who modeled wear by dependent renewal processes, and [12], who described the deterioration of a system by Markov models. As pointed out by Soyer [29], Gaver [10] was the first one who proposed modeling the failure rate as a stochastic process and introduced the notion of a randomly changing environment.

More formally [6] considered reliability of a system as a function of a stochastic process governing the dynamic environment. This notion was further developed in [7] who proposed models for dependence caused by a random environment. Özekici [19] developed maintenance policies for systems operating under random environments [21] considered a random environment to describe software failure behavior dependent on the operational profile of the software, and optimal testing strategies for software with an operational profile were presented in [20]. Network

A. Ay · R. Soyer (✉)
George Washington University, Washington, DC, USA
e-mail: aay@gwu.edu; soyer@gwu.edu

Y. Lio et al. (eds.), *Bayesian Inference and Computation in Reliability and Survival Analysis*, Emerging Topics in Statistics and Biostatistics,
https://doi.org/10.1007/978-3-030-88658-5_5

reliability assessment under a random environment was considered in [22]. A survey of stochastic processes for modeling reliability in dynamic environments is given in [28], and related statistical issues are discussed in [23].

It is important to note that the term "environment" is used in a loose sense in the reliability literature so that it represents any set of conditions that affect the deterioration and aging of the system in question. The notion is applicable to both discrete- and continuous-time changes in the failure characteristics of the system. For example [25] proposed a discrete-time hidden Markov process to describe changes in reliability of software as a result of modifications made to it during the debugging process. Landon et al. [14] considered a continuous-time Markov chain to describe the intensity of a Poisson process for software reliability analysis, whereas [16] used a gamma process to model the cumulative intensity of a nonhomogeneous Poisson process representing the rail track failures.

These processes have been of interest to statisticians because of the difficult inferential issues that they pose as a result of unobserved or hidden components they include. Advances in computational Bayesian methods and particularly in Monte Carlo-based approaches after 1990s have enhanced areas such as Bayesian inference in stochastic processes and Bayesian decision analysis in all fields including reliability analysis. A recent review of advances in Bayesian decision making in reliability and risk analysis can be found in [26].

In this chapter, our focus will be on recent methodological advances in Bayesian inference in stochastic processes with an emphasis on computational issues. In so doing, we consider Bayesian reliability modeling under random environments and present results for modulated Poisson processes and Markov modulated Markov processes. In Sect. 2, we present a Bayesian semi-parametric model for interval censored data coming from rail track inspections and discuss recent computational issues associated with the use of gamma process priors. In Sect. 3, we discuss Markov modulated Markov processes and illustrate how Bayesian inference can be developed for these processes using a modification of the exact Gibbs sampler proposed by Fearnhead and Sherlock [9]. In Sect. 4, we present two numerical illustrations implementing some of the methodology using actual reliability data from software engineering and power systems. Concluding remarks follow in Sect. 5.

2 Modulated Nonhomogeneous Poisson Processes for Rail Track Failures

Merrick and Soyer [16] considered railroad tracks that experience wear as a function of traffic usage, which is measured in millions of gross tons (MGTs). As noted by the authors, the wear causes a failure of a railroad track in the form of a crack in a rail section, and such a crack can possibly lead to a fracture if it is not repaired. Since the replacement of a whole rail track is very costly, it is preferred to repair such cracks. When a crack is found on the rail, a small piece of rail section around the crack is cut out and replaced with a new rail piece. Since this does not significantly change the performance of the rail section that can be miles in length, the rail sections are assumed to be minimally repaired. Thus, it is common practice to model the number of failures over MGT intervals as a nonhomogeneous Poisson process (NHPP).

A block replacement protocol with minimal repair (MR) in the sense of [2] was considered in [16], and optimal replacement policies were developed. In so doing, the authors considered a NHPP for $N_i(t)$, the number of failures over an MGT interval $[0, t)$ for rail section i, with cumulative intensity $\Lambda_i(t)$. Following [8], the cumulative intensity was defined by modulating a baseline cumulative intensity $\Lambda_0(t)$ with a function of covariates $\mathbf{Z}_i$ associated with rail section i as

$$\Lambda_i(t, \mathbf{Z}_i) = \Lambda_0(t)e^{\boldsymbol{\beta}^{\mathbf{T}}\mathbf{Z}_i}. \tag{1}$$

The model in (1) that takes into account both the time and the covariate effects on the failure intensity can be considered as a point process version of the proportional hazard models of Cox. It is important to note that in (1), the baseline cumulative intensity is assumed to be common for all rail sections and the differences between rail sections are represented by the covariate vector $\mathbf{Z}_i$ with unknown coefficient vector $\boldsymbol{\beta}$. If heterogeneity of rail sections cannot be fully captured by $\mathbf{Z}_i$'s, one can consider multiplicative random effects as in [30] or a semi-parametric Bayesian approach can be used with mixtures of Dirichlet processes following [17].

One strategy in Bayesian modeling of the cumulative intensity (1) is to assume a parametric form for the baseline cumulative intensity $\Lambda_0(t)$ and to specify a parametric prior for the coefficient vector $\boldsymbol{\beta}$. For example, a power law model can be specified as $\Lambda_0(t) = \alpha t^{\gamma}$. As an alternative strategy, we can use a nonparametric form for $\Lambda_0(t)$ and still use a parametric prior for $\boldsymbol{\beta}$. This gives us a *semi-parametric Bayesian* model. We can achieve this by treating the baseline cumulative intensity as a stochastic process and treat $\Lambda_0(t)$ as an unknown sample path of the stochastic process. This approach provides more flexibility than the parametric form since it allows for a wide variety of different forms for $\Lambda_0(t)$.

As pointed out by Merrick and Soyer [16], since $\Lambda_0(t)$ is a nondecreasing function taking values in $[0, \infty)$ and there is no restriction on the size of jumps of the $\Lambda_0(t)$, a suitable stochastic process for $\Lambda_0(t)$ is a gamma process. The choice of gamma process implies that all partitions of the sample path $\Lambda_0(t)$ are independent and have gamma distributions; see [30]. Following [16], we specify the gamma process prior for $\Lambda_0(t)$ as

$$(\Lambda_0(t)|D_0) \backsim G(cM(t), c), \tag{2}$$

where $M(t)$ is a best guess or the mean function and c is a precision parameter representing strength of belief about the choice of $M(t)$ given the prior history D_0. More specifically, (2) implies that

$$\begin{aligned} E[\Lambda_0(t)|D_0] &= M(t) \\ V[\Lambda_0(t)|D_0] &= M(t)/c. \end{aligned} \tag{3}$$

Note that $M(t)$ and c are specified in (2) where higher values of c describe a strong prior belief in the mean function $M(t)$. We can complete the specification of the Bayesian model by assuming a prior distribution for $\boldsymbol{\beta}$ that is typically assumed to be independent of $\Lambda_0(t)$ a priori.

2.1 Bayesian Analysis of the Modulated NHPP

Due to its conjugacy with the Poisson likelihood, the gamma process prior is a natural choice in the nonparametric Bayesian analysis of NHPPs. It is well known that if we assume a gamma process for the cumulative intensity function of an NHPP, then the posterior distribution for the cumulative intensity function is also a gamma process if all event times of the NHPP are observed; see, for example [13]. More specifically, if n event times are observed during the time interval $[0, t)$, then the posterior of $\Lambda_0(t)$ will be given by the gamma distribution

$$(\Lambda_0(t)|D_0, n) \backsim G(cM(t) + n, c + 1), \tag{4}$$

and for any subinterval $[s, \tau)$, i.e., $0 < s < \tau < t$, where we observe $n_{s,\tau} < n$ event times, the posterior distribution of $\Lambda_0(\tau) - \Lambda_0(s)$ will have a gamma distribution as

$$(\Lambda_0(\tau) - \Lambda_0(s)|D_0, n_{s,\tau}) \backsim G(c(M(\tau) - M(s)) + n_{s,\tau}, c + 1). \tag{5}$$

Due to the inspection process used for rail sections, exact times of failures will not be known. Inspections are typically performed using detection techniques such as visual image analysis. Detection equipment is placed in special cars that travel along the rail detecting and recording cracks (failures). The data is recorded in the form of the counts over a defined interval, that is, the data is interval censored. As a result, Bayesian analysis of modulated NHPPs using a gamma process prior is not straightforward for interval count data. Merrick and Soyer [16] point out that in the rail track failure data, different rail sections are inspected over different MGT intervals that typically overlap and as a result posterior process for $\Lambda_0(t)$ is no longer a gamma process. The authors proposed a data augmentation step within the Gibbs sampler to develop Bayesian analysis of modulated NHPPs with interval count data.

Following the notation of [16], we assume that for rail section i, the process $N_i(t)$ is observed at r_i MGT intervals with endpoints $(t_{i,1}, \ldots, t_{i,r_i})$, where $t_{i,1} < \ldots < t_{i,r_i}$. We denote the number of failures on the jth MGT interval $[t_{i,j-1}, t_{i,j})$ of rail i by $n_{i,j}$. In other words, $n_{i,j}$ is the realization of $N_i(t_{i,j}) - N_i(t_{i,j-1})$. We denote the observed data for rail section i by D_i defined as

$$D_i = \{n_{i,j}, \mathbf{Z}_i, j = 1, \ldots, r_i\}, \tag{6}$$

where $\mathbf{Z}_i$ is the covariate vector for rail section i. As noted by the authors, $\mathbf{Z}_i$ may include variables such as grinding level performed on the rail section, curvature of the rail section, and the weight and the speed limit for traffic traversing the rail.

Given data D_i on rail section i, using the independent increment property of the NHPP, we can write the likelihood function $L_i(\Lambda_0(t), \boldsymbol{\beta}; D_i)$ as

$$\prod_{j=1}^{r_i} \frac{\left(\left[\Lambda_0(t_{i,j}) - \Lambda_0(t_{i,j-1})\right] e^{\boldsymbol{\beta}^T \mathbf{Z}_i}\right)^{n_{i,j}}}{n_{i,j}!} \times \exp\left\{-\left(\left[\Lambda_0(t_{i,j}) - \Lambda_0(t_{i,j-1})\right] e^{\boldsymbol{\beta}^T \mathbf{Z}_i}\right)\right\}. \quad (7)$$

We assume that conditional on $\Lambda_0(t)$ and $\boldsymbol{\beta}$ the $N_i(t)$s are independent NHPPs. Given prior information and failure data from m rail sections as $D = (D_0, D_1, \ldots, D_m)$, the complete likelihood is obtained as a product of $L_i(\Lambda_0(t), \boldsymbol{\beta}; D_i)$'s, that is,

$$L(\Lambda_0(t), \boldsymbol{\beta}; D) = \prod_{i=1}^{m} L_i(\Lambda_0(t), \boldsymbol{\beta}; D_i). \quad (8)$$

Development of Bayesian analysis using the gamma process prior (2) for $\Lambda_0(t)$ and a standard parametric prior, such as multivariate normal, for $\boldsymbol{\beta}$ with the likelihood function (8) requires the use of Markov Chain Monte Carlo (MCMC) methods. Since one can easily draw samples from the full conditional posterior distribution of $\boldsymbol{\beta}$ using Metropolis–Hastings, an efficient sampling scheme is needed to draw from the full posterior conditional of $\Lambda_0(t)$, that is, from $p(\Lambda_0(t)|\boldsymbol{\beta}, D)$ for all partitions of t over $(0, \infty)$. Then one can use a Gibbs sampler to develop posterior and predictive analysis for rail failure data. Merrick and Soyer [16] proposed a data augmentation method to draw from $p(\Lambda_0(t)|\boldsymbol{\beta}, D)$, and we next discuss their approach.

2.1.1 Data Augmentation for Sampling from $p(\boldsymbol{\Lambda}_0(t)|\boldsymbol{\beta}, D)$

To illustrate the data augmentation algorithm, we first consider a few simple examples. Suppose that for rail section i failure data is observed for two intervals $[t_{1,1}, t_{1,2})$ and $[t_{1,2}, t_{1,3})$ such that $D_i = \{n_{1,1}, n_{1,2}, \mathbf{Z}_i\}$ as shown in Fig. 1.

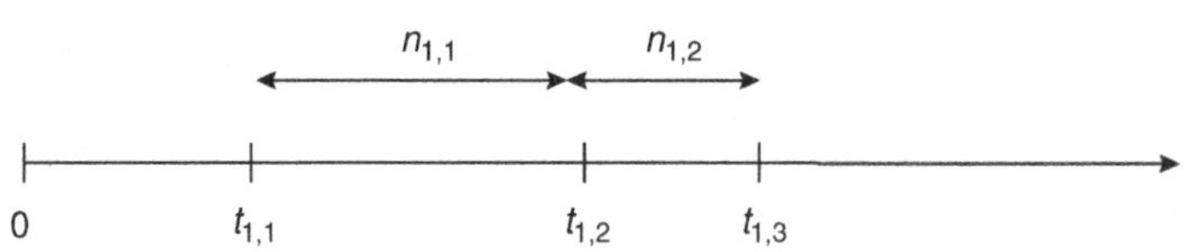

Fig. 1 Single rail section with two intervals

Using the independent increment property of the gamma process and the Bayes' rule, the full conditional posterior distribution of $\Lambda_0(t)$ can be obtained for the following MGT intervals:

$$
\begin{aligned}
(\Lambda_0(t)|\boldsymbol{\beta}, D_i) &\backsim G(cM(t), c), t \leq t_{1,1} \\
(\Lambda_0(t_{1,2}) - \Lambda_0(t_{1,1})|\boldsymbol{\beta}, D_i) &\backsim G(c(M(t_{1,2}) - M(t_{1,1})) + n_{1,1}, c + e^{\boldsymbol{\beta}^T \mathbf{z}_i}), t_{1,1} < t \leq t_{1,2} \\
(\Lambda_0(t_{1,3}) - \Lambda_0(t_{1,2})|\boldsymbol{\beta}, D_i) &\backsim G(c(M(t_{1,3}) - M(t_{1,2})) + n_{1,2}, c + e^{\boldsymbol{\beta}^T \mathbf{z}_i}), t_{1,2} < t \leq t_{1,3} \\
(\Lambda_0(t) - \Lambda_0(t_{1,3})|\boldsymbol{\beta}, D_i) &\backsim G(c(M(t) - M(t_{1,3})), c), t > t_{1,3}.
\end{aligned} \tag{9}
$$

We next consider the same scenario in Fig. 1 but focus on updating a subinterval as shown in Fig. 2. Assume that for prediction purposes or for evaluating a replacement strategy we need the posterior distribution of $\Lambda_0(t^*)$, where $t_{1,1} < t^* \leq t_{1,2}$, and n^* is the unknown number of failures between $t_{1,1}$ and t^*.

As pointed out by Merrick and Soyer [16], one can obtain the posterior distribution of $\Lambda_0(t^*)$ via data augmentation. If $N_i(t^*) - N_i(t_{1,1}) = n^*$ is known, then the distribution of $\Lambda_0(t^*)$ can be updated as the sum of independent gamma random variables $\left[\Lambda_0(t^*) - \Lambda_0(t_{1,1})\right] + \Lambda_0(t_{1,1})$, where $(\Lambda_0(t_{1,1})|D_i)$ is given from the first line of (9) and

$$
(\Lambda_0(t^*) - \Lambda_0(t_{1,1})|\boldsymbol{\beta}, D_i, n^*) \backsim G(c(M(t^*) - M(t_{1,1})) + n^*, c + e^{\boldsymbol{\beta}^T \mathbf{z}_i}). \tag{10}
$$

Similarly, we can obtain

$$
(\Lambda_0(t_{1,2}) - \Lambda_0(t^*)|\boldsymbol{\beta}, D_i, n^*) \backsim G(c(M(t_{1,2}) - M(t^*)) + (n_{1,1} - n^*), c + e^{\boldsymbol{\beta}^T \mathbf{z}_i}). \tag{11}
$$

Note that the distribution of $\Lambda_0(t_{1,3}) - \Lambda_0(t_{1,2})$ is still given by the third line of (9).

The final component of the Gibbs sampler is the conditional distribution of $\left(N_i(t^*) - N_i(t_{1,1})\right)$ given $\Lambda_0(t)$ and D_i. This distribution can be obtained using the properties of NHPPs as a binomial distribution given by

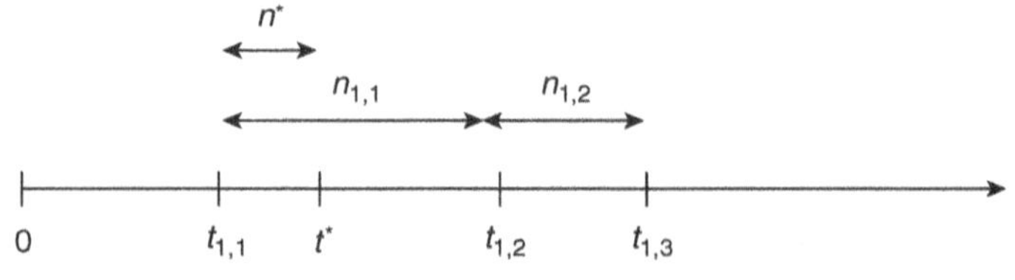

Fig. 2 Prediction in a single rail section

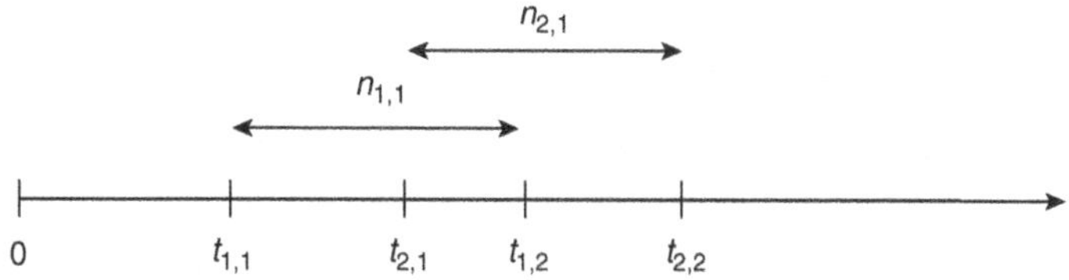

Fig. 3 Two rail sections with overlapping intervals

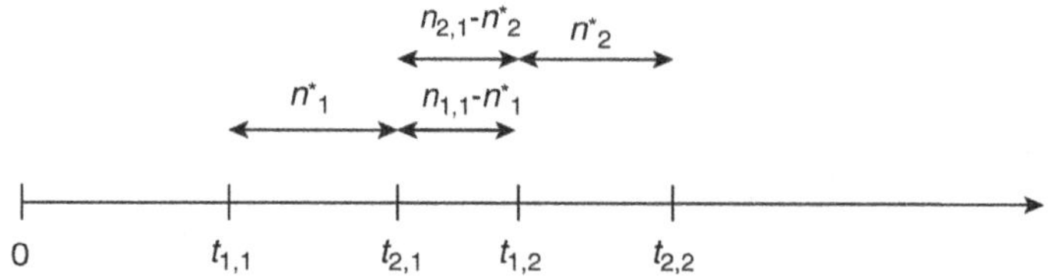

Fig. 4 Data augmentation for two rail sections

$$\left(N_i(t^*) - N_i(t_{1,1}) = n^* | \Lambda_0(t), D_i\right) \sim Bin\left(n_{1,1}, \frac{\Lambda_0(t^*) - \Lambda_0(t_{1,1})}{\Lambda_0(t_{1,2}) - \Lambda_0(t_{1,1})}\right). \tag{12}$$

It is also possible to have inspection data on two or more rail sections observed for overlapping MGT intervals. Figure 3 illustrates such a case with two rail sections. In this case, since the observed counts $n_{1,2}$ and $n_{2,2}$ are coming from overlapping intervals, $(\Lambda_0(t_{1,2}) - \Lambda_0(t_{1,1}))$ and $(\Lambda_0(t_{2,2}) - \Lambda_0(t_{2,1}))$ cannot be updated separately.

Similar to the prediction problem in a single rail section, we can data augment using unobserved counts n_1^* and n_2^* as shown in Fig. 4. We note that, conditional on the counts n_1^* and n_2^*, using the independent increment property of the gamma process, we can update the baseline cumulative intensity as

$$\begin{aligned}
&(\Lambda_0(t_{2,1}) - \Lambda_0(t_{1,1}) | \boldsymbol{\beta}, n_1^*, D) \backsim G\Big(c[M(t_{2,1}) - M(t_{1,1})] + n_1^*, c + e^{\boldsymbol{\beta}^T \mathbf{z}_1}\Big),\\
&(\Lambda_0(t_{1,2}) - \Lambda_0(t_{2,1}) | \boldsymbol{\beta}, n_1^*, n_2^*, D) \backsim G\Big(c[M(t_{1,2}) - M(t_{2,1})] + (n_{1,1} - n_1^*)\\
&\qquad\qquad + (n_{2,1} - n_2^*), c + \sum_i^2 e^{\boldsymbol{\beta}^T \mathbf{z}_i}\Big),\\
&(\Lambda_0(t_{2,2}) - \Lambda_0(t_{1,2}) | \boldsymbol{\beta}, n_2^*, D) \backsim G\Big(c[M(t_{2,2}) - M(t_{1,2})] + n_2^*, c + e^{\boldsymbol{\beta}^T \mathbf{z}_2}\Big).
\end{aligned} \tag{13}$$

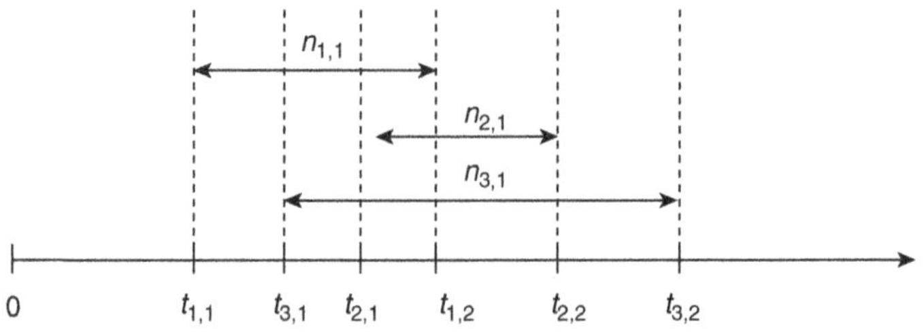

Fig. 5 A more general case

We can show that the full conditionals of latent counts can be obtained as independent binomial random variables given by

$$\left(N_1(t_{2,1}) - N_1(t_{1,1})|n_{1,1}, \frac{\Lambda_0(t_{2,1}) - \Lambda_0(t_{1,1})}{\Lambda_0(t_{1,2}) - \Lambda_0(t_{1,1})}\right) \backsim Bin\left(n_{1,1}, \frac{\Lambda_0(t_{2,1}) - \Lambda_0(t_{1,1})}{\Lambda_0(t_{1,2}) - \Lambda_0(t_{1,1})}\right)$$

$$\left(N_2(t_{2,2}) - N_2(t_{1,2})|n_{2,1}, \frac{\Lambda_0(t_{2,2}) - \Lambda_0(t_{1,2})}{\Lambda_0(t_{2,2}) - \Lambda_0(t_{2,1})}\right) \backsim Bin\left(n_{2,1}, \frac{\Lambda_0(t_{2,2}) - \Lambda_0(t_{1,2})}{\Lambda_0(t_{2,2}) - \Lambda_0(t_{2,1})}\right).$$

2.1.2 General Data Augmentation Algorithm

As noted by Merrick and Soyer [16], as the number of inspected rail sections and overlapping intervals increases, deciding which intervals upon which to data augment is more complicated and, therefore, requires a systematic approach. One alternative is to break the possible traffic usages into a partition defined by the endpoints of all intervals. This is illustrated in Fig. 5 for the case of three rail sections with overlapping intervals.

Merrick and Soyer [16] proposed a data augmentation algorithm to deal with the case of m rail sections with overlapping MGT intervals. In what follows we present the more general form of this data augmentation algorithm discussed by Kuzu and Soyer [13]. The first step in the algorithm is to determine the intervals that will be used for the data augmentation. Following [13], we define $t_1^* < t_2^* < \cdots < t_q^*$ as the q ordered values among the interval endpoints $t_{i,j}$ for $j = 1, \ldots, r_i$ and $i = 1, \ldots, m$.

Also, we define the unobserved number of failures in the interval $[t_k^*, t_{k+1}^*)$ for rail section i by $N_{i,k}^*$ and define $B_k^* = \{i : t_k^* \leq t_{i,j} < t_{k+1}^*\}$ for $k = 1, \ldots, q$, as the set of rail sections that have a failure count that spans the interval $[t_k^*, t_{k+1}^*)$. Let $S_{i,j}^* = \{t_k^* : t_{i,j-1} \leq t_k^* < t_{i,j}\}$ denote the set of all interval endpoints that fall in interval $[t_{i,j-1}, t_{i,j})$ and $m_{i,j}^* = |S_{i,j}^*|$ be the number of interval endpoints in this set. Furthermore, define the ordered list of members of $S^*_{i,j}$ by $\{\ell^1_{i,j}, \ldots, \ell^{m^*_{i,j}}_{i,j}\}$ with $\ell^{m^*_{i,j}+1}_{i,j} = t_{i,j}$.

As pointed out by Kuzu and Soyer [13], once these components are defined and $N^* = (N^*_{i,k}; i = 1, \ldots, m, k = 1, \ldots, q-1)$ are obtained, at each iteration of the Gibbs sampler we can draw from the full conditional distributions $p(\Lambda_0(t)|N^*, \boldsymbol{\beta}, D)$, $p(N^*|\Lambda_0(t), \boldsymbol{\beta}, D)$ and $p(\boldsymbol{\beta}|N^*, \Lambda_0(t), D)$. For drawing samples from $p(\Lambda_0(t)|N^*, \boldsymbol{\beta}, D)$, we can update $\Lambda_0(t^*_{k+1}) - \Lambda_0(t^*_k)$ by using the independent increment property of the gamma process. More specifically, given N^*, D and $\boldsymbol{\beta}$, a vector of covariate parameters, we can easily show that

$$(\Lambda_0(t^*_{k+1}) - \Lambda_0(t^*_k)\ |N^*, \boldsymbol{\beta}, D) \backsim G(c[M(t^*_{k+1}) - M(t^*_k)] + \sum_{i \in B^*_{k+1}} N^*_{i,k}, c + \sum_{i \in B^*_{k+1}} e^{\boldsymbol{\beta}^T \boldsymbol{Z}^*_{i,k}}) \tag{14}$$

for $k = 1, \ldots, q-1$, where $\boldsymbol{Z}^*_{i,k}$ denotes the covariate vector associated with rail sections that have a failure count spanning the interval $[t^*_k, t^*_{k+1})$.

To obtain the full conditional distribution of $N^*_{i,k}$'s, we consider the vector $\underline{N^*_{i,j}} = (N^*_{i,k} : t^*_k \in S^*_{i,j})$ containing $N^*_{i,k}$'s that lie in the interval $[t_{i,j-1}, t_{i,j})$ for rail section i. Given $\Delta = \{\Lambda(t^*_{k+1}) - \Lambda(t^*_k); k = 1, \ldots, q-1\}$, using the properties of NHPPs, we can obtain the full conditional of $\underline{N^*_{i,j}}$' as a multinomial given by

$$\left(\underline{N^*_{i,j}}|\Delta, D\right) \backsim Mult\left(n_{i,j}, p^*_{i,j,1}, \ldots, p^*_{i,j,m^*_{i,j}}\right), \tag{15}$$

where

$$p^*_{i,j,h} = \frac{\Lambda_0\left(\ell^{h+1}_{i,j}\right) - \Lambda_0\left(\ell^h_{i,j}\right)}{\Lambda_0\left(\ell^{m^*_{i,j}+1}_{i,j}\right) - \Lambda_0\left(\ell^1_{i,j}\right)}, \tag{16}$$

for $h = 1, \ldots, m^*_{i,j} - 1$. Obviously, if $m^*_{i,j} = 1$, then $N^*_{i,k} = n_{i,j}$. It is important to note that $\underline{N^*_{i,j}}$'s are drawn as independent multinomials across rail sections i and intervals $j = 1, \ldots, r_i$, for a given rail section.

The full conditional posterior distribution of $\boldsymbol{\beta}$ is not available in a familiar form, and therefore, a Metropolis–Hastings step can be used at each iteration of the Gibbs sampler to draw samples from $p(\boldsymbol{\beta}|N^*, \Lambda_0(t), D)$; see, for example [4].

Computation of posterior predictive distributions of the number of failures for new rail sections with different MGT intervals requires a minor modification of the data augmentation as discussed in [13].

3 Markov Modulated Markov Processes

Stochastic processes that are governed by Markov processes, which cannot be observed, are referred to as hidden Markov models (HMM) or Markov modulated Markov processes; see [29]. The term HMM is typically used to refer to discrete-time processes governed by Markov chains, whereas the term Markov modulated process is reserved for the case where the governing process is a continuous-time Markov chain (or Markov process). A semi-Markov process can also be used as the governing process as discussed in [24], but this will not be our focus in this section.

Ay et al. [1] consider a doubly stochastic Markov representation of the Markov modulated Markov processes (MMMPs) where the generator is also stochastic. In other words, the authors assume that the entries in the generator change with respect to the changing states of yet another Markov process that describes the random environment that the system operates in. This allows them to develop a Markovian analysis of the model and develop Bayesian inference using MCMC methods and consider special cases of MMMPs.

3.1 The Bivariate Markov Model

Following [1], we let $Z = \{Z_t; t \geq 0\}$ be a stochastic process such that Z_t representing the state of the system at time t. We assume that Z has a finite state space $F = \{1, 2, \cdots, N\}$ and it has a Markov structure. We define an environmental process $Y = \{Y_t; t \geq 0\}$ where Y_t represents the state of the environment at time t that has an effect on the process Z. Y is a continuous-time Markov process with a finite state space $E = \{1, 2, \cdots, K\}$ with generator

$$G_{ij} = \begin{cases} -\rho_i & \text{if} j = i \\ \rho_i P_{ij} & \text{if} j \neq i. \end{cases} \tag{17}$$

Equivalently, we can write $G_{ij} = \rho_i(P_{ij} - I_{ij})$ where I is the identity matrix. Note that the process Y spends an exponential amount of time with holding rate ρ_i in state i and, when it jumps, it randomly goes to state j with transition probability P_{ij} where $P_{ii} = 0$. Note that the environmental process Y is unobservable.

When state of the environment Y_t is $i \in E$, the observable process Z evolves as a Markov process with generator

$$A_i(x, y) = \begin{cases} -\lambda_i(x) & \text{if} y = x \\ \lambda_i(x) M_i(x, y) & \text{if} y \neq x \end{cases}. \tag{18}$$

The generator (18) implies that while the process Y is in state i, the process Z spends an exponential amount of time with holding rate $\lambda_i(x)$ in state x and, when it jumps, it randomly goes to state y with transition probability $M_i(x, y)$ where $M_i(x, x) = 0$. We refer to Z as a MMMP.

As noted by Ay et al. [1], the bivariate process $(Y, Z) = \{(Y_t, Z_t); t \geq 0\}$ is a Markov process with state space $E \times F$ where the generator Q of (Y, Z) is

$$Q_{(i,x),(j,y)} = \begin{cases} \rho_i P_{ij} & j \neq i, y = x \\ \lambda_i(x) M_i(x, y) & j = i, y \neq x \\ -(\rho_i + \lambda_i(x)) & j = i, y = x \end{cases} \tag{19}$$

for all $i, j \in E$ and $x, y \in F$. There are well-known processes that arise as special case of the bivariate process with generator (19). For example, Markov modulated Poisson process of [14] is a special case where $\lambda_i(x) = \lambda_i$ and $M_i(x, x + 1) = 1$. In the setting of [14], Z_t represents the total number of software failures until time t with initial state $Z_0 = 0$ and the state of Y process determines the failure intensity.

The Markov modulated birth–death process is another special case of the MMMP with $\lambda_i(x) = \gamma_i + \mu_i$ and

$$M_i(x, y) = \begin{cases} \dfrac{\gamma_i}{\gamma_i + \mu_i} & y = x + 1 \\ \\ \dfrac{\mu_i}{\gamma_i + \mu_i} & y = x - 1, \end{cases}$$

where γ_i and μ_i are the birth and death rates of the process and $M_i(0, 1) = 1$.

The MMMP reduces to a Markov modulated compound Poisson process when

$$Z_t = \sum_{k=1}^{N_t} W_k, \tag{20}$$

where N is a Poisson process with jump rate λ_i in environment i, W_k's are independent and identically distributed random variables representing the jump size, and $M_i(x, y)$ is the probability of having a jump with magnitude $(y - x)$ in environment i. One possibility is to assume that W_k's all have the binomial distribution with parameters n_i and p_i, while the jump occurs in environment i so that

$$M_i(x, x + z) = \binom{n_i}{z} p_i^z (1 - p_i)^{n_i - z} \tag{21}$$

for $z = 0, 1, 2, \cdots, n_i$. It is important to note that in the case of the compound Poisson process, the environmental process Y governs both the arrival rate of the Poisson process and the "success" probability of the binomial model (21). This is illustrated in Fig. 6 where the Y process occupies three different states over time.

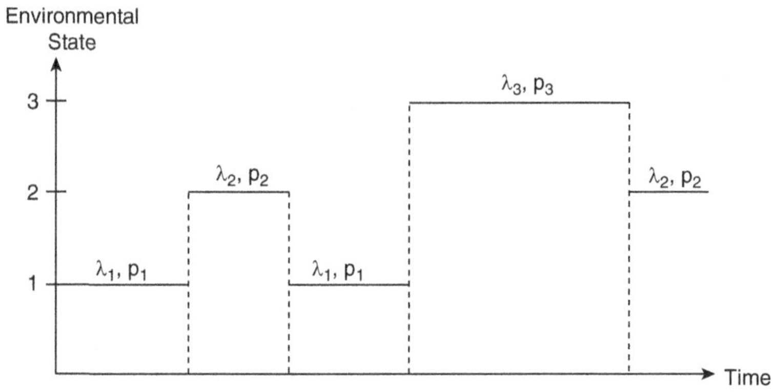

Fig. 6 Modulation in the compound Poisson process

Since (Y, Z) is a Markov process with generator matrix Q, its transition probability function

$$P_{(i,x),(j,y)}(t) = P[Y_t = j, Z_t = y | Y_0 = i, Z_0 = x] \tag{22}$$

is given by the exponential matrix form

$$P(t) = \exp(Qt) = \sum_{n=0}^{+\infty} \frac{t^n}{n!} Q^n. \tag{23}$$

Computationally tractable procedures for evaluation of the exponential matrix (23) is discussed in [18].

3.2 Bayesian Analysis of MMMPs

A Gibbs sampler based on data augmentation using the history of the environmental process Y was proposed by Fearnhead and Sherlock [9] for Bayesian analysis of Markov modulated Poisson processes. The exact Gibbs sampler proposed by the authors was implemented in [14] for software reliability analysis. Ay et al. [1] modified the Fearnhead–Sherlock algorithm for developing posterior inference for the MMMPs. In what follows, we will summarize the Ay et al. [1] modification.

The modified Gibbs sampler involves a three-stage process as in [9] to develop inference on all unknown parameters $\boldsymbol{\Theta}$ of the MMMP as well as the latent states of the Y process. Note that $\boldsymbol{\Theta} = (\boldsymbol{\rho}, \boldsymbol{P}, \boldsymbol{\lambda}, \boldsymbol{M})$, where $\boldsymbol{\rho} = \{\rho_i; i \in E\}$, the holding rates of the Y process, $\boldsymbol{P} = \{P_{ij}; i, j \in E\}$, transition probabilities of Y, $\boldsymbol{\lambda} = \{\lambda_i(x); i \in E, x \in F\}$, the holding rates of the Z process, and $\boldsymbol{M} = \{M_i(x, y); i \in E, x, y \in F\}$, its transition probabilities.

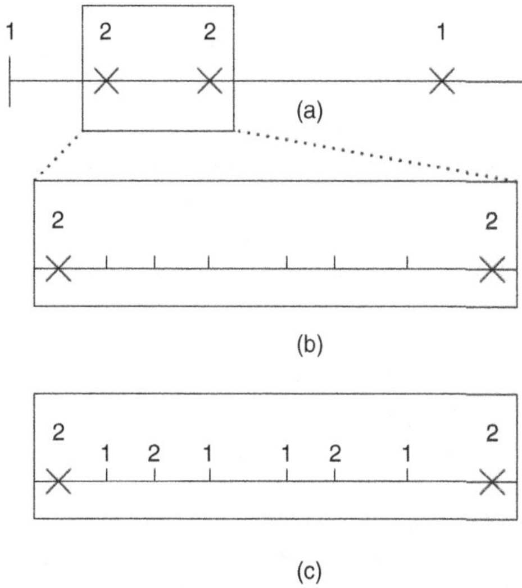

Fig. 7 Simulating the history of latent process Y

It is assumed that the process Z is observed completely until some time t_{obs}, while the process Y is latent. We suppose that the process Z changes its state a total of n times during $[0, t_{obs}]$, and we let $t^{(1)} < t^{(2)} < \cdots < t^{(n)}$ denote the jump times of the Z process. To simplify the notation, we will let $z^{(k)} = Z_{t^{(k)}}$ denote the observed state of Z after the kth change of state and $Y^{(k)} = Y_{t^{(k)}}$ denote the unobserved state the hidden Markov process at the kth time of change of the observed process Z.

Following [1], we also set $t^{(0)} = 0$, $t^{(n+1)} = t_{obs}$ for completeness and let $z^{(0)} = Z_0$ denote the initial observed state, while $z^{(n+1)} = z^{(n)}$ is the last state observed. Note that $\{t^{(k)}\}$ and $\{z^{(k)}\}$ are all contained in the data $\mathcal{D} = \{z_t; 0 \leq t \leq t_{obs}\}$, where z_t is the state of the MMMP observed at time t.

Given the entire path of the hidden Markov process, $\mathcal{F} = \{Y_t; 0 \leq t \leq t_{obs}\}$, it is possible to obtain the posterior distribution of the unknown parameters $p(\boldsymbol{\Theta}|\mathcal{F}, \mathcal{D})$. Since $\mathcal{F}$ is not observed, to evaluate the posterior distribution $p(\boldsymbol{\Theta}|\mathcal{D})$, we use a Gibbs sampler where we can simulate from the conditional posterior distributions $p(\boldsymbol{\Theta}|\mathcal{F}, \mathcal{D})$ and $p(\mathcal{F}|\boldsymbol{\Theta}, \mathcal{D})$ recursively by using the approach of [9].

The first stage of the modified algorithm involves simulating the state of the hidden Markov process at each of the times $t^{(1)}, t^{(2)}, \cdots, t^{(n)}$ given in the observed data set $\mathcal{D}$ and conditional on the parameters $\boldsymbol{\Theta}$. This is achieved by using the forward–backward algorithm [3] given the states at the start and end of the observation window. This is illustrated in part (a) of Fig. 7.

Given the simulated states of the Y process at each of our observation times $\{t^{(k)}\}$, we next simulate the entire hidden Markov process Y. To do this, we first simulate it over the interval $(t^{(0)}, t^{(1)})$, then $(t^{(1)}, t^{(2)})$ and so on until $(t^{(n)}, t^{(n+1)})$, where $t^{(n+1)} = t_{obs}$. The simulation over each interval is done using the uniformization of the Markov process Y assuming that $\rho = \max_{i \in E} \rho_i$ is finite. In doing so, the Markov process Y can be represented as a Markov chain $\hat{X}$ subordinated to a Poisson process $\hat{N}$ with arrival rate ρ so that $Y_t = \hat{X}_{\hat{N}_t}$ as discussed in [1]. Over any interval $(t^{(k-1)}, t^{(k)})$, given the simulated states $Y_{t^{(k-1)}} = s_{k-1}$ and $Y_{t^{(k)}} = s_k$ from stage 1, the number of arrivals from this process during $(t^{(k-1)}, t^{(k)})$ can be simulated. Finally, the states at these arrival times can be simulated recursively. The stage 2 of the algorithm is shown in parts (b) and (c) of Fig. 7.

Stage 3 of the algorithm involves simulating a new set of parameter values using the simulated history of the hidden Markov process and observed data. Since history $\mathcal{F}$ includes information on quantities such as the total time that the hidden Markov process Y spends in state i, the total amount of time that the modulated process Z spends in state x, while the state of Y is i, the number of times the hidden process Y makes a transition from state i to state j, and the number of times that the process Z jumps from state x to y while the hidden process Y is in state i, one can use conjugate priors for all unknown parameters. As a result, components of the posterior full conditional distribution $p(\boldsymbol{\Theta}|\mathcal{F}, \mathcal{D})$ can be obtained analytically. More specifically, one can use gamma priors for holding rates and Dirichlet priors for the transition probabilities as discussed in [1].

All details of the modified Gibbs sampler and related computational issues are given in [1]. The authors also discuss computation of marginal likelihood, in the sense of [4], to infer the number of states of the environmental process Y as well as treatment of different types of data.

4 Numerical Illustrations

In this section, we present two illustrations of Bayesian analysis of MMMPs using actual data. The first illustration involves Bayesian analysis of software failure data using a Markov modulated Poisson process, and the second illustration is on the use of a Markov modulated compound Poisson process to analyze power outages.

4.1 A Markov Modulated Poisson Process Model for Software Failures

We consider the "BDATA" of [11] on software testing. The data was observed over a period of $t_{obs} = 16{,}648$ units, and $n = 207$ failures were observed during this time.

We present results from the analysis of two-state Markov modulated Poisson process. We used proper but noninformative gamma priors for the arrival and holding rates with parameters $a_i^{\lambda} = b_i^{\lambda} = a_i^{\rho} = b_i^{\rho} = 0.01$ for $i = 1, 2$. After using a small burn-in sample, we collected 5000 simulations to obtain the posterior

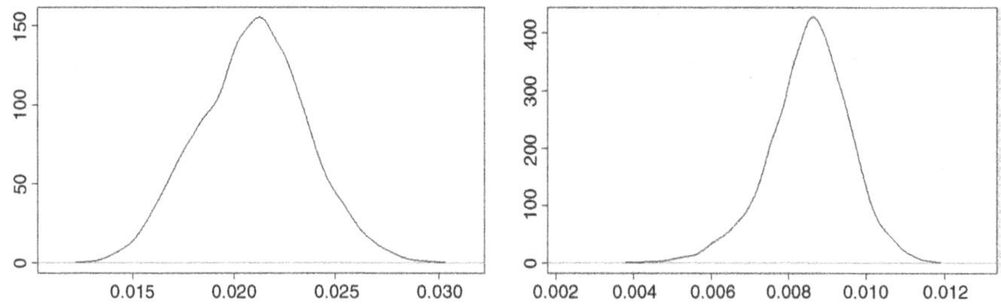

Fig. 8 Posterior densities of λ_1 and λ_2

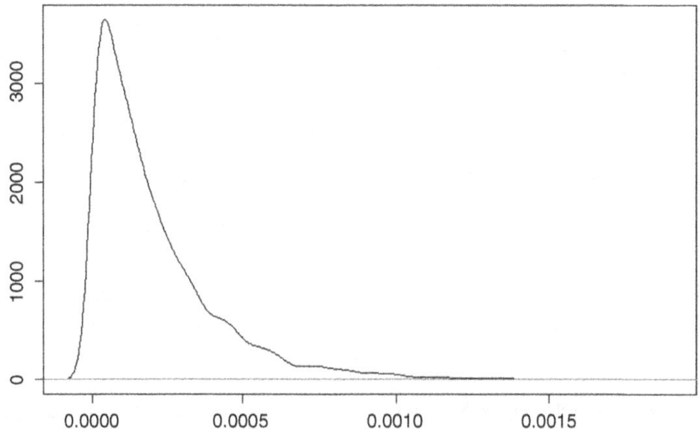

Fig. 9 Posterior density of ρ_1

distributions. The posterior distributions of λ_1 and λ_2 are given in Fig. 8, and the posterior density for ρ_1 is given in Fig. 9. The posterior means of λ_1 and λ_2 are given as $\lambda_1 = 0.021$ and $\lambda_2 = 0.0085$, and the posterior mean of ρ_1 is obtained as 0.0002.

Similar to the findings of [14] for a different set of software failure data, our analysis has shown that state 2 is acting like an absorbing state, that is, expected holding time is infinite. The process starts in state 1, stays there for a while, and then absorbed at state 2. We can also see this behavior by looking at the plot of actual and the expected time between failures using the holding rate of the environment with the higher posterior probability. This is shown in Fig. 10 where the red lines are the expected time between failures under the specific environments. Note that expected time between failures is higher under state 2, which has the lower failure rate, and the fact that the process is absorbed at state 2 suggests that the software debugging process has resulted in reliability improvement.

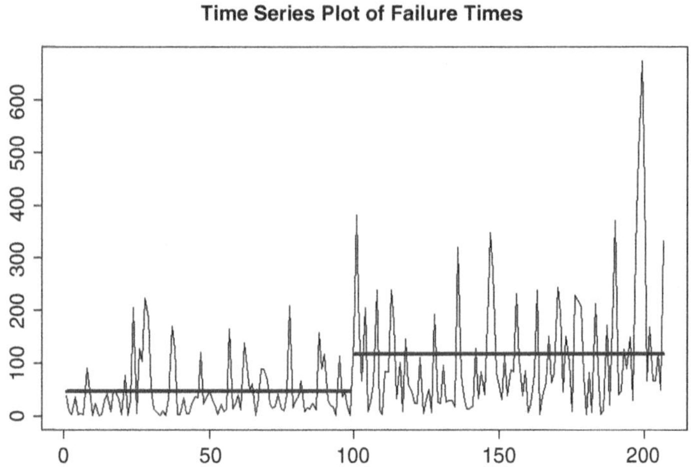

Fig. 10 Actual versus expected time between failures based on posterior modes of state distribution

4.2 A Markov Modulated Compound Poisson Process Model for Power Outages

In this section, we consider a Markov modulated compound Poisson process model for outage data from Loudoun County, Virginia, from May 1, 2014 to December 31, 2019 and the number of customers affected by each outage. The data consists of 1949 outages with the number of customers affected by each outage ranges from 1 to 1141. We use hours as the time unit in our analysis. We note that this data is different than the Stafford County, Virginia data considered in [1].

We consider a binomial model for representing the number of customers affected by each outage as in (21) but with $n_i = n$ representing the total number of customers (that is, households) that potentially could be affected by each outage. As in the previous section, we present results from the analysis using a two-state environmental process that now governs both the arrival and holding rates as well as the probabilities of the binomial model (21) process. We used proper but noninformative priors for all parameters. Specifically, gamma priors for the arrival and holding rates with $a_i^{\lambda} = b_i^{\lambda} = a_i^{\rho} = b_i^{\rho} = 0.01$ for $i = 1, 2$. We specified beta priors for binomial probabilities with $a_i^{p} = b_i^{p} = 0.01$ for $i = 1, 2$. Again, after using a small burn-in sample, we collected 5000 simulations to obtain the posterior distributions.

The posterior distributions of λ_1 and λ_2 are shown in Fig. 11 where the posterior means can be obtained as $\lambda_1 = 0.772$ and $\lambda_2 = 6.337$ implying that environment 2 is a more severe environment than environment 1. In other words, we expect to see more outages under environment 1.

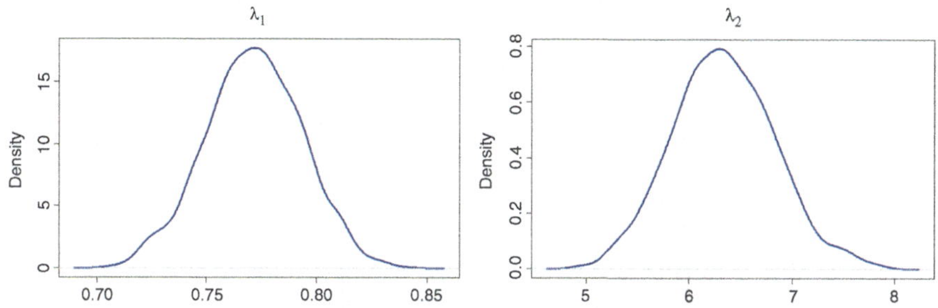

Fig. 11 Posterior density of λ's

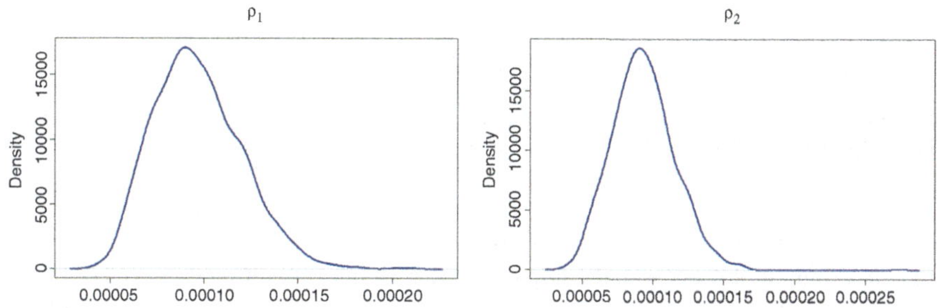

Fig. 12 Posterior density of ρ's

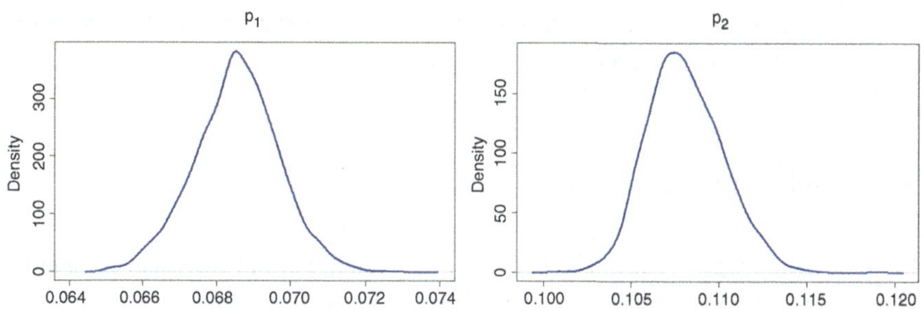

Fig. 13 Posterior density of p's

The posterior distributions of the holding rates ρ_1 and ρ_2 of the environmental process are given in Fig. 12. The posterior means of holding rates are very close given by $\rho_1 = 0.0000968$ and $\rho_2 = 0.0000934$ suggesting that the environmental process spends equal time in both states.

The posterior distributions of the binomial probabilities p_1 and p_2 are illustrated in Fig. 13. The posterior means of p_i's can be obtained as $p_1 = 0.068$ and $p_2 = 0.108$ suggesting that it is more likely that an household will be affected from an outage when the environmental process is in state 2. This is intuitive since state 2 represents a more severe environment in this case. We note that similar results were obtained in [1] for Stafford County, Virginia.

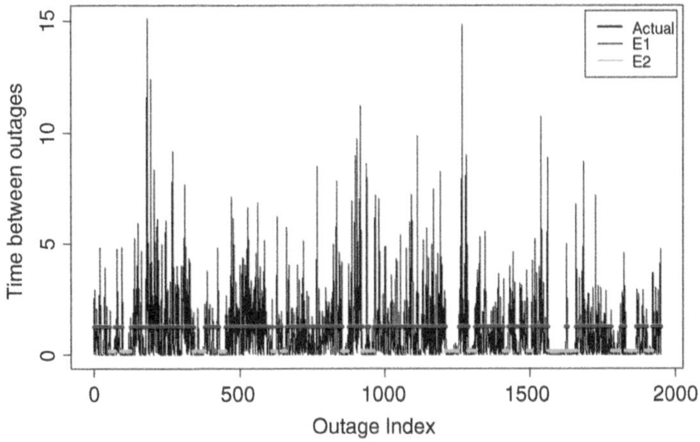

Fig. 14 Actual and expected time between outages based on the environmental state with the highest posterior probability

As we did in the previous illustration, we can also look at the state occupancies of the environmental process and compare them with the actual time between outages. We show in Fig. 14 the actual time between outages (in hours) in black and the expected time between outages in red when the posterior probability favors state 1. The expected time between outages when the posterior probability favors state 2 are shown in green. Again we see from the figure that the state 2, which is the more severe environment, is associated with shorter outage times.

5 Concluding Remarks

In this chapter, we have discussed some of the recent work in Bayesian computing in reliability analysis in dynamic environments. In doing so, first we have focused on Bayesian computations for semi-parametric NHPPs for analysis of interval count data and presented a data augmentation algorithm to alleviate difficulties associated with the use of gamma process priors. The second class of models considered was the MMMPs for which we discussed a modified algorithm based on the work of [9]. Although both classes of models were motivated from reliability problems, they have applications in other areas in operations such as call center modeling; see [30] and ticket queues; see [13].

References

1. Ay, A., Landon, J., Özekici, S.and Soyer, R.: Bayesian analysis of doubly stochastic Markov processes in reliability. Probab. Eng. Inf. Sci. **35**, 708–729 (2021)
2. Barlow, R.E., Hunter, L.: Optimum preventive maintenance policies. Oper. Res. **8**, 90–100 (1960)
3. Baum, L.E., Petrie, T., Soules, G., Weiss, N.: A maximisation technique occurring in the statistical analysis of probabilistic functions of Markov chains. Ann. Math. Stat. **41**, 164–171 (1970)
4. Chib, S.: Marginal likelihood from the Gibbs output. J. Am. Stat. Assoc. **90**, 1313–1321 (1995)
5. Chib, S., Greenberg, E.: Understanding the Metropolis–Hastings algorithm. Am. Stat. **49**, 327–335 (1995)
6. Çınlar, E.: Markov renewal theory. Adv. Appl. Probab. **1**, 123–187 (1969)
7. Çınlar, E., Özekici, S.: Reliability of complex devices in random environments. Probab. Eng. Inf. Sci. **1**, 97–115 (1987)
8. Cox, D.R.: The statistical analysis of dependencies in point processes. In: Lewis, P.A.W. (ed.) Stochastic Point Processes, pp. 55–66. Wiley, New York (1972)
9. Fearnhead, P., Sherlock, C.: An exact Gibbs sampler for the Markov-modulated Poisson process. J. R. Stat. Soc. Ser. B **68**, 767–784 (2006)
10. Gaver, D.P.: Random hazard in reliability problems. Technometrics **5**, 211–226 (1963)
11. Keiller, P.A., Mazzuchi, T.A.: Investigating a specific class of software reliability growth models. In: Proceedings of Annual Reliability and Maintainability Symposium, pp. 242–248 (2002)
12. Klein, M.: Inspection-maintenance-replacement schedules under Markovian deterioration. Manag. Sci. **9**, 25–32 (1962)
13. Kuzu, K. and Soyer, R.: Bayesian modeling of abandonments in ticket queues. Naval Research Logistics. **65**, 499–521 (2018)
14. Landon, J., Özekici, S., Soyer, R.: A Markov modulated poisson model for software reliability. Eur. J. Oper. Res. **229**, 404–410 (2013)
15. Mercer, A.: Some simple wear-dependent renewal processes. J. R. Stat. Soc. Ser. B **23**, 368–376 (1961)
16. Merrick, J.R., Soyer, R.: Semiparametric Bayesian optimal replacement policies: application to railroad tracks. Appl. Stoch. Models Bus. Ind. **33**, 445–460 (2017)
17. Merrick, J.R., Soyer, R., Mazzuchi, T.A.: Are maintenance practices for rail- road tracks effective? J. Am. Stat. Assoc. **100**, 17–25 (2005)
18. Moler, C., van Loan, C.: Nineteen dubious ways to compute the exponential of a matrix, twenty-five years later. SIAM Rev. **45**, 3–49 (2003)
19. Özekici, S.: Optimal maintenance policies in random environments. Eur. J. Oper. Res. **82**,283–294 (1995)
20. Özekici, S., Soyer, R.: Testing strategies for software with an operational profile. Nav. Res. Logist. **48**, 747–763 (2001)
21. Özekici, S., Soyer, R.: Reliability of software with an operational profile. Eur. J. Oper. Res. **149**, 459–474 (2003)
22. Özekici, S., Soyer, R.: Network reliability assessment in a random environment. Nav. Res. Logist. **50**, 574–591 (2003)
23. Özekici, S., Soyer, R.: Reliability modeling and analysis under random environments In: Soyer, R., Mazzuchi, T.A., Singpurwalla, N.D. (eds.) Mathematical Reliability: An Expository Perspective, pp. 249–273. Kluwer, Boston (2004)
24. Özekici, S., Soyer, R.: Semi-Markov modulated Poisson process: probabilistic and statistical analysis. Math. Methods Oper. Res. **64**, 125–144 (2006)
25. Pievatolo, A., Ruggeri, F., Soyer, R.: A Bayesian hidden Markov model for imperfect debugging. Reliab. Eng. Syst. Saf. **103**, 11–21 (2012)

26. Rios-Insua, D., Ruggeri, F., Soyer, R., Wilson, S.: Advances in Bayesian decision making in reliability. Eur. J. Oper. Res. **282**, 1–18 (2020)
27. Singpurwalla, N.D.: Survival in dynamic environments. Stat. Sci. **10**, 86–103 (1995)
28. Singpurwalla, N.D., Mazzuchi, T.A., Özekici, S., Soyer, R.: Stochastic process models for reliability in dynamic environments. In: Rao, C.R., Khattree, R. (eds.) Handbook of Statistics, vol. 22. Statistics in Industry, pp. 1109–1129. Elsevier, Amsterdam (2003)
29. Soyer, R.: Markov and hidden Markov models. In: Cochran, J.J. (ed.) Encyclopedia of Operations Research and Management Science, vol. 5, pp. 3034–3053. Wiley, New York (2011)
30. Soyer, R., Tarimcilar, M.M.: Modeling and analysis of call center arrival data: a Bayesian approach. Manag. Sci. **54**, 266–278 (2008)

Bayesian Analysis of Stochastic Processes in Reliability

Evans Gouno

Abstract In reliability, models involving complex stochastic processes play an important role. This type of model allows analysts to handle many problems such as the missing data or uncertain data problem. The Bayesian approach relying on prior belief or expertise appears to be a natural tool in such situations. Thus the Bayesian approach provides efficient methods for reliability analysis with stochastic processes. The objective of this chapter is to describe the main techniques to make Bayesian inference for stochastic processes.

1 Introduction

The literature on stochastic processes is plethoric. It is clear that the theory of stochastic processes contains many tools that can be applied to deal with different problems arising in the domain of reliability. Indeed reliability issues involve counting events or observing durations or to be general, non-negative random variables such as kilometers, the numbers of cycle, etc. The events of interest can be of different natures. Usually, they correspond to failures. Thus durations are times to failure or times elapsed between events. These elapsed times between events are often called *interarrivals*. Depending on the nature of the observation, the model will be different. In the case of interarrivals, renewal processes are the natural approach. When counting events, Poisson processes cover many situations since they are characterized by their intensities that can have many different forms.

Kijima and Shaked [37] gave a comprehensive overview of the applications and the concepts of stochastic processes theory in the field of reliability. They reviewed the use of the *first-passage time* concept in Markov chain and in some non-Markovian processes to deal with aging in maintenance issues. They describe

E. Gouno (✉)
Université Bretagne Sud, LMBA, Vannes, France
e-mail: evans.gouno@univ-ubs.fr

Y. Lio et al. (eds.), *Bayesian Inference and Computation in Reliability and Survival Analysis*, Emerging Topics in Statistics and Biostatistics,
https://doi.org/10.1007/978-3-030-88658-5_6

cumulative damage shock processes. They also display some results for comparison of repairable systems and replacement policies via point processes.

Ridgon and Basu [64] provided a general review of statistical methods for repairable systems. Kamranfar et al. [35] compare classical and Bayesian approaches for statistical analysis of a repairable sytem exposed to shocks. Nakagawa [55] surveyed basic stochastic processes with applications to reliability. Singpurwalla [69] proposed a road map to describe the stochastic process approach to failure models that displays the diversity of models from *Poisson* processes to *extended gamma* processes through *shot noise* processes. The book [70] provides a comprehensive overview of the use of stochastic processes for software reliability.

For this chapter, the goal is to give an overview of the Bayesian inference for some stochastic processes that are used in the context of reliability. The following section recalls the basic definitions and properties of stochastic processes. The intensity function is the fundamental object that characterizes a stochastic process. In Sect. 2, we propose a survey that displays various forms of intensity functions. After a short reminder of the principle of the Bayes analysis, we review applications of the Bayesian techniques for inference on various types of stochastic processes. This chapter is not intended to be an exhaustive review since hundreds of papers and entire books on the topic [5, 32] are available.

2 Stochastic Processes

A stochastic process can be viewed as a mathematical tool to describe a collection of points on the real line. One can be interested in the position of the points on the real line (dates) or in the number of points in a given interval (a time interval) or in the distance between two successive points (interarrival times). In practice, a point corresponds to an event (for example, a failure). Therefore, a stochastic process is described as a sequence $T_1, T_2, T_3, \ldots$ of dates, where T_i is the date of the i-th event, or as a sequence of interarrivals $X_1, X_2, \ldots$ with $X_i = T_i - T_{i-1}$, $i = 1, 2, \ldots$, $T_0 = 0$, or as $\{N(t), t \geqslant 0\}$, where $N(t)$ is the number of points in $[0, t]$. It seems natural to consider that the evolution of the process at a given time t might depend on the history of the process that is to say, the sequence $\mathscr{H}_t = \{t_1, t_2, \ldots t_{N(t^-)}\}$ or $\mathscr{H}_t = \{N(u); 0 \leqslant u \leqslant t^-\}$, where t_i is a realization of the random variables (r.v.) $T_i \mid T_{i-1}, \ldots, T_1$.

A classical procedure to characterize a stochastic process is to assume the following:

i. The numbers of events happening in disjoint intervals of time are independent.
ii. The probability of two or more events in an infinitesimal interval of length h is $o(h)$:

$$Pr\big(N(t, t + h) > 1 \mid \mathscr{H}_t\big) = o(h).$$

iii. The probability of exactly one event in an infinitesimal interval of length h is proportional to h with a coefficient $\lambda(t)$ depending on time

$$Pr\big(N(t, t+h) = 1 \mid \mathscr{H}_t\big) = \lambda(t)\, h + o(h), \tag{1}$$

where $o(h)$ is such that $o(h)/h$ goes to 0 when h goes to 0.

The coefficient $\lambda(t)$ is called the *intensity* of the process. It is the rate of occurrence of failures (ROCOF) in reliability. Since

$$\lim_{h\to 0} \frac{1}{h} Pr\big(N(t, t+h) = 1 \mid \mathscr{H}_t\big) = \lambda(t),$$

it is also called the *instantaneous failure rate* so that it is not confused with the *hazard rate*.

From the above assumptions, the distribution of the number of failures in the interval $[0, t]$ can be obtained as a Poisson distribution with parameter:

$$\Lambda(t) = \int_0^t \lambda(s)ds$$

and

$$Pr\big(N(t) = k\big) = \frac{\Lambda(t)^k}{k!}\, e^{-\Lambda(t)}, \ \forall k \in \mathbb{N},\ t \in \mathbb{R}^+. \tag{2}$$

Thus the expected number of failures at time t is

$$E[N(t)] = \Lambda(t).$$

$\Lambda(t)$ is called the *mean function* of the process. This characterization defines an important family of processes that is named *Poisson processes*. This family is very popular since according to the form of $\lambda(t)$, the intensity, Poisson processes cover many situations for practical applications.

In this family, processes can be classified into two categories according to the limiting behavior of $\Lambda(t)$ [40]. We distinguish processes such that $\lim_{t\to+\infty} \Lambda(t)$ is finite and processes where $\Lambda(t)$ goes to infinity when t goes to infinity.

2.1 Distributions Associated with Stochastic Processes

From (*i.*) and (2), one can write: for any $0 \leqslant s < t$

$$Pr\big(N(s, t) = k\big) = \frac{\big(\Lambda(t) - \Lambda(s)\big)^k}{k!}\, e^{-\left(\Lambda(t)-\Lambda(s)\right)}, \ \forall k \in \mathbb{N}.$$

Remark that: $Pr\big(N(t_{i-1}, t) = 0\big) = Pr(T_i > t \mid T_{i-1} = t_{i-1})$.
Therefore, $Pr(T_i > t \mid T_{i-1} = t_{i-1}) = \exp\big\{-\big(\Lambda(t) - \Lambda(t_i)\big)\big\}$, and taking the derivative, we obtain the probability density function (p.d.f.) of T_i given $T_{i-1} = t_{i-1}$:

$$f_{T_i|T_{i-1}=t_{i-1}}(t) = \lambda(t)\exp\big\{-\big(\Lambda(t) - \Lambda(t_i)\big)\big\},\ i = 1, \ldots, n.$$

Let us consider $\boldsymbol{T_n} = (T_1, T_2, \ldots, T_n)$ as a sample of dates with $T_1 < T_2 < \ldots < T_n$. Suppose that $\boldsymbol{T_n}$ admits a p.d.f. $f_{\boldsymbol{T_n}}(.)$.
This p.d.f. can be expressed as

$$f_{\boldsymbol{T}}(\boldsymbol{t}) = \prod_{i=1}^{n} f_{\boldsymbol{T}_i|\boldsymbol{T}_{i-1}=\boldsymbol{t}_{i-1}}(t_i),$$

where $\boldsymbol{T_i} = (T_1, T_2, \ldots, T_i)$, $\boldsymbol{t_i} = (t_1, t_2, \ldots, t_i)$.

A general expression for the marginal distribution of the i-th failure date, $i > 1$, can be proposed as

$$Pr(T_i \leqslant t) = Pr(N(t) \geqslant i) = \sum_{k=i}^{+\infty} \frac{\Lambda(t)^k}{k!}\, e^{-\Lambda(t)},\ i = 1, \ldots, n.$$

Taking the derivative, we have the p.d.f.

$$f_{T_i}(t) = \frac{\Lambda(t)^{i-1}}{(i-1)!}\, \Lambda'(t)\, e^{-\Lambda(t)},\ i = 1, \ldots, n.$$

For the distribution of $X_i = T_i - T_{i-1}$, the time elapsed between the $(i-1)$-th failure and the $i - th$ failure, we have

$$Pr(T_i - T_{i-1} > t \mid T_{i-1} = s) = Pr(N[s, s+t] = 0).$$

Therefore,

$$Pr(T_i - T_{i-1} > t \mid T_{i-1} = s) = \exp\{-[\Lambda(s+t) - \Lambda(s)]\}$$

and

$$\begin{aligned} Pr(X_i > t) &= \int_0^{+\infty} Pr(T_i - T_{i-1} > t \mid T_{i-1} = s)\ f_{T_{i-1}}(s)ds \\ &= \int_0^{+\infty} \exp\{-\Lambda(s+t)\}\, \frac{\Lambda(s)^{i-2}}{(i-2)!}\, d\Lambda(s). \end{aligned}$$

The previous expressions of the distributions of T_i and X_i depend on the mean function $\Lambda(t)$ and thus on the intensity function $\lambda(t)$. The next section is devoted to the various possible forms of intensity function.

3 Intensity Functions

As mentioned before, a stochastic process is characterized by its intensity function, that is to say this intensity function accounts for the behavior of event occurrences. This function needs to be an integrable function. In this section, we investigate the different possible forms of the intensity function.

A basic example is the situation where the rate is not depending on time that is $\lambda(t) = \lambda$. Then the process is the well-known *homogeneous Poisson process* (HPP). In this case, interarrivals are independent r.v. and follow an exponential distribution with rate parameter λ. The date of the i-th event has a gamma distribution with parameter (i, λ). The number of events occurring in an interval of length t follows a Poisson with parameter λt, and the expected number of failures is a linear function of t with a slope equal to λ. Therefore, performing Bayesian techniques in this case turns around performing Bayesian techniques for exponential distribution or Poisson distribution.

When the rate depends on time, the process is said to be a *non-homogeneous Poisson process* (NHPP). This family of Poisson processes is clearly a rich family, since one can imagine a vast number of forms for the intensity. That is the reason why it has been used in many fields from epidemiology to actuarial sciences (seismology, neurophysiology, software reliability). McCollin [48] described various forms of intensity for NHPP. Table 1 displays some classical expressions.

The choice of the shape intensity depends on the problem being investigated. For example, studying subway train doors reliability, Pievatolo et al. [60] suggest the following intensity function:

$$\lambda(t) = \alpha \frac{\log(1 + \beta t)}{1 + \beta}, \quad \alpha, \beta \geqslant 0,$$

where t are kilometers run by the train.

Table 1 Some classical examples of intensity function

Model	$\lambda(t)$
Exponential	λ_0
Polynomial	$\lambda_0 + \alpha t$ (linear ROCOF)
	$\lambda_0 + \alpha t + \beta t^2$ (quadratic ROCOF)
Duane [19]	$\alpha \beta t^{\beta - 1}$
Cox–Lewis [14]	$\exp\{\alpha + \beta t\}$, $\alpha,\ \beta > 0$
Goël–Okumoto [24]	$\alpha \beta e^{-\beta t}$, $\alpha,\ \beta > 0$
Musa–Okumoto [54]	$\alpha \beta / (1 + \beta t)$

When periodicity is involved (earthquakes), the following form can be considered:

$$\lambda(t) = \exp\{\alpha + \rho \sin(\omega t + \theta)\}.$$

Ruggeri and Sivaganesan [65] defined the general class of NHPPs described by an intensity function of the form $\lambda(t; M, \beta) = Mg(t, \beta)$, with $M, \beta > 0$. This formulation is very convenient to develop a Bayesian approach. One can see that the models in Table 1 belong to this class. Huang and Bier [31] considered an *exponential intensity* of the form $\lambda(t) = \lambda_0 e^{\beta t}$, $\beta \in \mathbb{R}$, which is again an element of this class.

Kuo and Yang [40] suggested an interesting categorization of NHPP models relying on general order statistics (GOS) model and record values statistic (RVS) model that unifies models used in software reliability and gives in the same time, a technique to generate different forms of intensity. The basic set-up for observation of a stochastic process is a time window $[0, C]$ where jumps of the process are recorded. We have a sequence of dates $t_1, t_2, \ldots, t_n$ such that $t_1 \leqslant t_2 \leqslant \ldots \leqslant t_n \leqslant C$ and n is the realization of a discrete r.v. N. This sequence can be interpreted as the first-order statistic from a random sample of n positive random variables $X_1, \ldots, X_n$. When the distribution of the X_i's is assumed to be of the form $\beta f(\beta t \mid \theta)$, this model is called the *general order statistics* (GOS) model [61]. If N has a Poisson distribution with parameter ρ, this model is equivalent to a NHPP with an intensity function $\lambda(t) = \rho f(\beta t)$, $(\rho > 0)$. If F is the cumulative distribution function (c.d.f.) associated to f, then the expected number of failures at t is $\Lambda(t) = \rho F(\beta t)$ and can be interpreted as ρ, the expected number of failures over $[0, +\infty)$ times a weight $F(t)$. These approaches generate a category of NHPPs that can be characterized by the fact that the expected number of failures at time t is such that $\lim_{t\to+\infty} \Lambda(t) < +\infty$. The NHPPs with such property are said to be NHPP-I [40]. Classical choices for f are exponential, Weibull and Pareto distributions. Remark that the exponential case corresponds to the Goël–Okumoto model. Kundu et al. [38] studied in more details the analogy between NHPP and GOS models in the context of software reliability.

Another elegant result given by Kuo and Yang [40] is to consider the sequence $t_1 \leqslant t_2 \leqslant \ldots \leqslant t_n$ as *record values*. Let us recall the definition of record values. Suppose $X_1, \ldots, X_n$ a n sample of independent and identically distributed random variables with p.d.f. f and c.d.f. F. We define the sequence of *record values* $\{T_n, n \geqslant 1\}$ and the *record times* R_k, $k \geqslant 1$, as follows [70]:

$R_1 = 1$,

$R_k = \min\{i : i > R_{k-1}, X_i > X_{R_{k-1}}\}$, for $k \geqslant 1$, and

$T_k = X_{R_k}$, for $k \geqslant 1$.

The sequence $\{T_k, k \geqslant 1\}$ can be associated to a NHPP via the following result from Dwass [20]:

Suppose that the date of events is described as the record values generated by a collection of independent and identically distributed random variables with a

common distribution F. Let $N(t)$ denote the number of events in times [0,t]. Then $\{N(t), t \geqslant \}$ can be described by a NHPP with mean value function $\Lambda(t) = \log\left(1/(1 - F(t))\right)$, and intensity function $\lambda(t) = f(t)/(1 - F(t))$, where $f(t)$ is the p.d.f. at t, if it exists [70].

This approach is particularly interesting in the context of software reliability where a repair might introduce new potential bugs. Therefore, the mean value function is no longer bounded. Indeed, in the RVS model, $\lim_{t \to +\infty} \Lambda(t) = +\infty$. The models from this family are said to be NHPP-II [40]. When f is the exponential p.d.f., we have a homogeneous Poisson process. When $f(x) = \alpha\beta^{\alpha}/(\beta + x)^{\alpha+1}$, a Pareto p.d.f., we have the Musa–Okumoto process. When $f(x) = \alpha\beta t^{\beta-1} e^{-\alpha t^{\beta}}$, a Weibull p.d.f., we have the PLP.

Thus, a large panel of intensity and process can be introduced providing model with a great flexibility.

For example, Vicini et al. [75] considered the generalized Gamma distribution leading to the following expression of the intensity:

$$\lambda(t) = \frac{1}{\Gamma(k)} \theta \beta^{k} \alpha t^{\alpha k - 1} \exp\left\{ - \beta t^{\alpha} \right\}.$$

Another example of intensity with high flexibility is given by Ramirez Cid et al. [63] who considered a p.d.f. from the *exponentiated Weibull* family [53] and studied the NHPP with an intensity function of the form:

$$\lambda(t) = \frac{\alpha\theta\left[1 - \exp\left(- (t/\sigma)^{\alpha}\right)\right]^{\theta-1} \exp\left(- (t/\sigma)^{\alpha}\right)(t/\sigma)^{\alpha-1}}{\sigma\left(1 - \left[1 - \exp\left(- (t/\sigma)^{\alpha}\right)\right]^{\theta}\right)},$$

which they named the *exponentiated Weibull intensity*.

If $\alpha \geqslant 1$ and $\theta \geqslant 1/\alpha$, $\lambda(t)$ is monotone increasing.
If $\alpha \leqslant 1$ and $\theta \leqslant 1/\alpha$, $\lambda(t)$ is monotone decreasing.
If $\alpha > 1$ and $\theta < 1/\alpha$, $\lambda(t)$ has a bathtub form ($0 < \theta < 1$).
If $\alpha < 1$ and $\sigma > 1/\alpha$, $\lambda(t)$ is unimodal.

The exponentiated-Weibull intensity has the advantage to cover many situations of monotonicity in particular it could be suitable for bathtub form. Bar-Lev et al. [2] developed a systematic method to build intensity function that also has this property. Their technique called *operator-based intensity* allows the construction of huge classes of non-monotonic intensity functions (convex or concave) for nonhomogeneous Poisson process, all of which convenient to modeling bath curve data.

More recently Bar-Lev and van der Duyn Schouten [3] studied in more detail the subclass of intensity generated by the operator-based intensity for which the base function is the intensity function of the power law. This special class is named *exponential power law process*.

Yang and Kuo [77] considered the superposition of NHPP that provides more flexibility on the rate of occurrence of failures. For example, the intensity of a process obtained by superposition a Musa–Okumoto process and a PLP has three possible types of shapes: increasing, decreasing, and bathcurve [29]. Yang and Kuo made Bayesian inference for this case using Markov Chain Monte Carlo (MCMC).

Another approach to generate flexible intensities is suggested by Ryan [62]. The basic idea is to "switch" from an intensity to another as t increases. For example, one can consider intensity of the form:

$$\lambda(t) = \big[1 - G\big((t-\omega)/\sigma\big)\big]\lambda_{PLP}(t) + G\big((t-\omega)/\sigma\big)\mu,$$

where $\lambda_{PLP}(t)$ is the intensity of a power law process (see Table 1), G is an arbitrary c.d.f., and ω, σ, μ parameters to be estimated.

An important family of intensity was introduced by Hawkes [26] defining self-exciting point processes (SEPP). A SEPP is a stochastic process such that the rate of failures at time t is not only depending on t but also on the number of failures $N(t^-)$ that occurs before t [71]. Thus the intensity is itself a stochastic process since it depends on the process $\{N(t), t \geqslant 0\}$. It is called the *intensity process*. Thus SEPP belongs to the family of doubly stochastic Poisson processes as introduced by Cox in 1955 [11]. With SEPP, the numbers of events in disjoint intervals are no longer independent. An example of SEPP is the classical birth and death process [36]. The intensity of a birth and death process is defined as a Markov process such that:

$$Pr\big(N(t+h) = j \mid N(t) = i\big) = \begin{cases} \lambda_i\, h + o(h), & j = i+1, \\ 1 - (\lambda_i + \mu_i)\, h + o(h), & j = i, \\ \mu_i\, h + o(h), & j = i-1, \\ o(h), & \text{otherwise}, \end{cases} \tag{3}$$

with $i = 0, 1, 2, \ldots$, $\lambda_i \geqslant 0$, $\mu_i \geqslant 0$ and $P\big(N(0) = n_0\big) = 1$, $n_0 \geqslant 0$. λ_i (the birth rate) and μ_i (the death rate) depend on i. When $\mu_i = 0,\ \forall i$, the process is a pure birth process. A classical choice for the birth rate is $\lambda_i = i\lambda$ (Yule's process). When $\lambda_i = 0$, we have a pure death process that moves from an initial state n_0 through state $n_0 - 1, n_0 - 2, \ldots, 2, 1$ until 0 (extinction). A classical choice for the death intensity is $\mu_i = (N - i)\mu$ to describe the extinction of a population where each individual has a probability μ to die. In the context of software reliability, the death process is underlying the Jelinski–Moranda model. This model assumes that N bugs are present in the software at the initial time. Each time a failure occurred, the bug is fixed without delay leading to a reliability growth. When all the bugs have been fixed, the intensity is zero.

Many stochastic processes can be interpreted as SEPP. Singpurwalla and Wilson [70] pointed out that *almost all of the proposed models for software reliability are special cases of the SEPP*. Chen et al. [10] used SEPP to unify software reliability models.

Table 2 Some examples of response functions

Response function	$g(t)$
Lomnitz formula	$\alpha e^{-\beta t},\ \alpha < \beta$
Omori formula	$K/(t+c)^p$
Laguerre type polynomial	$\sum_{k=0}^{m} a_k t^k e^{-bt}.$

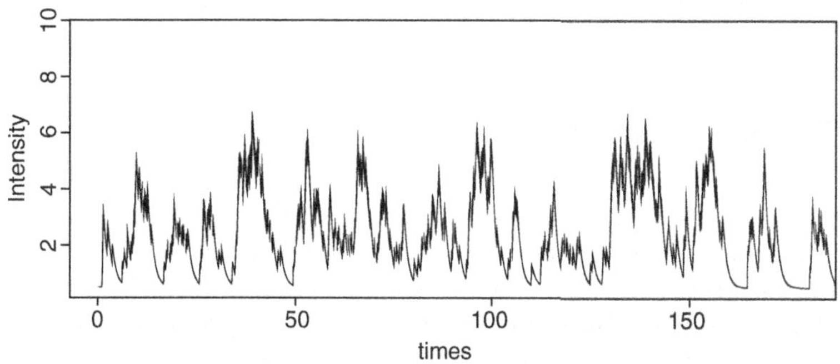

Fig. 1 Intensity of a SEPP for a Lomnitz response function with $\mu = 0.5$, $\alpha = 4$, and $\beta = 5$

In a seminal paper, Hawkes [26] considered the general following expression for the intensity:

$$\lambda(t) = \mu + \int_{-\infty}^{t} g(t-s)dN(s). \tag{4}$$

Before the first jump, the process behaves like a HPP and then each jump generates a modification of the rate of events. The function g is called the *response function* that has many possible forms. Table 2 displays some examples.

Let us consider an example of SEPP. Suppose that we observe a sample $t_1, \ldots, t_n$ of dates of events. The expression (4) is equivalent to $\lambda(t) = \mu$ before t_1 and

$$\lambda(t) = \mu + \sum_{j=1}^{i-1} g(t_j - t_{j-1}) + g(t - t_{i-1}), \text{ after } t_i.$$

Figure 1 displays the intensity of a SEPP for a Lomnitz response function with parameters $\mu = 0.5$, $\alpha = 4$, and $\beta = 5$.

To end this section on intensity, let us mention the Cox model [12] that suggests a relationship between the hazard rate and some covariates of the form:

$$\lambda\big(t; z)\big) = exp\big\{\boldsymbol{\beta}'\mathbf{z}(t)\big\}\lambda_0(t), \tag{5}$$

where $\mathbf{z}(t)$ is a p-dimensional vector describing the environment at time t; the component of $\mathbf{z}(t)$ could be constraints such as temperature, voltage, etc., $\boldsymbol{\beta}$ is a vector of unknown parameters to be estimated, and $\lambda_0(t)$ the baseline, the hazard rate, in the standard conditions. As we mentioned before, the intensity should not be confused with the failure rate (hazard rate) but a stochastic with an intensity of the form (5) worth to be investigated [13]. Merrick et al. [51] considered an intensity of such form with $\lambda_0(t) = \alpha\gamma t^{\gamma-1}$ to study the effect of a maintenance practice on railroad tracks. The components of the vector $\mathbf{z}$ are the amount of grinding that is applied on rail fatigue defects and some other physical characteristics of the rail.

4 Bayesian Inference

The basic principle for a Bayesian approach of statistical inference is to assume a prior distribution for the unknown parameter of the statistical model and to consider an update of this prior through the observation called the posterior distribution. The procedure relies on the Bayes formula. Let $f(x \mid \theta)$ be the distribution of X (in practice, $f(x \mid \theta)$ is often inaccurately called *the likelihood*) and $\pi(\theta)$, a prior distribution of θ. The posterior distribution of θ given x is

$$\pi(\theta \mid x) = f(x \mid \theta)\pi(\theta)/f(x),$$

where $f(x) = \int_{\Theta} f(x \mid \theta)\pi(\theta)d\theta$, the commonly named the *predictive distribution*.

Different strategies are available to define Bayes estimators. Very often, the expectation associated to the posterior distribution or its mode is retained. For an extended complete coverage of Bayesian analysis, the book of Berger [4] is a reference book. In order to develop Bayesian techniques for inference on stochastic process, we need to express the likelihood associated with the observation of this latter. Then choices for the prior distribution are to be made. Different expressions for the likelihood are obtained depending on the form of the observation. Roughly speaking, the observation is usually a total number of events accompanied by a sample of dates. We have remarked previously that many processes can be interpreted as SEPP. Therefore, we choose to write the likelihood for a SEPP with an intensity function denoted $\lambda(t, \mathscr{H}_t)$ to be general.

Let us consider $\{t_1, t_2, \ldots, t_{N(C)}\}$ a sequence of dates in a time window $[0, C]$. A general expression for the likelihood [16] can be obtained as

$$L\big(\theta \mid N(C)\big) = \prod_{i=1}^{N(C)} \lambda(t_i, \mathscr{H}_{t_i}; \theta) \exp\left\{-\int_0^C \lambda(s, \mathscr{H}_s; \theta)ds\right\}, \tag{6}$$

and the log-likelihood is

$$\log L(\theta \mid N(C)) = \left\{ \int_0^C \log\left(\lambda(t, \mathscr{H}_t; \theta)\right) dN(t) - \int_0^C \lambda(s, \mathscr{H}_s; \theta) ds \right\}. \quad (7)$$

In some situation, $N(C)$ is predetermined; it is a fixed number n that is to say the observation stops after the n-th events. In this case, the likelihood is

$$\log L(\theta \mid N(C)) = \sum_{i=1}^{n} \log \lambda(t_i, \mathscr{H}_{t_i}; \theta) - \int_0^{t_n} \lambda(s, \mathscr{H}_s; \theta) ds. \quad (8)$$

Here the parameter of interest is θ that is an element of a subset Θ of $\mathbb{R}^q$. Let us recall that the intensity is itself a stochastic process. A nonparametric point of view can be adopted assuming a prior for the stochastic process $\{\lambda(t, \mathscr{H}_t), t \geq 0\}$ or the mean value function. Lo [46] proved that a gamma process is a conjugate prior for the Poisson process model. This approach leads to interesting theoretical development relying on measure theory.

The expression of the likelihood displayed in (6) is general. Every hypothesis of intensity will generate a particular form. Therefore, the choices of prior distribution for the parameters needed in order to perform a Bayesian inference for stochastic processes will depend on the nature of the stochastic process.

In the following, we review some classical stochastic process examples that are useful in the context of reliability.

5 Homogeneous Poisson Process

The parameter of interest for a HPP is the constant intensity λ. We have the following results:

- The expected number of failures at time t is proportional to λ: $\Lambda(t) = \lambda t$.
- The interarrivals have an exponential distribution with parameter λ (a HPP with intensity λ is a renewal with independent exponential interarrivals with parameter λ).
- The i-th failure date has a gamma distribution with parameters (i, λ).

Thus deriving a Bayesian approach for a HPP boils down to consider Bayesian inference for a Poisson distribution or an exponential or a gamma distribution depending on the observation considered (the numbers of events, times between failures, dates of failure). The literature on the topic is considerable. The Poisson distribution and the exponential distribution are classical basic examples used to illustrate the Bayesian paradigm. They are also interesting to investigate and illustrate the problem of prior parameters elicitation; examples and references are given in [32].

In the following section, we investigate some classical examples of nonhomogeneous Poisson process. We begin with the PLP.

6 The Power Law Process

For a HPP, the expected number of failures is a linear function: $\Lambda(t) = \lambda t$. A natural generalization is to consider a function of the form:

$$\Lambda(t) = \lambda t^{\beta}, \beta > 0.$$

In this case, we have a NHPP with intensity $\lambda\beta t^{\beta-1}$. This model is clearly more flexible than the HPP model and covers different possible evolutions for the expected number of failures (growth, decay). A stochastic process with such intensity function is called a *power law process* (PLP). Others denominations can be found in the literature: Duane process, Weibull process, etc. The PLP is very popular because of its mathematical tractability, and the literature on this process is extensive. Another common parametrization is

$$\lambda(t) = \frac{\beta}{\alpha^{\beta}} t^{\beta-1}, \alpha > 0, \beta > 0,$$

called *the Weibull intensity* [21].

The denomination Weibull process is misleading since some authors call *Weibull process*, the renewal process with Weibull independent interarrivals [72, 73]. For a PLP, only the time to the first failure has a Weibull distribution. The distribution of the time T_i to the i-th failure given the time t_{i-1} of the $(i-1)$-th failure is a left-truncated Weibull distribution with support $[t_{i-1}, +\infty[$. Suppose that we observe n events $t_1 < \ldots < t_n$ in a time window $[0, C]$. Taking into account the fact that no failure occurs between t_n and C, the writing of the likelihood is straightforward:

$$\begin{aligned} L(\alpha, \beta) &= f(t_1) f(t_2 \mid t_1) f(t_3 \mid t_2, t_1) \cdots f(t_n \mid t_{n-1} \cdots t_1) P\big(N(t_n, C) = 0\big) \\ &= \frac{\beta^n}{\alpha^{n\beta}} \prod_{i=1}^{n} t_i^{\beta-1} \exp\left\{-\left(\frac{C}{\alpha}\right)^{\beta}\right\}. \end{aligned} \tag{9}$$

The same expression can be obtained by applying (6).

We review in the following Bayesian approach for inference on the PLP.

Considering the parametrization $\lambda(t) = \lambda\beta t^{\beta-1}$ and assuming that the observation stops at t_n, Higgins and Tsokos [27] suggested what they refer to as a *quasi-Bayes* strategy to estimate the value of the intensity at the n-th failure date that is $\nu_n = \lambda\beta t_n^{\beta}$. They computed a pseudo-likelihood for ν_n as a parameter, considered a gamma prior distribution for ν_n, and obtained the quasi-Bayes posterior mean as a Bayesian estimate of ν_n. They compared maximum likelihood estimates and quasi-Bayes estimates through simulations that demonstrate results quite favorable to the quasi-Bayes estimates.

Kyparisis and Singpurwalla [41] analyzed both interval and event truncation data by employing informative priors on α and β and derived prediction distributions of future jumps and the number of jumps in some future time interval. Their predictive and posterior distributions generally require complicated numerical computations.

Assuming a sample $t_1, \ldots, t_n$, successive occurrence times of failures from a PLP process, Guida et al. [25] proposed Bayes estimators considering different types of priors. They considered: **1.** a non-informative prior for the two parameters, **2.** a combination of informative and non-informative priors, and **3.** an informative case. For illustration, the obtained estimators are displayed hereafter. They do not have closed-form expression and require numerical computations:

1. Non-informative prior
   $\pi(\alpha, \beta) \propto \dfrac{1}{\alpha\beta}$
   Bayes estimators
   $$\widehat{\beta} = \frac{1}{n-1}\sum_{i=1}^{n} \log(t_n/t_i)$$
   $$\widehat{\alpha} = \frac{t_n z^{n-1}}{\Gamma(n)\Gamma(n-1)} \int_0^{+\infty} \beta^{n-2} w^{\beta} \Gamma(n - 1/\beta) d\beta$$
2. Informative/non-informative
   $\pi(\beta) \propto \mathscr{U}[\beta_1, \beta_2]$
   $\pi(\alpha) \propto \dfrac{1}{\alpha}, \ \alpha > 0$
   Bayes estimators
   $$\widehat{\beta} = \frac{I(\beta_1, \beta_2; n)}{I(\beta_1, \beta_2; n-1)}$$
   $$\tilde{\alpha} = \frac{t_n}{\Gamma(n)} \frac{I(\beta_1, \beta_2; n)}{I(\beta_1, \beta_2; n-1)},$$
   where $I(\beta_1, \beta_2; k) = \displaystyle\int_{\beta_1}^{\beta_2} \beta^k w^{\beta} d\beta.$
3. Informative
   $\pi(\alpha \mid \beta) = \beta b^a C^{\beta} \alpha^{-\beta-1} \exp\big[-b(C/\alpha)^{\beta}\big]/\Gamma(a)$
   $\pi(\beta) \propto \mathscr{U}[\beta_1, \beta_2]$
   Bayes estimators
   $$\widehat{\beta} = \frac{I_2(\beta_1, \beta_2; n+1)}{I_2(\beta_1, \beta_2; n)}$$
   with $I_2(\beta_1, \beta_2; k) = \displaystyle\int_{\beta_1}^{\beta_2} \beta^k w_C^{\beta}\big[(t_n/C)^{\beta} + b\big]^{-n-a} d\beta$
   $$\widehat{\alpha} = \frac{C}{\Gamma(n+a)} \frac{I_3(\beta_1, \beta_2; n)}{I_2(\beta_1, \beta_2; n)}$$
   with $I_3(\beta_1, \beta_2; k) = \displaystyle\int_{\beta_1}^{\beta_2} \beta^n w_C^{\beta}\big[(t_n/c)^{\beta} + b\big]^{-n-a+1/\beta} \Gamma(n + a - 1/\beta) d\beta$

Calabria et al. [6] derived predictive distributions for future failure times using both informative and non-informative priors and noted the numerical equivalence with classical methods when non-informative priors are used. The above three references usually assume that the prior distributions on α and β are independent.

Alternatively, they consider independent priors on α and the mean value function $\Lambda(t)$, with t fixed. Both scenarios can be handled in the same manner and result in the same type of posterior inference on α and β in contrast to the frequency approach in which each case must be treated separately and different types of results are obtained. Yu et al. [78] developed Bayesian techniques for predictive inference on the PLP. Bar-Lev et al. [1] considered a non-informative prior of the form $(\alpha\beta^{\nu})^{-1}$. They expressed the posterior distributions and present techniques for making prediction on the number of failures in times intervals and prediction on future failure times. From the same form of non-informative prior, Sen [67] showed that the posterior inference of current intensity yields closed-form results. He considered various loss functions to calculate the Bayes estimators of $\lambda(t)$. The expressions have the form of the MLE times a weight and can be seen as generalization of some classical frequentist estimators.

An important issue is the elicitation of the hyperparameters, that is to say the determination of the prior parameter values. De Oliveira et al. [17] proposed a reparametrization of the likelihood considering $\eta = (C/\alpha)^{\beta}$ in (9). The parametrization has the advantage to facilitate the prior elicitation since the parameters have a simple operational interpretation. Indeed, η is the expected number of failures and β is the elasticity of this number.

Huang and Bier [30], among others [9, 17, 18], developed conjugate prior distribution for the parameters of the PLP.

Relying on [30], Do and Gouno [18] defined the Huang–Bier (H–B) distribution as a natural conjugate prior distribution. It is a bivariate distribution with 4 parameters.

Definition 1 A bivariate r.v. $(X, Y) \in \mathbb{R}^+ \times \mathbb{R}^+$ has a Huang–Bier distribution with parameters (a, b, c, d) where $a, b, c, d > 0$ and such that $c < d^a$, denoted $(X, Y) \sim HB(a, b, c, d)$, if it has a p.d.f. of the form:

$$f_{X,Y}(x, y) = K\ (xy)^{a-1} c^y \exp\{-bd^y x\}, \tag{10}$$

where $K = [b \log(d^a/c)]^a / \Gamma(a)^2$.

Figures 2, 3, and 4 display the density and contour plots for Huang–Bier distribution with different parameter values.

The following theorem provides the conditional distribution of X.

Theorem 1 *Let $(X, Y) \sim HB(a, b, c, d)$. Then:*

(i) Y has a gamma distribution with parameters $\Big(a, log(d^a/c)\Big)$.
(ii) X given $Y = y$ has a gamma distribution with parameters (a, bd^y).

This theorem allows to compute the expectation of X:

$$E(X) = \frac{a}{b}\left[\frac{\log(d^a/c)}{\log(d^{a+1}/c)}\right]^a, \tag{11}$$

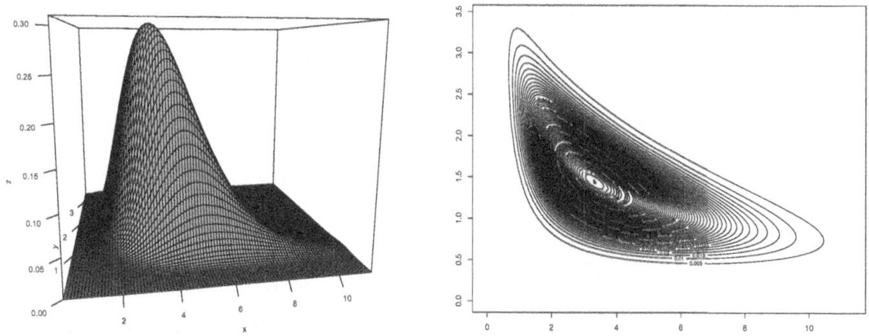

Fig. 2 Density plot and contour plot of the HB(10, 1, 2, 1, 10)

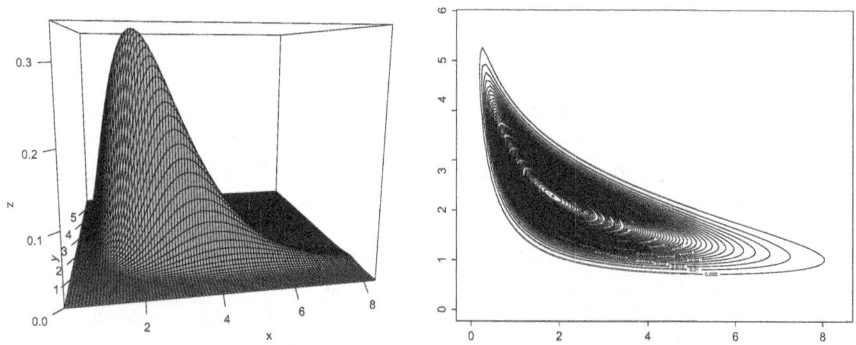

Fig. 3 Density plot and contour plot of the HB(10, 10, 2, 1, 10)

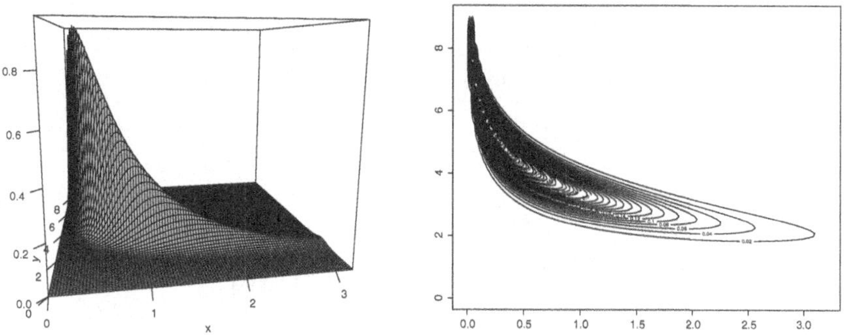

Fig. 4 Density plot and contour plot of the HB(10, 100, 2, 1, 10)

and the expectation of Y:

$$E(Y) = \frac{a}{\log(d^a/c)}. \tag{12}$$

The variances are

$$Var(X) = \frac{a}{b^2}\left[\frac{\log(d^a/c)}{\log(d^{a+1}/c)}\right]^a \text{ and } Var(Y) = \frac{a}{\left[\log(d^a/c)\right]^2}.$$

It is interesting to remark that when $d = 1$, X and Y are independent and have gamma distributions.

We have the following theorem:

Theorem 2 *Let* $(X, Y) \sim H - B(a, b, c, 1)$. *Then* X *and* Y *are independent,* X *has a gamma distribution with parameters* (a, b), *and* Y *has a gamma distribution with parameters* $(a, \log(1/c))$.

Thus when $d = 1$, the expectations and the variances are easily obtained.

$E(X) = a/b$, $Var(X) = a/b^2$, $E(Y) = a/\log(1/c)$, and $Var(Y) = a/[\log(1/c)]^2$. The following theorem claims that the HB distribution is a natural conjugate prior for the PLP Bayesian inference.

Theorem 3 *Let* $\mathbf{t} = (t_1, \ldots, t_n)$ *be the jump dates of a PLP with intensity* $\lambda\beta t^{\beta-1}$. *Then a Huang–Bier distribution with parameters* (a, b, c, t_n) *is a natural conjugate prior, and the posterior distribution is a Huang–Bier distribution with parameters* $(n + a, 1 + b, c\prod_{i=1}^{n} t_i, t_n)$.

Assuming a quadratic loss, the Bayes estimators are the expectation of the posterior distributions. Therefore, from (11) and (12), we have

$$\widehat{\beta} = \frac{n+a}{\log\left[t_n^{a+n}/(c\prod_{i=1}^{n} t_i)\right]} \tag{13}$$

and

$$\widehat{\lambda} = \frac{n+a}{1+b}\left[\frac{\log\left[t_n^{a+n}/(c\prod_{i=1}^{n} t_i)\right]}{\log\left[t_n^{a+n+1}/(c\prod_{i=1}^{n} t_i)\right]}\right]^{n+a}. \tag{14}$$

7 Software Reliability Models

Software reliability is a domain where stochastic processes play a central role. Many models suggested in this domain have an inherent Bayesian flavor. Soyer [74] gave an overview of the state of art in software reliability. The book of Gaudoin and Ledoux [22] and the book of Singpurwalla and Wilson [70] are major contributions on the topic that give a complete framework to handle problems involved in the domain. In this section, we review some traditional models and their Bayesian analysis.

7.1 Jelinski–Moranda Model

The famous Jelinski–Moranda model (J–M model) is an application of the classical extinction processes well known in population studies and in biology. Suppose a population of size n, and consider the process $\{N(t), t \geqslant 0\}$, and the number of remaining individuals in the population ($N(0) = n$). A jump of this process is interpreted as a death. $\{N(t), t \geqslant 0\}$ can be interpreted as a Markov process whose state space is $0, 1, \ldots, n$ and for which:

i. $P\big(N(t+h) = j-1 \mid N(t) = j\big) = \lambda_j h + o(h), i = 1, \ldots, n.$
ii. $P\big(N(t+h) = j \mid N(t) = j\big) = 1 - \lambda_j h + o(h), i = 1, \ldots, n.$
iii. $P\big(N(t+h) > j \mid N(t) = j\big) = 0, j = 0, 1, \ldots, n.$

The transposition to software reliability is straightforward by assuming that $N(0) = n$ bugs are contained in a given code at the initial time; each time a failure occurs a bug is detected and corrected without delay and the process $\{N(t), t \geqslant 0\}$ decreases of one unit. Axiom *i.* means that, at any time, the probability of more than one fault in an interval of length h with h close to 0 is proportional to a constant depending on the number of remaining bugs in the code. Jelinski and Moranda [33] suggested a dependency of the form:

$$\lambda_j = (n - j + 1)\phi.$$

This is the *Jelinski–Moranda model*. This model is a linear death process, and applying classical properties of this model family, we have that the distribution of $N(t)$ given $N(0) = n$ is a binomial distribution with parameters $\big(n, e^{-\phi t}\big)$. Let T be the time where all the faults have been removed from the software, and we have

$$P(T \leqslant t) = P\big(N(t) = 0 \mid N(0) = n\big) = \big(1 - e^{-\phi t}\big)^n.$$

Remark that the linear death process arises when considering n independent lifetimes associated to the bugs from an exponential distribution with parameter ϕ. Then it can be shown that the time elapsed between the $(j-1)$-th fault and the j-th fault, T_j, follows an exponential distribution with rate parameter $(n - j + 1)\phi$, i.e.,

$$P(T_i \geqslant t) = \exp\big\{-(n - j + 1)\phi t\big\}.$$

Therefore, the failure rate between bugs is a constant. Furthermore, a bug contributes the same amount ϕ to the rate, and when a bug is detected, it is perfectly repaired. The model is simple but relies on unrealistic assumptions. Alternative models have been proposed. If the model is considered as a SEPP, modifications can be done through the response function.

Indeed, the J-M model is a SEPP with a failure rate $\mu = n\phi$ before the first bug and with a response function $g(t) = -\phi$, that is to say each time a failure occurs, the failure decreases of an amount ϕ. After the detection of the n bugs contained in the program, the failure rate is 0. We have

$$\lambda(t) = n\phi - \sum_{i=1}^{N(t^-)} \phi = \big(n - N(t^-)\big)\phi.$$

Thus the failure rate is a linear function of the remaining bugs in the software. In this case, the response function is a constant and does not depend neither on t nor on the number of failures occurred previously. This model does not take into account the uncertainty in the removal of a bug.

Moranda [52] suggested a model where the failure rate is still constant between failures but decreasing geometrically:

$$\lambda(t) = \rho^{N(t^-)}\phi,\ 0 < \rho < 1.$$

This model can be interpreted as a SEPP where the response function depends on the number of failures and is defined as

$$g(t) = -\rho^{N[(t+a)^-]}(1-\rho)\phi\ \mathbb{1}_{[a,+\infty[}(t),\ a \in \mathbb{R}.$$

Starting with a rate ϕ, the occurrence of the i-th failure results in a decrease of $\rho^{i-1}(1-\rho)\phi$ of the failure rate.

There are two unknown parameters in the J-M model: n and ϕ. Meinhold and Singpurwalla [50] considered two choices of prior distributions. A first choice is: n has a Poisson distribution with a given parameter and ϕ is degenerated at a known quantity. The second choice is: n has a Poisson distribution with a given parameter and ϕ has a gamma distribution. In both case they compute the posterior distributions. Kuo and Yang [39] developed the previous results considering a hierarchical model and using Gibbs and Metropolis algorithms to deal with computations issues.

A generalization of the J-M model is suggested by Washburn [76] who considers a negative binomial prior distribution for the number of faults remaining with a gamma prior for ϕ. Jewell [34] calculated the predictive distribution of not detected error at the end of the software testing.

To override the hypothesis of perfect repairs inherent in the J-M model, Goel and Okumoto [23] suggested an *imperfect debugging model* introducing a proportion p

such that after i bugs detected, a proportion $p \times i$ of the failures have been perfectly repaired. The model becomes:

$$\lambda(t) = \big(n - pN(t^-)\big)\varphi(t).$$

Schick and Wolverton [68] considered the model where $\varphi(t) = \phi t$.

Remark that as a death process is considered to model the evolution of the number of bugs in the software, a birth and death process might be an interesting model to characterize the fact that new bugs can be introduced in the program. In the definition of the birth and death process (3), the rate of death $\lambda(t)$ will be the rate of occurrences of failures due to bugs and the rate of birth $\mu(t)$ will be the rate of news bugs introduced in the software. Dauxois [15] investigated the Bayesian analysis of this process in a general context.

7.2 *Littlewood–Verrall Model*

Littlewood [44] reconsidered the J–M model assuming that each failure does not have the same contribution to the intensity. He turns the parameter ϕ from the J-M model into a parameter ϕ_i, a failure rate associated to the failure i that is considered to be a r.v. from a gamma distribution. Littlewood and Verrall [45] extended the previous model by assuming the following:

1. The interarrival times $t_1, \ldots, t_n$ are conditionally independent, and t_i given λ_i has an exponential distribution with parameter Λ_i:

$$f(t_i \mid \Lambda_i) = \Lambda_i \exp\big\{ - \Lambda_i t_i \big\}.$$

2. The Λ_i's are independent and have a gamma distribution with parameter $(\alpha, \psi(i))$

$$g(\Lambda_i \mid \alpha, \psi(i)) = \frac{\psi^\alpha}{\Gamma(\alpha)} \Lambda_i^{\psi(i)-1} \exp\big\{ - \psi(i)\Lambda_i \big\},$$

where ψ is a function from $\mathbb{N}$ to $\mathbb{R}$.

From these assumptions, the distribution of t_i can be deduced as a Pareto distribution with parameters $\big(\alpha, \Phi(i+1)\big)$.

The intensity of Littlewood–Verrall model (L–V model) is

$$\lambda(t) = \frac{\alpha}{\psi(N(t^- + 1) + t - T_{N(t^-)}}.$$

If the function ψ is chosen to be increasing, then the intensity is decreasing implying a "reliability growth." A classical choice for ψ is a linear function $\beta_0 + \beta_1 i$.

Littlewood [43] suggested the form $\beta_0 i + \beta_1 i^2$. Kuo and Yang [39] considered a polynomial: $\psi(i) = \beta_0 + \beta_1\, i + \beta_2\, i^2 + \cdots + \beta_k\, i^k$. For inference, Littlewood and Verrall proposed an hybrid approach. The parameter α is estimated via a Bayesian method, and a maximum likelihood method is used for the coefficients β_0 and β_1. Mazzuchi and Soyer [47] considered a hierarchical model and applied Lindley's approximation to compute the moment of the posterior distribution. Their work is extended by Kuo and Yang [39] to polynomial curves. They developed Gibbs sampling techniques to obtain the posterior moments. Langberg and Singpurwalla [42] suggested that adopting a Bayesian point of view on the J-M model enables a unification of many models in software reliability. They emphasized the link between J-M, L-V, Goël-Okumoto (G-O) models through adequate choices of prior distributions.

7.3 Goël–Okumoto Model

The Goël–Okumoto model (G–O model) [24] is characterized by an intensity of the form: $\alpha\beta e^{-\beta t}$. Applying (6), the likelihood is

$$L(\alpha, \beta) = \left(\prod_{i=1}^{n} \alpha\beta e^{-\beta t_i}\right) \exp\left\{ -\alpha(1 - e^{-\beta t})\right\}.$$

Kuo and Yang [39] assumed that α and β are independent, and consider gamma distributions as prior: $\alpha \sim \mathcal{G}(a, b)$ and $\beta \sim \mathcal{G}(c, d)$. Setting $N' = N - n$, they suggest the following Gibbs algorithm:

$$N' \mid \alpha, \beta \sim \mathcal{P}(\alpha e^{-\beta t_i})$$
$$\alpha \mid N', \beta \sim \mathcal{G}\big(a + n + N', b + 1\big)$$
$$\beta \mid N', \alpha \sim \mathcal{G}\big(c + n, d + tN' + \textstyle\sum_{i=1}^{n} t_i\big)$$

Assuming that n bugs have been detected by a time t, McDaid and Wilson [49] computed the joint distribution of (α, β) given $n, t_1, \ldots, t_n, t$ and described some elicitation strategies.

7.4 Musa-Okumoto Model

Musa and Okumoto [54] considered a NHPP where the expected number of failures at t has a logarithmic form leading to an intensity of the form:

$$\lambda(t) = \frac{\alpha\beta}{1 + \beta t}.$$

Campodónico and Singpurwalla [7, 8] performed the Bayesian analysis for this model introducing expert opinion in the construction of the prior distribution of (α, β). Hirata et al. [28] presented a unified MCMC algorithm based on the Metropolis–Hastings algorithm. Their algorithm can be applied to many software reliability models and is implemented as a Java-based tool. Okamura et al. [57, 58] investigated a variational Bayesian approach of inference for NHPP in software reliability model. This approach provides closed analytical forms for approximations of the posterior distributions that have almost the same accuracy than MCMC but are much lower in terms of computational complexity.

8 Self-Exciting Point Processes

As we mentioned before, many of the stochastic processes described previously can be interpreted as SEPPs. The form of SEPPs intensity allows to cover many situations encountered in "real life." Chen and Singpurwalla [10] proposed a unification of software reliability models via self-exciting point processes.

Developing a Bayesian methodology to analyze the time evolution of earthquake activity, Peruggia and Santner [59] considered the epidemic-type model [56]

$$\lambda^*(t) = \mu + \sum_{t_i < t} e^{\omega(m_i - M_r)} \beta e^{-\alpha(t-t_i)},$$

where t_i, $i = 1, \ldots, n$, are the occurrence times, m_i, $i = 1, \ldots, n$, are the magnitude of events, and M_r is a structural parameter given by experts, a threshold (prespecified).

The parameters (ω, α, β) characterize the aftershock and are the parameters to be estimated with μ that characterize the main shock.

Peruggia and Santner [59] chose gamma distributions for prior on the parameters assuming independence except for ω for which they considered a gamma distribution given α, β. They developed Markov Chain Monte Carlo algorithms to compute the posterior distributions.

Another example of Bayesian strategy for SEPP is presented by Ruggeri and Soyer [66] in the context of software reliability. They introduced a SEPP model where the intensity increases each time a bug is attempted to be fixed. The maintenance introduces new bugs and so on. The repair is imperfect. They suggested the following expression for the intensity:

$$\lambda^*(t) = \mu(t) + \sum_{j=1}^{N(t^-)} Z_j \, g_j(t - t_j).$$

Occurrences of bugs are basically described as a power law process with intensity $\mu(t) = M\beta t^{\beta-1}$. Z_j is a Bernoulli r.v. with parameter p_j.

$Z_j = 1$ if the repair of the j-th failure (bug) introduced a new bug and 0 otherwise. The response function $g_j(t)$ is supposed to be positive.

Suppose we observe a sequence of jumps $t_1, \ldots, t_n$, denoted $\mathbf{t}$, in a time window $[0, C]$ and $Z_1, \ldots, Z_n$, denoted $\mathbf{Z}$. The distribution of the observation is

$$
\begin{aligned}
f(\mathbf{t} \mid \mathbf{Z}; M, \alpha, \beta) &= \prod_{i=1}^{n} \Big[\mu(t_i) + \sum_{j=1}^{i-1} Z_j g(t_i - t_j)\Big] \\
&\quad \times \exp\Big\{ - \int_0^C \mu(t)dt - \sum_{j=1}^{N(t^-)} Z_j \int_O^{C-t_j} g_j(t)dt \Big\} \\
&= M^n \beta^n \prod_{i=1}^{n} A_i(\beta, \mathbf{Z}_{i-1})\, exp\Big\{ - M\ B(\beta, \mathbf{Z}_n)\Big\},
\end{aligned}
$$

where $\mathbf{Z}_i = (Z_1, \ldots, Z_i)$, $A_i(\beta, \mathbf{Z}_{i-1}) = t_i^{\beta-1} + \sum_{j=1}^{i-1} Z_j(t_i - t_j)$

and $B(\beta, \mathbf{Z}_n) = C^\beta + \sum_{j=1}^{N(C^-)} Z_j(C - t_j)^\beta$.

Ruggeri and Soyer [66] proposed the following choices for the prior distributions:

$M \sim \mathscr{G}(\alpha, \delta)$.
$\beta \sim \mathscr{G}(\rho, \lambda)$.
$p_j \sim \mathscr{B}eta(\mu_j, \sigma_j)$, $j = 1, \ldots, n$.

And the following conditional posterior distributions are obtained:

- $M \mid \beta, \mathbf{Z}, \mathbf{p} \sim \mathscr{G}\big(\alpha + n, \delta + B(\beta, \mathbf{Z})\big)$.
- $\beta \mid M, \mathbf{Z}, \mathbf{p} \propto \beta^{\rho+n} \prod_{i=1}^{n} A_i(\beta, \mathbf{Z}_{i-1})\, e^{-MB(\beta,\mathbf{Z})-\lambda\beta}$.
- $p_j \mid M, \beta, \mathbf{Z}, p_{-j} \sim \mathscr{B}eta\big(\mu_j + Z_j, \sigma_j + (1 - Z_j)\big)$, where $p_{-j} = (p_1, \ldots, p_j, p_{j+1}, \ldots, p_n)$.

MCMC methods are used to make inference on the parameters.

9 Conclusion

This chapter has provided an overview of the Bayesian modeling of stochastic processes in the context of reliability. It shows the diversity of the techniques combining issues in modeling and computation and attempts to be a guideline, not exactly a comprehensive state of art, to help the reader who may wish to go further.

We have described some principles of the methods for Bayesian parameter estimation. The MCMC techniques allow to avoid the untractability computational issues that usually arise from the Bayesian paradigm. The use of stochastic process is everywhere in reliability, from accelerated life test (ALT) to degradation model. The Bayesian approach offers a great flexibility to assess model in each of these various topics.

References

1. Bar-Lev, S.K., Lavi, I., Reiser, B.: Bayesian inference for the power law process. Ann. Inst. Stat. Math. **44**(4), 623–639 (1992)
2. Bar-Lev, S.K., Bshouty, D., van der Duyn Schouten, F.A.: Operator-based intensity functions for the nonhomogeneous Poisson process. Math. Methods Statist. **25**(2), 79–98 (2016)
3. Bar-Lev, S.K., van der Duyn Schouten, F.A.: The exponential Power-Law Process for the nonhomogeneous Poisson process and bathtub data. Int. J. Reliab. Qual. Saf. Eng. **27**(04), 2050011 (2020)
4. Berger, J.: Statistical decision theory and Bayesian analysis. Springer Series in Statistics (2010)
5. Broemeling, L.D.: Bayesian Inference of Stochastic Processes. CRC Press, Boca Raton (2018)
6. Calabria, R., Guida, M., Pulcini, G.: Bayesian estimation of prediction intervals for a power law process. Commun. Stat. Theory Methods **19**, 3023–3035 (1990)
7. Campodónico, S., Singpurwalla, N.D.: A Bayesian analysis of the logarithmic-Poisson execution time model based on expert opinion and failure data. IEEE Trans. Softw. Eng. **20**(9), 677–683 (1994)
8. Campodónico, S., Singpurwalla, N.D.: Inference and predictions from Poisson point processes incorporating expert knowledge. J. Am. Stat. Assoc. **90**(429), 220–226 (1995)
9. Chen, Z.: Empirical Bayes analysis on the power law process with natural conjugate priors. J. Data Sci. **8**, 139–149 (2010)
10. Chen, Y., Singpurwalla, N.D.: Unification of software reliability models by self-exciting point processes. Adv. Appl. Probab. **29**, 337–352 (1997)
11. Cox, D.R.: Some statistical methods connected with series of events. J. R. Stat. Soc. B, **17**, 129–164 (1955)
12. Cox, D.R.: Regression models and life-tables. J. R. Stat. Soc. B **34**, 187–2020 (1972)
13. Cox D.R.: The statistical analysis of dependencies in point processes. In Lewis, P.A.W. (ed.) Stochastic Point Processes, pp. 55–56, Wiley, Hoboken (1972)
14. Cox, D.R., Lewis, P.A.: Statistical Analysis of Series of Events. Methuen, London (1966)
15. Dauxois, J.-Y.: Bayesian inference for linear growth birth and death processes. J. Stat. Plan. Infer. **121**, 1–19 (2004)
16. Daley, D.J., Vere Jones, D.: An Introduction to the Theory of Point Processes. Springer, Berlin (2003)
17. de Oliveira, M.D., Colosimo, E.A., Gilardoni, G.L.: Bayesian inference for power law process with application in repairable systems. J. Stat. Plan. Infer. **5**, 1151–1160 (2012)
18. Do, V.C., Gouno, E.: A conjugate prior for Bayesian analysis of the power-law process. In: Applied Mathematics in Engineering and Reliability, pp. 3–8. CRC Press, Balkema (2016)
19. Duane, J.T.: Learning curve approach to reliability monitoring. IEEE Trans. Aerosp. Electron. Syst. **2**, 563–566 (1964)
20. Dwass, M.: Extremal processes. Ann. Math. Stat. **35**, 1718–1725 (1964)
21. Finkelstein, J. M.: Confidence bounds on the parameters of the Weibull process. Technometrics **18**, 115–117 (1976)
22. Gaudoin, O., Ledoux, J.: ModṔelisation aléatoire en fiabilité des logiciels. Ed. Lavoisier (2007)

23. Goel, A.L., Okumoto, K.: An analysis of recurrent software failures on a real-time control system. In: Proceedings of ACM Conference, Washington, pp. 496–500 (1978)
24. Goel, A.L., Okumoto, K.: Time-dependent error detection rate model for software reliability and other performance measure. IEEE Trans. Reliab. **R-28**, 206–211 (1979)
25. Guida, M., Calabria, R., Pulcini, G.: Bayes inference for a non-homogeneous Poisson process with power intensity law. IEEE Trans. Reliab. **38**, 603–609 (1989)
26. Hawkes, A.G.: Spectra of some self-exciting and mutually exciting point processes. Biometrika **58**(1), 83–90 (1971)
27. Higgins, J.J., Tsokos, C.P.: A quasi-Bayes estimate of the failure intensity of a reliability-growth model. IEEE Trans. Reliab. **30**, 471–475 (1981)
28. Hirata, T., Okamura, H., Dohi, T.: A Bayesian inference tool for NHPP-based software reliability assessment. Fut. Gen. Inf. Technol. **5899**, 225–236 (2009)
29. Hjorth, U.: A reliability distribution with increasing, decreasing, constant, and bathtub-shaped failure rates. Technometrics **22**, 99–107 (1980)
30. Huang, Y.S., Bier, V.M.: A natural conjugate prior for the non-homogeneous Poisson process with a power law intensity function. Commun. Stat. Simul. Comput. **27**, 525–551 (1998)
31. Huang, Y.S., Bier, V.M.: A natural conjugate prior for the non-homogeneous Poisson process with an exponential law intensity. Commun. Stat. Theory Methods **25**, 1479–1509 (1999)
32. Insua, R.D., Ruggeri, F., Wiper, M.P.: Bayesian Analysis of Stochastic Process Models. Wiley, Hoboken (2012)
33. Jelinski, Z., Moranda, P.: Software reliability research. In: Freiburger, W. (ed.) Statistical Computer Performance Evaluation, pp. 465–484. Academic Press, New York (1972)
34. Jewell, W.S.: Bayesian extension to a basic model of software reliability. IEEE Trans. Softw. Eng. **11**, 1465–1471 (1985)
35. Kamranfar, H., Etminan, J., Chankandi, M.: Statistical inference for a repairable system subject to shocks: classical vs. Bayesian. J. Stat. Comput. Simul. **90**(1), 112–137 (2020)
36. Keiding, N.: Maximum likelihood estimation in the birth-and-death process. Ann. Stat. **3**(2), 363–372 (1975)
37. Kijima, M., Li, H., Shaked, M.: Stochastic processes in reliability. Handbook Stat. **19**, 471–510 (2001)
38. Kundu, S., Nayak, T.K., Bose, S.: Are nonhomogeneous Poisson process models preferable to general-order statistics models for software reliability estimation? In: Statistical Models and Methods for Biomedical and Technical Systems, pp. 137–152 (2008)
39. Kuo, L., Yang, T.Y.: Bayesian computation of software reliability. J. Comput. Graph. Stat. **4**(1), 65–82 (1995)
40. Kuo, L., Yang, T.Y.: Bayesian computation for nonhomogeneous Poisson processes in software reliability. J. Am. Stat. Assoc. **91**, 763–773 (1996)
41. Kyparisis, J., Singpurwalla, N.D.: Bayesian inference for the Weibull process with applications to assessing software reliability growth and predicting software failures. Comput. Sci. Stat. 57–64 (1985)
42. Langberg, N., Singpurwalla, N.D.: A unification of some software reliability models. SIAM J. Sci. Stat. Comput. **6**, 781–790 (1985)
43. Littlewood, B.: The Littlewood-Verrall model for software reliability compared with some rivals. J. Syst. Softw. **1**, 251–258 (1980)
44. Littlewood, B.: Stochastic reliability growth: a model for fault-removal in computer program and hardware designs. IEEE Trans. Reliab. **R-40**(4), 313–320 (1981)
45. Littlewood, D., Verrall, J.L.: A Bayesian reliability growth model for computer software. J. R. Stat. Soc.: Ser. C: Appl. Stat. **22**(3), 332–346 (1973)
46. Lo, A.Y.: Bayesian nonparametric statistical inference for Poisson processes. Zeitschrift für Wahrscheinlichkeitstheorie und Verwandte Gebiete **59**, 55–66 (1982)
47. Mazzuchi, T.A., Soyer, R.: A Bayes empirical-Bayes model for software reliability. IEEE Trans. Reliab. **37**(2), 248–254 (1988)

48. Mc Collin, C.: Intensity functions for nonhomogeneous Poisson processes. In: Ruggieri, F., Kenett, K., Faltin, F. (eds.) Encyclopedia of Statistics in Quality and Reliability, pp. 861–868. John Wiley & Sons, Hoboken (2007)
49. McDaid, K., Wilson, S.P.: Deciding how long to test software. J. R. Stat. Soc. Ser. D (Stat.) **50**(2), 117–134 (2001)
50. Meinhold, R.J., Singpurwalla, N.D.: Bayesian analysis of a commonly used model for describing software failures. Statistician **32**, 168–173 (1983)
51. Merrick, J.R., Soyer, R., Mazzuchi, T.A.: Are maintenance practices for railroad track effective? J. Am. Stat. Assoc. **100**(469), 17–25 (2005)
52. Moranda, P.B.: Prediction of software reliability and its applications. In: Proceedings of the Annual Reliability and Maintainability Symposium, Washington, pp. 327–332 (1975)
53. Mudholkar, G.S., Srivastava, D.K., Friemer, M.: The exponentiated-Weibull family: a reanalysis of the bus-motor failure data. Technometrics **37**, 436–445 (1995)
54. Musa, J.D., Okumoto, K.: A logarithmic Poisson execution time model for software reliability measurement. In: Proceedings of Seventh International Conference on Software Engineering, Orlando, pp. 230–238 (1984)
55. Nakagawa, T.: Stochastic processes with applications to reliability theory. In: Springer Series in Reliability Engineering. Springer, Berlin (2011)
56. Ogata, Y.: Statistical models for earthquake occurrences and residual analysis for point processes. Ann. Instit. Stat. Math. **83**, 9–27 (1988)
57. Okamura, H., Sakoh, T., Dohi, T.: Variational Bayesian approach for exponential software reliability model. In: Proceeding 10th IASTED International Conference on Software Engineering and Applications, pp. 82–87 (2006)
58. Okamura, H., Grottke, M., Dohi, T., Trivedi, K.S.: Variational Bayesian approach for interval estimation of NHPP-based software reliability models. In: Proceeding of the International Conference on Dependable Systems and Networks, pp. 698–707 (2007)
59. Peruggia, M., Santner, T.: Bayesian analysis of time evolution of earthquakes. J. Am. Stat. Assoc. **91**, 1209–1218 (1996)
60. Pievaloto, A., Ruggeri, F., Argiento, R.: Bayesian analysis and prediction of failures in underground trains. Qual. Reliab. Eng. Int. **19**, 327–336 (2003)
61. Raftery, A.E.: Inference and prediction for a general order statistic model with unknown population size. J. Am. Stat. Assoc. **82**(400), 1163–1158 (1987)
62. Ryan, K.J.: Some flexible families of intensities for non-homogeneous Poisson process models and their Bayes inference. Qual. Reliab. Eng. Int. **19**(2), 171–181 (2003)
63. Ramirez Cid, J.E., Achcar, J.A.: Bayesian inference for nonhomogeneous Poisson processes in software reliability models assuming nonmonotonic intensity functions. Comput. Stat. Data Anal. **32**, 147–159 (1999)
64. Ridgon, S.E., Basu, A.P.: Statistical Methods for the Reliability of Repairable Systems. John Wiley and Sons, Inc. New-York (2000)
65. Ruggeri, F., Sivaganesan, S.: On modeling change points in non-homogeneous Poisson processes. Stat. Infer. Stoch. Process **8**, 311–329 (2005)
66. Ruggeri, F., Soyer, R.: Advances in Bayesian software reliability modelling. In: Bedford, T., Quigley J., Walls L., Alkali, B., Daneshkhah, A., Hardman, G. (eds.) Advances in Mathematical Modeling for Reliability. IOS Press, Amsterdam, pp. 165–176 (2008)
67. Sen, A.: Bayesian estimation and prediction of the intensity of the power law process. J. Stat. Comput. Simul. **72**, 613–631 (2002)
68. Shick, G.J., Wolverton, R.W.: Assessment of software reliability. In: Proceedings in Operations Research, pp. 395–422. Physica-Verlag, Vienna (1978)
69. Singpurwalla, N.: Survival in dynamic environments. Stat. Sci. **1**, 86–103 (1995)
70. Singpurwalla, N., Wilson, S.P.: Statistical Method in Software Engineering, vol. 1, pp. 86–103. Springer, New York (1999)
71. Snyder, D.L., Miller, M.L.: Random Point Processes in Time and Space. Springer, Berlin (1991)

72. Soland, R.M.: Bayesian analysis of Weibull process with unknown scale and its application to acceptance sampling. IEEE Trans. Reliab. **17**(4), 84–90 (1968)
73. Soland, R.M.: Bayesian analysis of Weibull process with unknown scale and shape parameters. IEEE Trans. Reliab. **18**(4), 181–184 (1969)
74. Soyer, R.: Software reliability. Wiley Interdisciplinary Reviews: Computational Statistics, vol. 3, pp. 269–281 (2011)
75. Vicini, L., Hotta, L.K., Achcar J.A.: Non-homogeneous Poisson processes applied to count data: a Bayesian approach considering different prior distributions. J. Environ. Protect. **3**, 1336–1345 (2012)
76. Washburn, A: A sequential Bayesian generalization of the Jelinski–Moranda software reliability model. Nav. Res. Logist. **53**, 354–362 (2005)
77. Yang, T.A., Kuo, L.: Bayesian computation for the superposition of nonhomogeneous Poisson processes. Can. J. Stat. **27**(3), 547–556 (1999)
78. Yu, J.W., Tian, G.L., Tang, M.L.: Predictive analysis for nonhomogeneous Poisson processes with power law using Bayesian approach. Comput. Stat. Data Anal. **51**, 4254–4258 (2007)

Bayesian Analysis of a New Bivariate Wiener Degradation Process

Ancha Xu

Abstract Copula functions are often used to describe the dependence between two performance characteristics of a system. However, the reliability of the system has no analytic form when using copula method, and choosing a suitable copula function can be hard. In this chapter, we propose a new bivariate degradation model, which could describe the unit-to-unit variation and dependence simultaneously. The reliability functions of the system and the residual lifetime have analytic forms and are presented in this chapter. Statistical inference is conducted by data augmentation and Bayesian methods. Weak informative priors are considered, and Gibbs sampling method is utilized to draw sample for the evaluation of the unknown parameters. A simulated example is used for illustration purpose.

1 Introduction

Traditionally, accelerated life testing (ALT) was the main way to collect the failure data of a product, and the collected data was used to assess the reliability of the product. Many statistical models and methods of ALT have been widely used in practice and summarized for reference. See [15] for more details. However, as the products become more and more reliable, collecting failure data by ALT becomes harder. Under this situation, if a product has a quality characteristic or performance characteristic (PC) that degenerates with time, and the PC is related with the life of the product, then we could monitor the degradation of PC to assess the reliability of the product. Fortunately, most of the commercial products have at least one PC. For example, operating current is the PC of laser device [15], and light intensity is the PC of a light-emitting diode (LED) product [12]. In such a case, the failure threshold level will be specified in advance, and if the degradation of PC exceeds the threshold level, the product is considered to have failed. There are two main kinds of models

A. Xu (✉)
Department of Statistics, Zhejiang Gongshang University, Zhejiang, China
e-mail: xuancha2011@aliyun.com

Y. Lio et al. (eds.), *Bayesian Inference and Computation in Reliability and Survival Analysis*, Emerging Topics in Statistics and Biostatistics,
https://doi.org/10.1007/978-3-030-88658-5_7

for fitting the degradation data of the PC. The first one is the degradation path model, which was first proposed by Lu and Meeker [14]. The model is actually the mixed-effect model, taking the unit-to-unit variation of the products into consideration. For further details about this kind of models, see [1, 27, 38] and the references therein. The second kind of models is stochastic process. Three commonly used stochastic processes are Wiener process [12, 17, 21, 31, 37], gamma process [10, 13, 18], and inverse Gaussian process [23, 28, 34]. This chapter will not introduce these models in detail, and hence readers can refer [35] for more information.

All the above literature only considered the system with one PC. However, complex systems usually have two or multiple PCs. For example, heavy machine tools [22] have two performance indicators: positioning accuracy and output power. The rubidium consumption and the light intensity are the two PCs of a rubidium discharge lamp, and the lamp is considered to have failed if the degradation value of one of the PCs exceeds the specified threshold level. The literature on bivariate or multiple degradation paths are rare compared with those on one degradation path. Huang and Askin [6] considered an electronic device with two failure modes, one of which is a catastrophic failure and the other is a degradation failure, and they assumed that the two failure modes are independent. Bagdonavicius et al. [2] and [3] studied the problem of multiple failure modes with degradation data when the failure modes were also assumed to be independent. To the best of our knowledge, the study by Sari [26] was the first to consider the dependence among the multiple degradation paths, and the dependence of the degradation paths was described by a copula function. Pan and Balakrishnan [16] considered a system with two PCs, and the degradation process of each PC followed a stationary gamma process. Then, the reliability function of the system can be approximated by a bivariate Birnbaum–Saunders distribution and its marginal distributions. Using the copula method, bivariate degradation process models based on Wiener process, gamma process, and inverse Gaussian process are considered by [19, 20, 22, 30], and [29]. Although the copula method is commonly used to describe the dependence between two random variables, there are several drawbacks for modeling bivariate degradation process: (1) Copula functions are difficult to select. Usually, the authors choose several Archimedean copulas and use Akaike information criterion (AIC) to pick the best one. However, the reason for choosing these copula functions or Archimedean family is hard to justify, which still is an open question. (2) Copula method models dependency on the increments of the two assumed stochastic processes, which means that the correlation coefficient or Kendall's tau is constant for any time interval. This assumption may be a little strong and is hard to verify, because the means and variances of the increments are dependent on time. Jin and Matthews [9] proposed a bivariate Wiener process that models the dependence of increments of the two PCs by assuming that the diffusion parameters of the Wiener processes are correlated. However, the model also fails to describe the dynamic changes of the correlation coefficient. (3) The reliability function of the system usually has no analytic form using copula method. Recently, Xu et al. [33] proposed a bivariate Wiener degradation by assuming that the degradation of the two PCs is affected by a common frailty factor. However, their model is only suitable for the case that a common random factor affects the degradation of two PCs simultaneously. In this chapter, we propose a new bivariate Wiener degradation process for analyzing the degradation data of two PCs. The new model will include the model of [33] as a special case. Based on the new model, a dynamic correlation coefficient between two processes can be shown intuitively and the reliability function of the system has an analytic form. Besides, statistical inference based on the proposed model is very flexible.

This chapter is organized as follows. In Sect. 2, a new bivariate Wiener degradation process with time-scale transformation is introduced. We derive the correlation coefficient function between the bivariate Wiener process and the reliability function of the system. In Sect. 3, we propose data augmentation and Bayesian method to estimate the model parameters when the observed data are available. In Sect. 4, an artificial data is analyzed for illustration. Finally, we give a conclusion of this chapter.

2 Bivariate Degradation Model

2.1 Model

Assume that a system has two PCs and that the degradation process of the s-th PC is modeled as follows:

$$Y_s(t) = \alpha_s h_s(t, \beta_s) + \sigma_s B_s(h_s(t, \beta_s)),\ s = 1, 2, \tag{1}$$

where α_s and σ_s denote the drift parameter and the diffusion parameter, respectively, $h_s(t, \beta_s)$ is a non-decreasing function of time with $h_s(0, \beta_s) = 0$, and $B_s(t)$ is a standard Brownian motion. Thus, $Y_s(t)$ follows a Brownian motion with time-scale transformation. We assume that $B_1(t)$ and $B_2(t)$ are independent of each other. Due to some endogenous and exogenous factors, the products may have heterogeneities. To describe the unit-to-unit variation among the products, we assume that α_s is random, and

$$\alpha = (\alpha_1, \alpha_2)' \sim \boldsymbol{N}_2(\mu, \Sigma),\ \mu = \begin{pmatrix}\mu_{\alpha_1}\\ \mu_{\alpha_2}\end{pmatrix} \text{ and } \Sigma = \begin{pmatrix}\sigma_{\alpha_1}^2 & \rho\sigma_{\alpha_1}\sigma_{\alpha_2}\\ \rho\sigma_{\alpha_1}\sigma_{\alpha_2} & \sigma_{\alpha_2}^2\end{pmatrix}, \tag{2}$$

where $\boldsymbol{N}_2(\mu, \Sigma)$ denotes the bivariate normal distribution with mean μ and variance–covariance matrix Σ. We can rewrite the model (1) as follows:

$$Y_s(t) = \gamma_s \mu_{\alpha_s} h_s(t, \beta_s) + \sigma_s B_s(h_s(t, \beta_s)),\ s = 1, 2,$$

where $(\gamma_1, \gamma_2)' \sim \boldsymbol{N}_2((1,1)', \Sigma_\gamma)$, and $\Sigma_\gamma = \begin{pmatrix} \sigma_{\alpha_1}^2/\mu_{\alpha_1}^2 & \rho\sigma_{\alpha_1}\sigma_{\alpha_2}/(\mu_{\alpha_1}\mu_{\alpha_2}) \\ \rho\sigma_{\alpha_1}\sigma_{\alpha_2}/(\mu_{\alpha_1}\mu_{\alpha_2}) & \sigma_{\alpha_2}^2/\mu_{\alpha_2}^2 \end{pmatrix}$. If $\sigma_{\alpha_1}^2/\mu_{\alpha_1}^2 = \sigma_{\alpha_2}^2/\mu_{\alpha_2}^2$ and $\rho = 1$, then the model is reduced to the model of [33].

Assume that conditions on α, $Y_1(t)$, and $Y_2(t)$ are independent. Thus, the joint probability density function (pdf) of $(Y_1(t), Y_2(t), \alpha)$ is

$$
\begin{aligned}
& f(Y_1(t), Y_2(t), \alpha) \\
& = (2\pi)^{-1}|\Sigma|^{-\frac{1}{2}} \exp\left\{ -\frac{(\alpha-\mu)'\Sigma^{-1}(\alpha-\mu)}{2} \right\} \\
& \times (2\pi)^{-1}\left(\sqrt{\sigma_1^2 h_1(t,\beta_1)\sigma_2^2 h_2(t,\beta_2)}\right)^{-1} \\
& \times \exp\left\{ -\frac{(y_1(t)/h_1(t,\beta_1)-\alpha_1)^2}{2\sigma_1^2/h_1(t,\beta_1)} - \frac{(y_2(t)/h_2(t,\beta_2)-\alpha_2)^2}{2\sigma_2^2/h_2(t,\beta_2)} \right\}.
\end{aligned}
$$

After integrating out α, the joint pdf of $Y_1(t)$ and $Y_2(t)$ is a bivariate normal distribution and

$$
\left(\frac{Y_1(t)}{h_1(t,\beta_1)}, \frac{Y_2(t)}{h_2(t,\beta_2)}\right)' \sim \boldsymbol{N}_2\left(\begin{pmatrix}\mu_{\alpha_1} \\ \mu_{\alpha_2}\end{pmatrix}, \Sigma + \begin{pmatrix} \sigma_1^2/h_1(t,\beta_1) & 0 \\ 0 & \sigma_2^2/h_2(t,\beta_2)\end{pmatrix}\right).
$$

Let

$$
H = \begin{pmatrix} h_1(t,\beta_1) & 0 \\ 0 & h_2(t,\beta_2)\end{pmatrix}, \quad \mu_H = \begin{pmatrix}\mu_{\alpha_1} h_1(t,\beta_1) \\ \mu_{\alpha_2} h_2(t,\beta_2)\end{pmatrix},
$$

$$
\Sigma_1 = \Sigma + \begin{pmatrix} \sigma_1^2/h_1(t,\beta_1) & 0 \\ 0 & \sigma_2^2/h_2(t,\beta_2)\end{pmatrix}.
$$

Then, we have

$$
\begin{pmatrix} Y_1(t) \\ Y_2(t) \end{pmatrix} \sim \boldsymbol{N}_2(\mu_H, H'\Sigma_1 H). \tag{3}
$$

The variance–covariance matrix of $Y_1(t)$ and $Y_2(t)$ is not diagonal. Thus, they are correlated. The correlation coefficient between $Y_1(t)$ and $Y_2(t)$ at time t is

$$
\rho(t) = \mathrm{corr}(Y_1(t), Y_2(t)) = \frac{\rho\sigma_{\alpha_1}\sigma_{\alpha_2}}{\sqrt{\sigma_{\alpha_1}^2 + \sigma_1^2/h_1(t,\beta_1)}\sqrt{\sigma_{\alpha_2}^2 + \sigma_2^2/h_2(t,\beta_2)}}.
$$

For the copula method, the dependence between $Y_1(t)$ and $Y_2(t)$ is reflected by the increments of the degradation observations of the two PCs, and the dependent structure between $Y_1(t)$ and $Y_2(t)$ at a certain time is hard to explain. However, in our model, the correlation coefficient function $\rho(t)$ between $Y_1(t)$ and $Y_2(t)$

changes with time and is a non-increasing or non-decreasing function of time t when $\rho < 0$ or $\rho > 0$. Before the product being put into use, $\rho(t) = 0$, while as $t \to \infty$, $\rho(t) \to \rho$. Therefore, we can see that as the product begins to be used, the two PCs degenerate correspondingly, which leads to the changes of dependence between the two PCs. Thus, the new model can reflect that the two PCs influence each other dynamically and intuitively.

Denote that the threshold level of $Y_s(t)$ is τ_s, $s = 1, 2$. Let $\tau = (\tau_1, \tau_2)'$. The lifetime of the s-th PC is defined as

$$T_s = \inf\{t : Y_s(t) \geq \tau_s\}.$$

Then, conditioned on α_s, the pdf of T_s is [36]

$$f_s(t_s|\alpha_s) = \frac{\tau_s}{\sqrt{2\pi\sigma_s^2(h_s(t_s,\beta_s))^3}} \exp\left\{-\frac{(\tau_s - \alpha_s h_s(t_s,\beta_s))^2}{2\sigma_s^2 h_s(t_s,\beta_s)}\right\} \frac{dh_s(t_s,\beta_s)}{dt_s}. \tag{4}$$

Thus, the joint pdf of T_1 and T_2 is

$$\begin{aligned}
&f(t_1,t_2)\\
&= \iint f_1(t_1|\alpha_1) f_2(t_2|\alpha_2) f(\alpha_1,\alpha_2)\mathrm{d}\alpha_1\mathrm{d}\alpha_2\\
&= \frac{\tau_1\tau_2}{(h_1(t_1,\beta_1)h_2(t_2,\beta_2))^2}(2\pi)^{-1}|\Sigma_1|^{-\frac{1}{2}} \exp\left\{-\frac{(\tau_H-\mu)'(\Sigma_1)^{-1}(\tau_H-\mu)}{2}\right\}\\
&\times \frac{dh_1(t_1,\beta_1)}{dt_1}\frac{dh_2(t_2,\beta_2)}{dt_2}.\\
&= \frac{(2\pi)^{-1}|\Sigma_1|^{-\frac{1}{2}}\tau_1\tau_2}{(h_1(t_1,\beta_1)h_2(t_2,\beta_2))^2} \exp\left\{-\frac{1}{|\Sigma_1|}[(\frac{\tau_1}{h_1(t_1,\beta_1)} - \mu_{\alpha_1})^2(\sigma_{\alpha_2}^2 + \sigma_2^2/h_2(t_2,\beta_2))\right.\\
&- 2\rho\sigma_{\alpha_1}\sigma_{\alpha_2}\left(\frac{\tau_1}{h_1(t_1,\beta_1)} - \mu_{\alpha_1}\right)\left(\frac{\tau_2}{h_2(t_2,\beta_2)} - \mu_{\alpha_2}\right) + \left(\frac{\tau_2}{h_2(t_2,\beta_2)} - \mu_{\alpha_2}\right)^2\\
&\left.\times (\sigma_{\alpha_1}^2 + \sigma_1^2/h_1(t_1,\beta_1))]\right\}\frac{dh_1(t_1,\beta_1)}{dt_1}\frac{dh_2(t_2,\beta_2)}{dt_2},
\end{aligned}$$

where

$$\tau_H = \begin{pmatrix}\tau_1/h_1(t_1,\beta_1)\\ \tau_2/h_2(t_2,\beta_2)\end{pmatrix},\quad |\Sigma_1| = [\sigma_{\alpha_1}^2 + \sigma_1^2/h_1(t_1,\beta_1)][\sigma_{\alpha_2}^2 + \sigma_2^2/h_2(t_2,\beta_2)] - \rho^2\sigma_{\alpha_1}^2\sigma_{\alpha_2}^2.$$

The cumulative distribution function (cdf) of T_s given α_s is

$$F_{T_s}(t_s|\alpha_s) = \Phi\left(\frac{\alpha_s h_s(t_s,\beta_s) - \tau_s}{\sigma_s\sqrt{h_s(t_s,\beta_s)}}\right) + \exp\left\{\frac{2\alpha_s\tau_s}{\sigma_s^2}\right\}\Phi\left(\frac{-\tau_s - \alpha_s h_s(t_s,\beta_s)}{\sigma_s\sqrt{h_s(t_s,\beta_s)}}\right). \tag{5}$$

Before giving the joint cdf of T_1 and T_2, we need to introduce some notations. Let

$$C_1 = \begin{pmatrix} -\tau_1/(\sigma_1\sqrt{h_1(t_1,\beta_1)}) \\ -\tau_2/(\sigma_2\sqrt{h_2(t_2,\beta_2)}) \end{pmatrix},\ \nu = \begin{pmatrix} 2\tau_1/\sigma_1^2 \\ 2\tau_2/\sigma_2^2 \end{pmatrix},\ D_1 = \begin{pmatrix} \sqrt{h_1(t_1,\beta_1)}/\sigma_1 & 0 \\ 0 & \sqrt{h_2(t_2,\beta_2)}/\sigma_2 \end{pmatrix},$$

$$D_2 = \begin{pmatrix} \sqrt{h_1(t_1,\beta_1)}/\sigma_1 & 0 \\ 0 & -\sqrt{h_2(t_2,\beta_2)}/\sigma_2 \end{pmatrix},\ D_3 = \begin{pmatrix} -\sqrt{h_1(t_1,\beta_1)}/\sigma_1 & 0 \\ 0 & \sqrt{h_2(t_2,\beta_2)}/\sigma_2 \end{pmatrix},$$

and $D_4 = -D_1$. Then, the joint cdf of T_1 and T_2 can be rewritten as

$$\begin{aligned} F(t_1,t_2) =& \iint F_{T_1}(t_1|\alpha_1)F_{T_2}(t_2|\alpha_2)f(\alpha_1,\alpha_2)d\alpha_1 d\alpha_2 \\ =& A_1 + A_2 + A_3 + A_4, \end{aligned} \tag{6}$$

where $A_1 = \Phi_2((D_1\Sigma D_1 + I_2)^{-\frac{1}{2}}(C_1 + D_1\mu))$, $A_2 = \exp\left(\frac{2\tau_2\mu_{\alpha_2}}{\sigma_2^2} + \frac{4\tau_2^2}{(1-\rho^2)\sigma_{\alpha_2}^2\sigma_2^4}\right)\cdot$ $\Phi_2((D_2\Sigma D_2 + I_2)^{-\frac{1}{2}}(C_1 + D_2\mu))$, $A_3 = \exp\left(\frac{2\tau_1\mu_{\alpha_1}}{\sigma_1^2} + \frac{4\tau_1^2}{(1-\rho^2)\sigma_{\alpha_1}^2\sigma_1^4}\right)$ $\Phi_2((D_3\Sigma D_3 + I_2)^{-\frac{1}{2}}(C_1 + D_3\mu))$, and $A_4 = \exp\left(\nu'\mu + \frac{\nu'\Sigma^{-1}\nu}{2}\right)\Phi_2((D_4\Sigma D_4 + I_2)^{-\frac{1}{2}}(C_1 + D_4\mu))$, where $\Phi_2((x_1,x_2)') = \Phi(x_1)\Phi(x_2)$ and $\Phi(\cdot)$ is the cdf of standard normal distribution. I_p denotes the p-dimensional identity matrix. The derivation of (6) is given in Appendix.

2.2 Reliability Function

The lifetime of the product is defined as

$$T = \min(T_1, T_2).$$

The reliability of the product at time t can be computed as follows:

$$\begin{aligned} R(t) = P(T > t) =& P(T_1 > t, T_2 > t) \\ =& P(T_1 < t, T_2 < t) + 1 - P(T_1 < t) - P(T_2 < t) \\ =& F(t,t) + 1 - F_{T_1}(t) - F_{T_2}(t), \end{aligned} \tag{7}$$

where $F_{T_s}(t)$ is the cdf of T_s, and its analytic form is

$$F_{T_s}(t) = \int F_{T_s}(t|\alpha_s) f(\alpha_s) \mathrm{d}\alpha_s$$
$$= \Phi\left(\frac{\mu_{\alpha_s} h_s(t,\beta_s) - \tau_s}{\sqrt{\sigma_{\alpha_s}^2 (h_s(t,\beta_s))^2 + \sigma_s^2 h_s(t,\beta_s)}}\right) +$$
$$\exp\left\{\frac{2\mu_{\alpha_s}\tau_s}{\sigma_s^2} + \frac{2\sigma_{\alpha_s}^2 \tau_s^2}{\sigma_s^4}\right\} \Phi\left(-\frac{2\sigma_{\alpha_s}^2 \tau_s h_s(t,\beta_s) + \sigma_s^2(\mu_{\alpha_s} h_s(t,\beta_s) + \tau_s)}{\sigma_s^2 \sqrt{\sigma_{\alpha_s}^2 (h_s(t,\beta_s))^2 + \sigma_s^2 h_s(t,\beta_s)}}\right),$$

where $f(\alpha_s)$ is the marginal pdf of α_s.

The residual life $L_k^{(s)}$ of the $s-$th PC at time t_k is defined as

$$L_k^{(s)} = \inf\{l : Y_s(l + t_k) \geq \tau_s | Y_s(t_j) < \tau_s, j = 1, 2, \cdots, k\},\ s = 1, 2, \tag{8}$$

where $t_1, \ldots, t_k$ are the measurement times. The cdf of $L_k^{(s)}$ given α_s is

$$F_{L_k^{(s)}}(l_s|\alpha_s) = \Phi\left(\frac{\alpha_s h_s(l_s,\beta_s) - (\tau_s - Y_s(t_k))}{\sigma_s \sqrt{h_s(l_s,\beta_s)}}\right) +$$
$$\exp\left\{\frac{2\alpha_s(\tau_s - Y_s(t_k))}{\sigma_s^2}\right\} \Phi\left(\frac{(Y_s(t_k) - \tau_s) - \alpha_s h_s(l_s,\beta_s)}{\sigma_s \sqrt{h_s(l_s,\beta_s)}}\right).$$

After obtaining the observations of

$$Y = \{Y_1(t_1), \ldots, Y_1(t_k), Y_2(t_1), \ldots, Y_2(t_k)\},$$

the joint cdf of α is also updated. Let

$$h_{sk} = h_s(t_k, \beta_s), \quad H = \begin{pmatrix} \sigma_1^2/h_{1k} & 0 \\ 0 & \sigma_2^2/h_{2k} \end{pmatrix}, \quad Y_k = \begin{pmatrix} Y_1(t_k)/h_{1k} \\ Y_2(t_k)/h_{2k} \end{pmatrix}.$$

Using Bayesian theory, we can obtain that given the current observations Y, the joint cdf of α is

$$\alpha | Y \sim \boldsymbol{N}_2(\tilde{\mu}, \tilde{\Sigma}),$$

where $\tilde{\mu} = (\Sigma^{-1} + H^{-1})^{-1}(\Sigma^{-1}\mu + H^{-1}Y_k) = (\mu_{1l}, \mu_{2l})'$, $\tilde{\Sigma} = (\Sigma^{-1} + H^{-1})^{-1} = \begin{pmatrix} \tilde{\sigma}_{11} & \tilde{\sigma}_{12} \\ \tilde{\sigma}_{21} & \tilde{\sigma}_{22} \end{pmatrix}$. Then, the joint cdf of $(L_k^{(1)}, L_k^{(2)})'$ is

$$\begin{aligned} F_L(l_1, l_2) = & \iint F_{L_k^{(1)}}(l_1|\alpha_1) F_{L_k^{(2)}}(l_2|\alpha_2) f(\alpha_1, \alpha_2|Y) d\alpha_1 d\alpha_2 \\ = & B_1 + B_2 + B_3 + B_4, \end{aligned} \tag{9}$$

where $B_1 = \Phi_2((D_{1l}\tilde{\Sigma}D_{1l} + I_2)^{-\frac{1}{2}}(C_{1l} + D_{1l}\tilde{\mu}))$,
$B_2 = \exp\left(\frac{2(\tau_2 - Y_2(t_k))\mu_{2l}}{\sigma_2^2} + \frac{4(\sigma_2^2 + h_{2k}(1-\rho^2)\sigma_{\alpha_2}^2)(\tau_2 - Y_2(t_k))^2}{(1-\rho^2)\sigma_{\alpha_2}^2\sigma_2^6}\right)\Phi_2((D_{2l}\tilde{\Sigma}D_{2l} + I_2)^{-\frac{1}{2}}(C_{1l} + D_{2l}\tilde{\mu}))$,
$B_3 = \exp\left(\frac{2(\tau_1 - Y_1(t_k))\mu_{1l}}{\sigma_1^2} + \frac{4(\sigma_1^2 + h_{1k}(1-\rho^2)\sigma_{\alpha_1}^2)(\tau_1 - Y_1(t_k))^2}{(1-\rho^2)\sigma_{\alpha_2}^2\sigma_1^6}\right)\Phi_2((D_{3l}\tilde{\Sigma}D_{3l} + I_2)^{-\frac{1}{2}}(C_{1l} + D_{3l}\tilde{\mu}))$, and
$B_4 = \exp\left(\nu_l'\tilde{\mu} + \frac{\nu_l'\tilde{\Sigma}^{-1}\nu_l}{2}\right)\Phi_2((D_{4l}\tilde{\Sigma}D_{4l} + I_2)^{-\frac{1}{2}}(C_{1l} + D_{4l}\tilde{\mu}))$, C_{1l}, ν_l, D_{1l}, D_{2l}, D_{3l}, and D_{4l} are C_1, ν, D_1, D_2, D_3, and D_4, where τ_s and t_s are replaced by $\tau_s - Y_s(t_k)$ and l_s, respectively. The derivation of (9) is similar to (6), and thus we omit it.

Assume that the s-th PC does not exceed the threshold τ_s at current time t_k. Then, the residual life of the product is defined as

$$L_k = \min(L_k^{(1)}, L_k^{(2)}). \tag{10}$$

Similarly, the reliability function of L_k at time l can be computed as follows:

$$R_{L_k}(l) = F_L(l, l) + 1 - F_{L_k^{(1)}}(l) - F_{L_k^{(2)}}(l), \tag{11}$$

where $F_{L_k^{(s)}}(l)$ is the cdf of $L_k^{(s)}$, and its analytical form is

$$\begin{aligned} F_{L_k^{(s)}}(l) = \Phi & \left(\frac{\mu_{sl}h_s(l, \beta_s) - (\tau_s - Y_s(t_k))}{\sqrt{\tilde{\sigma}_{ss}(h_s(l, \beta_s))^2 + \sigma_s^2 h_s(l, \beta_s)}}\right) + \\ & \exp\left\{\frac{2\mu_{sl}(\tau_s - Y_s(t_k))}{\sigma_s^2} + \frac{2\tilde{\sigma}_{ss}(\tau_s - Y_s(t_k))^2}{\sigma_s^4}\right\} \times \\ & \Phi\left(-\frac{2\tilde{\sigma}_{ss}(\tau_s - Y_s(t_k))h_s(l, \beta_s) + \sigma_s^2(\mu_{sl}h_s(l, \beta_s) + (\tau_s - Y_s(t_k)))}{\sigma_s^2\sqrt{\tilde{\sigma}_{ss}(h_s(l, \beta_s))^2 + \sigma_s^2 h_s(l, \beta_s)}}\right). \end{aligned}$$

3 Statistical Inference

Assume that there are n products tested in an experiment. For the i-th product, let y_{isj} be the j-th measured value of the s-th PC at the measurement time t_{isj},

$s = 1, 2, j = 1, 2, \ldots, m_{is}$. Here we do not require the two PCs measured at the same time, and the number of measurement times could be different. Let $y_{is0} = 0$, $z_{isj} = y_{isj} - y_{is(j-1)}$, and $g_{isj}(\beta_s) = h_s(t_{isj}, \beta_s) - h_s(t_{is(j-1)}, \beta_s)$, $s = 1, 2, i = 1, 2, \ldots, n, j = 1, 2, \ldots, m_{is}$. For the sake of notation simplification, we denote $g_{isj} = g_{isj}(\beta_s)$. Then, for the i-th product, we have the model $z_{isj}|\alpha_{is} \sim \boldsymbol{N}(\alpha_{is} g_{isj}, \sigma_s^2 g_{isj})$, and $\alpha_i = \binom{\alpha_{i1}}{\alpha_{i2}} \sim \boldsymbol{N}_2(\mu, \Sigma), s = 1, 2, \; j = 1, 2, \ldots, m_{is}$. Let $z = \{z_{isj}, \; s = 1, 2, i = 1, 2, \ldots, n, j = 1, 2, \ldots, m_{is}\}$ and $\theta = \{\mu, \Sigma, \sigma_1^2, \sigma_2^2, \beta_1, \beta_2\}$. The likelihood function of the observed data z is

$$
\begin{aligned}
L(z|\theta) \\
&= \prod_{i=1}^{n} \iint \prod_{s=1}^{2} \prod_{j=1}^{m_{is}} \frac{1}{\sqrt{2\pi\sigma_s^2 g_{isj}}} \exp\left\{-\frac{(z_{isj} - \alpha_{is} g_{isj})^2}{2\sigma_s^2 g_{isj}}\right\} \\
&\times (2\pi)^{-1} |\Sigma|^{-\frac{1}{2}} \exp\left\{-\frac{(\alpha_i - \mu)' \Sigma^{-1} (\alpha_i - \mu)}{2}\right\} d\alpha_{i1} d\alpha_{i2} \\
&= \prod_{i=1}^{n} \left\{ \left[\prod_{s=1}^{2} \prod_{j=1}^{m_{is}} \frac{1}{\sqrt{2\pi\sigma_s^2 g_{isj}}} \exp\left\{-\frac{z_{isj}^2}{2\sigma_s^2 g_{isj}}\right\}\right] \exp\left\{\frac{y_{i1m_{i1}}^2}{2\sigma_1^2 h_{i1m_{i1}}} + \frac{y_{i2m_{i2}}^2}{2\sigma_2^2 h_{i2m_{i2}}}\right\} \right. \\
&\left. \times \sqrt{\frac{2\pi\sigma_1^2\sigma_2^2}{h_{i1m_{i1}} h_{i2m_{i2}}}} |\Sigma + H_i|^{-1/2} \exp\left\{-\frac{(\bar{y}_i - \mu)'(\Sigma + H_i)^{-1}(\bar{y}_i - \mu)}{2}\right\}\right\},
\end{aligned} \tag{12}
$$

where $h_{ism_{is}} = h_s(t_{ism_{is}}, \beta_s)$, $H_i = \begin{pmatrix} \sigma_1^2/h_{i1m_{i1}} & 0 \\ 0 & \sigma_2^2/h_{i2m_{i2}} \end{pmatrix}$, $\bar{y}_i = \binom{y_{i1m_{i1}}/h_{i1m_{i1}}}{y_{i2m_{i2}}/h_{i2m_{i2}}}$. (12) is too complicated and is hard to get reasonable solutions using optimization. Considering that α_i is a latent variable and is unobservable, EM algorithm can be used in such a case. However, the interval estimates of the parameters are not easy to compute using EM algorithm. Alternatively, Bayesian method can obtain point estimates and interval estimates simultaneously using Markov chain Monte Carlo (MCMC) and thus is preferred in this chapter.

3.1 Prior Specification

Prior information plays an important role in Bayesian statistics, where the parameters in the model are treated as random variables. Prior distribution can be specified by several ways, e.g., noninformative priors, conjugate priors, and hierarchical priors. Noninformative priors are typically elicited from some well-defined rules and principles, such as the principle of maximum entropy [7], the Jeffrey's rule [8], and the Kullback–Liebler divergence [4]. We need to check the posterior property of the model parameters, as noninformative priors are usually improper. For the proposed bivariate Wiener degradation model, both the derivation of the noninformative priors and the proof of the posterior property are not easy. Conjugate priors are the most commonly used because the prior and posterior distributions are from the same distribution family, and the hyper-parameters can be easily explained. The hyper-parameters in prior distribution can be elicited by experts' experience or some historical information. If neither of these information are available, we can elicit the conjugate prior with large variance by choosing proper hyper-parameters, so that the impact of the prior distribution would be weak. The rationality of the method of hyper-parameter specification has been justified by many authors; see [11, 32] for more details. The priors for the parameters in this chapter are as follows:

1. The conditional conjugate prior for μ is assumed to be bivariate normal distribution with mean μ_0 and variance–covariance matrix Σ_0; that is, $\mu \sim \boldsymbol{N}_2(\mu_0, \Sigma_0)$. The hyper-parameter μ_0 is chosen as $(1, 1)'$, Σ_0 is a 2×2 symmetric positive-definite matrix, and we let $\Sigma_0 = 10^2 \cdot I_2$. The large variance means the weak belief on the μ_0, which can make data information play the main role in the Bayesian analysis.
2. We assume that Σ follows the inverse Wishart distribution $\boldsymbol{IW}(\Psi, v)$ with pdf

$$\frac{|\Psi|^{v/2}}{2^v \pi^{1/2} \Gamma(v/2) \Gamma((v-1)/2)} |\Sigma|^{-(v+3)/2} \exp\{-tr(\Psi \Sigma^{-1})\},$$

where Ψ is a 2×2 symmetric positive-definite scale matrix, v is the degrees of freedom, $v > 1$, and $\Gamma(\cdot)$ is the gamma function. Similarly, we let $v = 2$ and $\Psi = I_2$ in the data analysis. In fact, the inverse-gamma distribution is a special case of inverse Wishart distribution for the one-dimensional case.
3. The prior for σ_s^2 is specified as inverse-gamma distribution $\boldsymbol{IG}(a_s, b_s)$ with pdf

$$\frac{b_s^{a_s}}{\Gamma(a_s)} \left(\sigma_s^2\right)^{-a_s-1} \exp\{-b_s/\sigma_s^2\}.$$

The prior for β_s is specified as gamma distribution $\boldsymbol{G}(c_s, d_s)$ with mean c_s/d_s and variance c_s/d_s^2. We set $a_s = b_s = c_s = d_s = 0.01$ to reflect that we are lacking the knowledge about the parameters. This setting makes the shape of the inverse-gamma prior or gamma prior flat and can be regarded as noninformative prior.

3.2 Gibbs Sampling

Notice that α_i is unobservable, and using the likelihood function (12) is intractable for posterior analysis. Thus, we use data augmentation method to do the Bayesian analysis. Let $\alpha_0 = (\alpha_1, \ldots, \alpha_n)$. The likelihood function of the complete data (α_0, z) is

$$L(\alpha_0, z|\theta) = \prod_{i=1}^{n}\Bigg\{\prod_{s=1}^{2}\prod_{j=1}^{m_{is}} \frac{1}{\sqrt{2\pi\sigma_s^2 g_{isj}}} \exp\left\{-\frac{(z_{isj} - \alpha_{is} g_{isj})^2}{2\sigma_s^2 g_{isj}}\right\} \times (2\pi)^{-1}|\Sigma|^{-\frac{1}{2}} \exp\left\{-\frac{(\alpha_i - \mu)'\Sigma^{-1}(\alpha_i - \mu)}{2}\right\}\Bigg\}. \tag{13}$$

Based on the priors specified above and (13), the full conditional posterior distributions of the parameters can be obtained as follows.

1. Conditioned on the parameters θ and z, the posterior distribution of α_i is the bivariate normal distribution with mean $\tilde{\mu}_i$ and variance–covariance matrix $\tilde{\Sigma}_i$, where $\tilde{\mu}_i = (\Sigma^{-1} + H_i^{-1})^{-1}(\Sigma^{-1}\mu + H_i^{-1}\bar{y}_i)$, $\tilde{\Sigma}_i = (\Sigma^{-1} + H_i^{-1})^{-1}$, $i = 1, \ldots, n$.
2. Given z, α_0, and θ_μ (θ except for μ), the posterior distribution of μ is also the bivariate normal distribution with mean $\tilde{\mu}$ and variance–covariance matrix $\tilde{\Sigma}$, where $\tilde{\mu} = (\Sigma_0^{-1} + n\Sigma^{-1})^{-1}(\Sigma_0^{-1}\mu_0 + n\Sigma^{-1}\bar{\alpha})$, $\bar{\alpha} = \frac{1}{n}\sum_{i=1}^{n}\alpha_i$, and $\tilde{\Sigma} = (\Sigma_0^{-1} + n\Sigma^{-1})^{-1}$.
3. Given z, α_0, and θ_Σ, the posterior distribution of Σ is the inverse Wishart distribution $\boldsymbol{IW}\left(\sum_{i=1}^{n}(\alpha_i - \mu)(\alpha_i - \mu)' + \Psi, n + v\right)$.
4. Given z, α_0, and $\theta_{\sigma_s^2}$, the posterior distribution of σ_s^2 is the inverse-gamma distribution $\boldsymbol{IG}\left(\sum_{i=1}^{n} m_{is} + a_s,\ \frac{1}{2}\sum_{i=1}^{n}\sum_{j=1}^{m_{is}} (z_{isj} - \alpha_{is} g_{isj})^2/g_{isj} + b_s\right)$, $s = 1, 2$.
5. Given z, α_0, and θ_{β_s}, the posterior density function of β_s is proportional to

$$\prod_{i=1}^{n}\prod_{s=1}^{2}\prod_{j=1}^{m_{is}} \frac{1}{\sqrt{g_{isj}}} \exp\left\{-\frac{(z_{isj} - \alpha_{is} g_{isj})^2}{2\sigma_s^2 g_{isj}}\right\} (\beta_s)^{c_s - 1} \exp\{-d_s\beta_s\}.$$

   Unlike the other parameters, the full conditional posterior distribution of β_s is related to the analytic form of $h_s(t, \beta_s)$. Metropolis–Hastings algorithm can be used to get the posterior samples of β_s.

After getting the full conditional posteriors of the parameters, the Gibbs sampling algorithm can be implemented correspondingly. For example, we run the Gibbs sampling iteration K times, and check the convergence of the Gibbs sampling algorithm by ergodic mean. The burn-in period K' will be also determined when the ergodic means become stationary. For other methods for checking the convergence of MCMC, please refer to [5, 24]. After discarding the burn-in samples, we monitor the autocorrelation functions of the posterior samples and choose a sampling lag L after which the corresponding autocorrelation is small enough. Then the length of the thinning interval can be chosen as L. Finally, the number of kept posterior samples is $(K - K')/L$, which will be used for estimating the parameters.

4 Data Analysis

The original data from [15] present the growth of fatigue crack with measurement frequency 0.01 million of cycles up to 0.09 million of cycles. There are totally 21 units in the experiment. The initial crack length of each unit is 0.9 inches. For the illustration of bivariate degradation analysis, the authors of [20, 26], and [29] selected 20 units and divided them into two parts equally. One part represents the degradation of the first PC, and the other part denotes the degradation of the second PC. The artificial data are showed in Fig. 1. The failure threshold levels for the two PCs are 1.3 inches and 1.6 inches, respectively. Similar to [20] and [29], we assume that the two PCs are dependent on each other. Two time-scale transformations $h_s(t, \beta_s) = t^{\beta_s}$ and $h_s(t, \beta_s) = \exp\{\beta_s t\} - 1$ are considered. However, we compare the two time-scale transformations, and it shows that $h_s(t, \beta_s) = t^{\beta_s}$ is substantially better than the other model in terms of the AIC for model selection. Thus, we just list the detailed results of the model with the time-scale transformations $h_s(t, \beta_s) = t^{\beta_s}$.

The iteration number of Gibbs sampling is 100,000. The ergodic means of each parameters are shown in Fig. 2. As we can see in Fig. 2, the ergodic means become stationary very fast, and thus we discard the first 4000 iterations as the burn-in period. For the rest of the posterior samples, autocorrelation functions are computed and listed in Table 1. According to Table 1, we can see that the posterior samples are heavily correlated. The autocorrelations of posterior samples of σ_1^2, σ_2^2, $\sigma_{\alpha_1}^2$, $\sigma_{\alpha_2}^2$, and ρ are not significant when the lag is 30, while the lag should be 60 for the other parameters. Such a phenomenon is very common for data augmentation method (see [25] for more details). Thus, the length of thinning interval is taken to be 60. Finally, $(100{,}000 - 4000)/60 = 1600$ posterior samples are kept for further

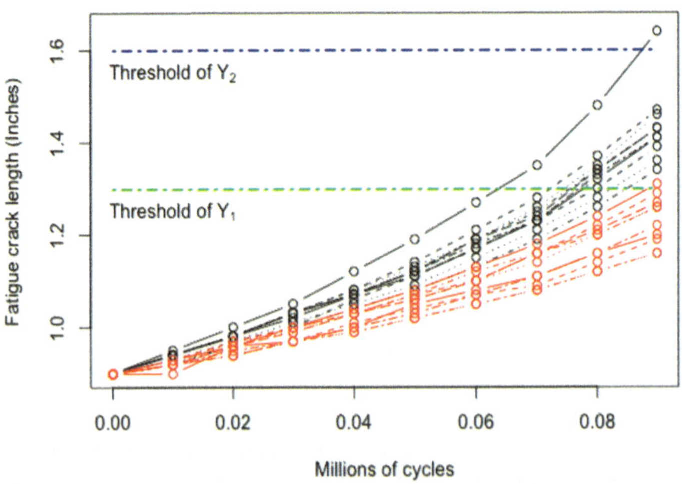

Fig. 1 The artificial fatigue crack data

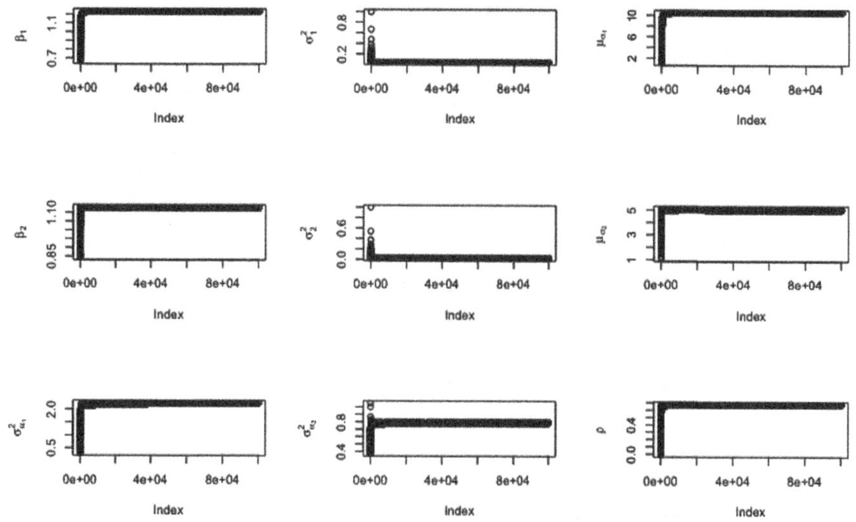

Fig. 2 Ergodic means of the posterior samples of the model parameters

Table 1 Autocorrelations based on different lags

Lag	β_1	β_2	σ_1^2	σ_2^2	μ_{α_1}	μ_{α_2}	$\sigma_{\alpha_1}^2$	$\sigma_{\alpha_2}^2$	ρ
30	0.301	0.239	0.021	1.51×10^{-3}	0.263	0.203	0.021	0.0161	1.79×10^{-3}
50	0.142	0.103	4.23×10^{-3}	9.68×10^{-4}	0.125	0.087	6.41×10^{-3}	6.59×10^{-3}	7.05×10^{-3}
60	0.090	0.077	3.01×10^{-3}	-2.04×10^{-4}	0.079	0.062	1.30×10^{-3}	2.54×10^{-3}	-4.64×10^{-5}

parameter estimation. The results of posterior means and 95% credible intervals of the parameters are listed in Table 2, where the estimates of the parameters for the independent case are also listed, and "SD" denotes the standard deviation. The model assumption implies that the drift parameters of the degradation process should be positive, and the probability of the improper feature $\Pr\{\alpha_1 \leq 0, \alpha_2 \leq 0\}$ is estimated to be 2×10^{-16}, which is negligible. In Table 2, we can see that the posterior means of the parameters are very close to each other for the dependent and independent cases. This result is similar to [29]. The reason may be that the dependence between the two PCs is not strong enough. Although the posterior mean of ρ is 0.667, as we have pointed out in the previous section, the correlation coefficient between $Y_1(t)$ and $Y_2(t)$ is a function of time, and when the time goes to infinity, the correlation coefficient will be ρ. Figure 3 shows the curve of correlation coefficient function between $Y_1(t)$ and $Y_2(t)$. When the million of cycles is less than 0.05, the correlation coefficient function $\rho(t)$ is very small, even less than 0.4.

Based on the posterior means of the parameters, we draw the reliability functions of the system and the two PCs according to (7). Figure 4 shows the three reliability functions, and we can see that the reliability before 0.08 millions of cycles is very close to 1 and will decrease fast after that. Based on (11), we select one of the

Table 2 Estimation of the model parameters

Parameters	Dependent case			Independent case		
	Mean	SD	95% credible interval	Mean	SD	95% credible interval
μ_{α_1}	10.474	1.056	(8.506, 12.667)	10.860	1.180	(8.430, 13.043)
σ_1^2	0.0398	4.736×10^{-3}	(0.0316, 0.0501)	0.0399	4.864×10^{-3}	(0.0317, 0.0507)
β_1	1.235	0.0369	(1.161, 1.306)	1.264	0.0394	(1.159, 1.314)
μ_{α_2}	5.011	0.645	(3.674, 6.285)	4.914	0.654	(3.610, 6.269)
σ_2^2	0.0163	1.872×10^{-3}	(0.0129, 0.0202)	0.0165	1.969×10^{-3}	(0.0131, 0.0208)
β_2	1.125	0.0472	(1.020, 1.205)	1.119	0.0480	(1.021, 1.219)
$\sigma_{\alpha_1}^2$	1.813	1.430	(0.563, 4.606)	2.908	2.415	(0.531, 9.078)
$\sigma_{\alpha_2}^2$	0.662	0.459	(0.175, 1.883)	0.811	0.650	(0.209, 2.425)
ρ	0.667	0.225	(0.106, 0.923)	–	–	–

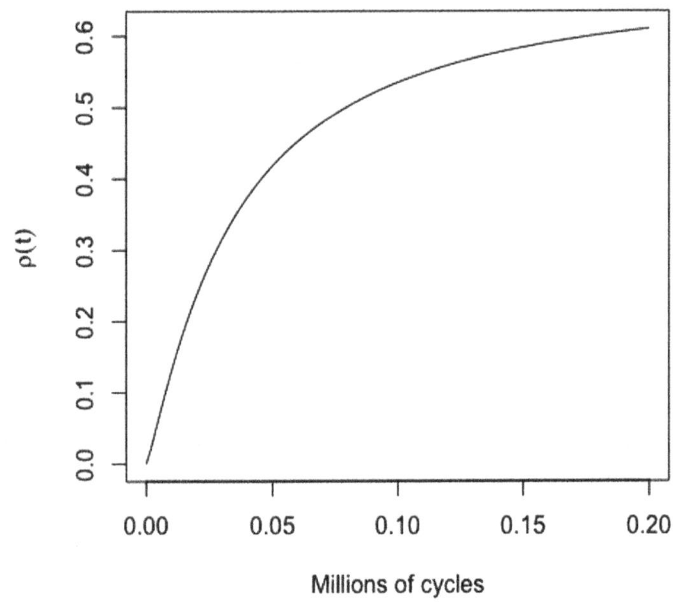

Fig. 3 The correlation coefficient function between $Y_1(t)$ and $Y_2(t)$

tested systems, and the reliability of residual life of the system at different time is shown in Fig. 5. Figure 5 shows that the more we use the system, the less reliable the system will be. Figure 6 shows the normal quantile–quantile plot of the standardized residual of the model, where the straight lines indicate that the model fits the data well. As a comparison, we also draw the estimated mean degradation paths $\hat{\mu}_{\alpha_s} t^{\hat{\beta}_s}$ of the models of [20] and [29] in Fig. 7, where "the empirical mean" denotes the empirical mean of degradation process. We can see that the model of [20] and the proposed model seem to fit the data better than the model of [29]. For fitting the data

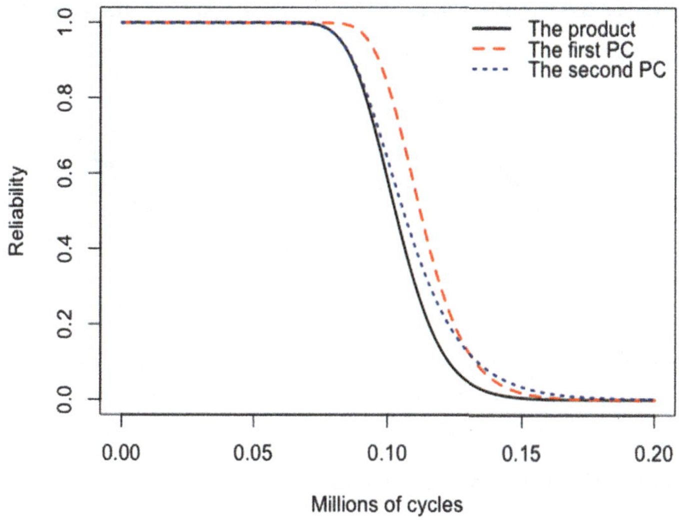

Fig. 4 The reliability of the product, PC 1 and PC 2

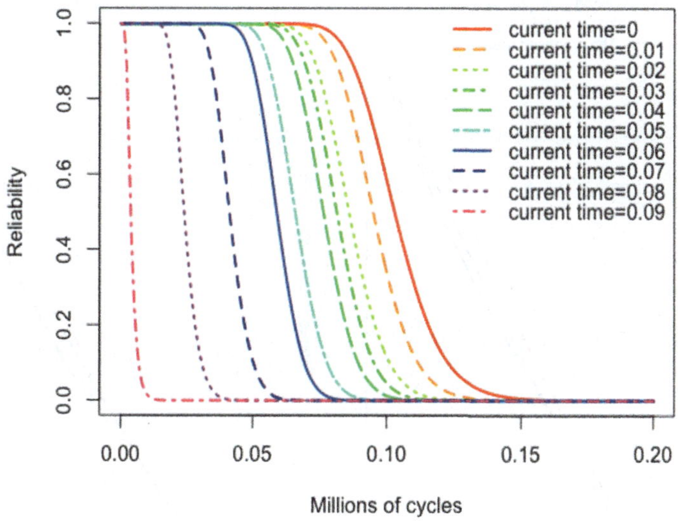

Fig. 5 The reliability of residual life of the system at different times

of the first PC, the proposed model performs better than the model of [20], while for fitting the data of the second PC, the results of the two models are very close to each other.

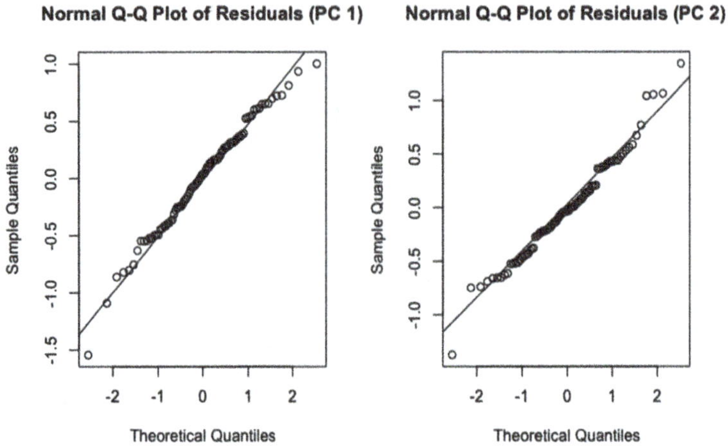

Fig. 6 Normal Q–Q plot of residuals based on the proposed model

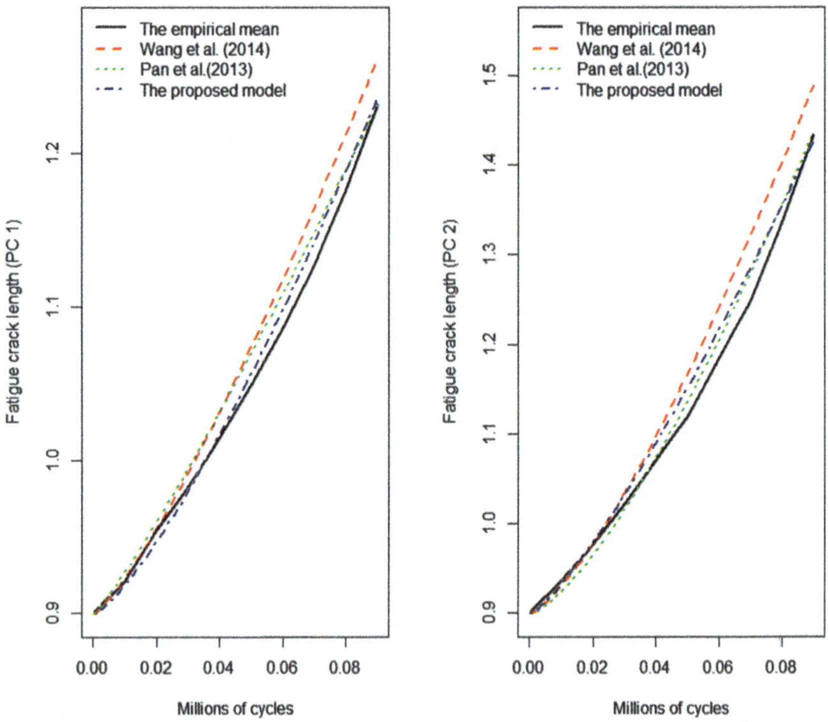

Fig. 7 Model comparison

5 Conclusion

In this chapter, a new bivariate Wiener degradation process has been proposed to characterize the system with two PCs, and the dependence between two PCs is described by a bivariate normal distribution. The reliability functions of the system and the residual lifetime are derived under the proposed model. Bayesian methods are used to obtain the estimation of the model parameters. Finally, the proposed model is illustrated by a simulated example.

Appendix

Lemma 1 *1. If* $Y = (y_1, \ldots, y_p)' \sim \boldsymbol{N}_p(\mu, \Sigma)$*, then for any* $C \in R^p$, $D \in R^{p\times p}$, $\mathrm{E}[\Phi_p(C + DY)] = \Phi_p\left((D\Sigma D' + I_p)^{-\frac{1}{2}}(C + D\mu)\right)$, *where* $\Phi_p(Y) = \prod_{i=1}^{p} \Phi(y_i)$.

2. If $Y \sim \boldsymbol{N}_p(\mu, \Sigma)$*, and* $v, C \in R^p$, $D \in R^{p\times p}$*, then*
$\mathrm{E}[\exp(v'Y)\Phi_p(C + DY)] = \exp(v'\mu + \frac{v'\Sigma^{-1}v}{2})\Phi_p\left((I_p + D\Sigma D')^{-\frac{1}{2}}(C + D\mu + D\Sigma v)\right)$.

Proof of (1):
Using the property of conditional expectation, we have

$$
\begin{aligned}
\mathrm{E}[\Phi_p(C + DY)] &= \mathrm{E}[\mathrm{E}(I_{\{Z\le C+DY\}})|Y] = P(Z \le C + DY) \\
&= P(Z - DY - C < 0) = \Phi_p\left((D\Sigma D' + I_p)^{-\frac{1}{2}}(C + D\mu)\right),
\end{aligned}
$$

where $I_{\{.\}}$ denotes the indicator function, $Z \sim \boldsymbol{N}_p(0, I_p)$, and Z and Y are independent. Then, $Z - DY - C \sim \boldsymbol{N}_p(-C - D\mu, I_p + D\Sigma D')$.

Proof of (2):

$$E[\exp(v'Y)\Phi_m(C+DY)] =$$

$$(2\pi)^{-\frac{m}{2}}|\Sigma|^{-\frac{1}{2}}\int \exp\Big\{-\frac{(Y-\mu)'\Sigma^{-1}(Y-\mu)}{2}\Big\}\exp(v'Y)\Phi_m(C+DY)dY$$

$$=(2\pi)^{-\frac{m}{2}}|\Sigma|^{-\frac{1}{2}}\int \exp\Big\{-\frac{(Y-(\mu+\Sigma v))'\Sigma^{-1}(Y-(\mu+\Sigma v))}{2}\Big\}$$

$$\exp\Big\{v'\mu+\frac{v'\Sigma^{-1}v}{2}\Big\}\Phi_m(C+DY)dY$$

$$=\exp\Big\{v'\mu+\frac{v'\Sigma^{-1}v}{2}\Big\}\int \phi_m(\Sigma^{-\frac{1}{2}}[Y-(\mu+\Sigma v)])\Phi_m(C+DY)dY$$

$$=\exp\Big\{v'\mu+\frac{v'\Sigma^{-1}v}{2}\Big\}\int \phi_m(z)\Phi_m(C+D\mu+D\Sigma v+D\Sigma^{\frac{1}{2}}z)dz$$

$$=\exp\Big\{v'\mu+\frac{v'\Sigma^{-1}v}{2}\Big\}\Phi_m((I_m+D\Sigma D')^{\frac{1}{2}}(C+D\mu+D\Sigma v)).$$

Proof of the joint cdf of T_1 and T_2

$$\begin{aligned}F(t_1,t_2)=&\iint F_{T_1}(t_1|\alpha_1)F_{T_2}(t_2|\alpha_2)f(\alpha_1,\alpha_2)d\alpha_1 d\alpha_2\\ =&A_1+A_2+A_3+A_4.\end{aligned}$$

Using (5) and Lemma 1, we have

$$\begin{aligned}A_1=&\iint\prod_{s=1}^{2}\Phi\left(\frac{\alpha_s h_s(t_s,\beta_s)-\tau_s}{\sigma_s\sqrt{h_s(t_s,\beta_s)}}\right)f(\alpha_1,\alpha_2)d\alpha_1 d\alpha_2\\ =&E_\alpha[\Phi_2(C_1+D_1\alpha)]=\Phi_2((D_1\Sigma D_1+I_2)^{-\frac{1}{2}}(C_1+D_1\mu)),\end{aligned}$$

where

$$C_1=-\begin{pmatrix}\tau_1/\sigma_1\sqrt{h_1(t_1,\beta_1)}\\ \tau_2/\sigma_2\sqrt{h_2(t_2,\beta_2)}\end{pmatrix},\quad D_1=\begin{pmatrix}\sqrt{h_1(t_1,\beta_1)}/\sigma_1 & 0\\ 0 & \sqrt{h_2(t_2,\beta_2)}/\sigma_2\end{pmatrix}.$$

$$
\begin{aligned}
A_2 = & \iint \Phi_1\left(\frac{\alpha_1 h_1(t_1,\beta_1)-\tau_1}{\sigma_1\sqrt{h_1(t_1,\beta_1)}}\right)\exp\left\{\frac{2\alpha_2\tau_2}{\sigma_2^2}\right\}\times \\
& \Phi\left(\frac{-\tau_2-\alpha_2 h_2(t_2,\beta_2)}{\sigma_2\sqrt{h_2(t_2,\beta_2)}}\right) f(\alpha_1,\alpha_2)d\alpha_1 d\alpha_2 \\
= & E_\alpha[\exp(v_1'\alpha)\Phi_2(C_1+D_2\alpha)] \\
= & \exp\left(\frac{2\tau_2\mu_{\alpha_2}}{\sigma_2^2}+\frac{2\tau_2^2}{(1-\rho^2)\sigma_{\alpha_2}^2\sigma_2^4}\right)\Phi_2((D_2\Sigma D_2+I_2)^{-\frac{1}{2}}(C_1+D_2\mu)),
\end{aligned}
$$

where

$$
v_1=\begin{pmatrix}0\\ 2\tau_2/\sigma_2^2\end{pmatrix},\quad D_2=\begin{pmatrix}\sqrt{h_1(t_1,\beta_1)}/\sigma_1 & 0\\ 0 & -\sqrt{h_2(t_2,\beta_2)}/\sigma_2\end{pmatrix},
$$

$$
\Sigma^{-1}=\frac{1}{1-\rho^2}\begin{pmatrix}\frac{1}{\sigma_{\alpha_1}^2} & -\frac{\rho}{\sigma_{\alpha_1}\sigma_{\alpha_2}}\\ -\frac{\rho}{\sigma_{\alpha_1}\sigma_{\alpha_2}} & \frac{1}{\sigma_{\alpha_2}^2}\end{pmatrix}.
$$

$$
\begin{aligned}
A_3 = & \iint \Phi_2\left(\frac{\alpha_2 h_2(t_2,\beta_2)-\tau_2}{\sigma_2\sqrt{h_2(t_2,\beta_2)}}\right)\exp\left\{\frac{2\alpha_1\tau_1}{\sigma_1^2}\right\}\times \\
& \Phi\left(\frac{-\tau_1-\alpha_1 h_1(t_1,\beta_1)}{\sigma_1\sqrt{h_1(t_1,\beta_1)}}\right) f(\alpha_1,\alpha_2)d\alpha_1 d\alpha_2 \\
= & E_\alpha[\exp(v_2'\alpha)\Phi_2(C_1+D_3\alpha)] \\
= & \exp\left(\frac{2\tau_1\mu_{\alpha_1}}{\sigma_1^2}+\frac{2\tau_2^2}{(1-\rho^2)\sigma_{\alpha_1}^2\sigma_1^4}\right)\Phi_2((D_3\Sigma D_3+I_2)^{-\frac{1}{2}}(C_1+D_3\mu)),
\end{aligned}
$$

where

$$
v_2=\begin{pmatrix}2\tau_1/\sigma_1^2\\ 0\end{pmatrix},\quad D_3=\begin{pmatrix}-\sqrt{h_1(t_1,\beta_1)}/\sigma_1 & 0\\ 0 & \sqrt{h_2(t_2,\beta_2)}/\sigma_2\end{pmatrix}.
$$

$$
\begin{aligned}
A_4 = & \iint \exp\left(\frac{2\tau_1\alpha_1}{\sigma_1^2} + \frac{2\tau_2\alpha_1}{\sigma_2^2}\right) \Phi\left(\frac{-\tau_1 - \alpha_1 h_1(t_1, \beta_1)}{\sigma_1\sqrt{h_1(t_1, \beta_1)}}\right) \times \\
& \Phi\left(\frac{-\tau_2 - \alpha_2 h_2(t_2, \beta_2)}{\sigma_2\sqrt{h_2(t_2, \beta_2)}}\right) f(\alpha_1, \alpha_2) d\alpha_1 d\alpha_2 \\
= & E_\alpha[\exp(\nu'\alpha)\Phi(C_1 + D_4\alpha)] \\
= & \exp\left(\nu'\mu + \frac{\nu'\Sigma^{-1}\nu}{2}\right) \Phi_2((D_4\Sigma D_4 + I_2)^{-\frac{1}{2}}(C_1 + D_4\mu)),
\end{aligned}
$$

where

$$
\nu = \begin{pmatrix} 2\tau_1/\sigma_1^2 \\ 2\tau_2/\sigma_2^2 \end{pmatrix}, \quad D_4 = \begin{pmatrix} -\sqrt{h_1(t_1, \beta_1)}/\sigma_1 & 0 \\ 0 & -\sqrt{h_2(t_2, \beta_2)}/\sigma_2 \end{pmatrix} = -D_1,
$$

$$
\nu'\mu + \frac{\nu'\Sigma^{-1}\nu}{2} = 2\sum_{s=1}^{2} \frac{\tau_s \mu_{\alpha_s}}{\sigma_s^2} + \frac{2}{1-\rho^2}\left[\frac{\tau_1^2}{\sigma_{\alpha_1}^2\sigma_1^4} - 2\frac{\rho\tau_1\tau_2}{\sigma_{\alpha_1}\sigma_{\alpha_2}\sigma_1^4\sigma_2^4} + \frac{\tau_2^2}{\sigma_{\alpha_2}^2\sigma_2^4}\right].
$$

References

1. Bae, S., Kuo, W., Kvam, P.: Degradation models and implied lifetime distributions. Reliab. Eng. Syst. Saf. **92**(5), 601–608 (2007)
2. Bagdonavicius, V., Bikelis, A., Kazakevicius, V.: Statistical analysis of linear degradation and failure time data with multiple failure modes. Lifetime Data Anal. **10**(1), 65–81 (2004)
3. Bagdonavicius, V., Bikelis, A., Kazakevicius, V., Nikulin, M.: Analysis of joint multiple failure mode and linear degradation data with renewals. J. Stat. Plan. Infer. **137**(7), 2191–2207 (2007)
4. Bernardo, J.: Reference posterior distributions for Bayesian inference (with discussion). J. R. Stat. Soc. B **41**, 113–147 (1978)
5. Brooks, S., Gelman, A.: General methods for monitoring convergence of iterative simulation. J. Comput. Graph. Stat. **7**, 434–455 (1998)
6. Huang, W., Askin, R.: Reliability analysis of electronic devices with multiple competing failure modes involving performance aging degradation. Qual. Reliab. Eng. Int. **19**, 241–254 (2003)
7. Jaynes, E.: Prior probabilities. IEEE Trans. Syst. Sci. Cybern. **4**, 227–241 (1968)
8. Jeffreys, H.: Theory of Probability. Oxford University Press, London (1961)
9. Jin, G., Matthews, D.: Measurement plan optimization for degradation test design based on the bivariate Wiener process. Qual. Reliab. Eng. Int. **30**, 1215–1231 (2014)
10. Lawless, J., Crowder, M.: Covariates and random effects in a gamma process model with application to degradation and failure. Lifetime Data Anal. **10**(3), 213–227 (2004)
11. Lawson, A.: Bayesian Disease Mapping: Hierarchical Modeling in Spatial Epidemiology. Chapman & Hall/CRC, Boca Raton (2009)
12. Liao, C., Tseng, S.: Optimal design for step-stress accelerated degradation tests. IEEE Trans. Reliab. **55**(1), 59–66 (2006)
13. Ling, M., Tsui, K., Balakrishnan, N.: Accelerated degradation analysis for the quality of a system based on the gamma process. IEEE Trans. Reliab. **64**(1), 463–472 (2015)
14. Lu, C., Meeker, W.: Using degradation measures to estimate a time-to-failure distribution. Technometrics **35**(2), 161–174 (1993)

15. Meeker, W.Q., Escobar, L.A.: Statistical Methods for Reliability Data. Wiley & Sons, New York (1998)
16. Pan, Z., Balakrishnan, N.: Reliability modeling of degradation of products with multiple performance characteristics based on gamma processes. Reliab. Eng. Syst. Saf. **96**(8), 949–957 (2011)
17. Park, C., Padgett, W.J.: New cumulative damage models for failure using stochastic processes as initial damage. IEEE Trans. Reliab. **54**(3), 530–540 (2005)
18. Park, C., Padgett, W.J.: Stochastic degradation models with several accelerating variables. IEEE Trans. Reliab. **55**(2), 379–390 (2006)
19. Pan, Z., Balakrishnan, N., Sun, Q.: Bivariate constant-stress accelerated degradation model and inference. Commun. Stat. Simul. Comput. **40**(2), 259–269 (2011)
20. Pan, Z., Balakrishnan, N., Sun, Q., Zhou, J.: Bivariate degradation analysis of products based on Wiener processes and copulas. J. Stat. Comput. Simul. **83**(7), 1316–1329 (2013)
21. Peng, C.Y., Tseng, S.T.: Mis-specification analysis of linear degradation models. IEEE Trans. Reliab. **61**(2), 444–455 (2009)
22. Peng, W., Li, Y., Yang, Y., Zhu, S., Huang, H.: Bivariate analysis of incomplete degradation observations based on inverse Gaussian processes and copulas. IEEE Trans. Reliab. **65**(2), 624–639 (2016)
23. Peng, W., Li, Y., Yang, Y., Mi, J., Huang, H.: Bayesian degradation analysis with inverse Gaussian process models under time-varying degradation rates. IEEE Trans. Reliab. **66**(1), 84–96 (2017)
24. Raftery, A., Lewis, S.: One long run with diagnostics: implementation strategies for Markov chain Monte Carlo. Stat. Sci. **7**, 493–497 (1992)
25. Robert, C., Casella, G.: Monte Carlo Statistical Methods (2nd edn.) Springer, New York (2005)
26. Sari, J., Newby, M., Brombacher, A., Tang, L: Bivariate constant stress degradation model: LED lighting system reliability estimation with two-stage modelling. Qual. Reliab. Eng. Int. **25**, 1067–1084 (2009)
27. Shiau, J., Lin, H.: Analyzing accelerated degradation data by nonparametric regression. IEEE Trans. Reliab. **48**(2), 149–158 (1999)
28. Wang, X., Xu, D.: An inverse Gaussian process model for degradation data. Technometrics **52**(2), 188–197 (2010)
29. Wang, X., Guo, B., Cheng, J.: Residual life estimation based on bivariate Wiener degradation process with time-scale transformations. J. Stat. Comput. Simul. **84**(3), 545–563 (2014)
30. Wang, X., Balakrishnan, N., Guo, B., Jiang, P.: Residual life estimation based on bivariate non-stationary gamma degradation process. J. Stat. Comput. Simul. **85**(2), 405–421 (2015)
31. Whitmore, G.A., Schenkelberg, F.: Modelling accelerated degradation data using Wiener diffusion with a time scale transformation. Lifetime Data Anal. **3**(1), 27–45 (1997)
32. Xu, A., Basu, S., Tang, Y.: A full Bayesian approach for masked data in step-stress accelerated life testing. IEEE Trans. Reliab. **63**(3), 798–806 (2014)
33. Xu, A., Shen, L., Wang, B., Tang, Y.: On modeling bivariate Wiener degradation process. IEEE Trans. Reliab. **67**(3), 897–906 (2018)
34. Ye, Z.S., Chen, N.: The inverse Gaussian process as a degradation model. Technometrics **56**(3), 302–311 (2014)
35. Ye, Z.S., Xie, M.: Stochastic modelling and analysis of degradation for highly reliable products. Appl. Stoch. Models Bus. Ind. **31**, 16–32 (2015)
36. Ye, Z.S., Wang, Y., Tsui, K., Pecht, M.: Degradation data analysis using Wiener processes with measurement errors. IEEE Trans. Reliab. **62**(4), 772–780 (2013)
37. Ye, Z.S., Chen, N., Shen, Y.: A new class of Wiener process models for degradation analysis. Reliab. Eng. Syst. Saf. **139**, 58–67 (2015)
38. Yuan, X., Pandey, M.: A nonlinear mixed-effects model for degradation data obtained from in-service inspections. Reliab. Eng. Syst. Saf. **94**(2), 508–519 (2009)

Bayesian Estimation for Bivariate Gamma Processes with Copula

Yu-Jau Lin, Tzong-Ru Tsai, and Yuhlong Lio

Abstract Gamma stochastic process has been proposed to replace Brownian motion and geometric Brownian motion to characterize the degradation measurements from an accelerated degradation test (ADT). Tsai et al. [27] applied bivariate Gamma process to model the two-variable ADT under the independent assumption. In this chapter, we consider three bivariate Gamma processes utilizing the Clayton, Frank, and Gumbel copulas to describe the dependence characteristics of bivariate Gamma variables. Owing to the complex structure of modeling, the differentiation-based likelihood estimation of the copulas are not always tractable. Bayesian analysis using Markov chain Monte Carlo method is an effective alternative to implement parameter estimation and model comparisons. Extensive simulation studies that calculate the mean square errors (MSEs) of the derived estimates are conduced to show the efficiency of the proposed method. Three data sets from the Clayton, Frank, and Gumbel copulas are analyzed and used for the demonstration of model selections via Bayesian approach.

1 Introduction

An accelerated degradation test (ADT) is one of the effective procedures in reliability engineering to obtain the lifetime-related degradation information from highly reliable systems within a relatively short time for reliability inference that

---

Y.-J. Lin
Applied Mathematics Department, Chung Yuan Christian University, Taoyuan City, Taiwan
e-mail: yujaulin@cycu.edu.tw

T.-R. Tsai (✉)
Department of Statistics, Tamkang University, New Taipei City, Taiwan
e-mail: tzongru@gms.tku.edu.tw

Y. Lio
Department of Mathematical Sciences, University of South Dakota, Vermillion, SD, USA
e-mail: Yuhlong.Lio@usd.edu

Y. Lio et al. (eds.), *Bayesian Inference and Computation in Reliability and Survival Analysis*, Emerging Topics in Statistics and Biostatistics,
https://doi.org/10.1007/978-3-030-88658-5_8

includes the prediction of the mean time to failure or lifetime percentiles of products based on the degradation information of test products under high stress-loading conditions. Lim and Yum [14], Padgett and Tomlinson [18], Park and Padgett [19], and Tsai et al. [24] had provided comprehensive introduction about ADT. Because of using s-normal distribution to model the increments of degradation in consecutive periods at an original scale and logarithmic transformation, Brownian motion (BM) and geometric Brownian motion (GBM) processes had been easy and widely applied to model the degradation of products under ADT over time. For more detailed information, the reader can refer Liao and Tseng [13], Lim and Yum [14], Tsai et al. [24]), Tsai et al. [25], and Whitmore [29]. However, the flow of BM and GBM processes for the modeling of the degradation of items under the ADT is that these two processes allow the degradation process that has negative increments. It is not true for numerous realistic cases that have shown the cumulative damage of a product is always monotonically increasing over time; for example, the LED Lumen degradation studied by Tsai et al. [24] as well as fatigue crack growth data discussed by Gertsbackh and Kordonskiy [10] and studied by Lu and Meeker [16]. Therefore, the Gamma process is more suitable to model a degradation process for performing reliability assessment than the BM and GBM processes due to the positive output from Gamma process. Boulanger and Escobar [1], Guan, and Tang [11], Park and Padgett [19], Park and Padgett[20], Park and Padgett [21], Peng [22], Tsai et al. [26], and Tseng et al. [28] have more comprehensive information about the Gamma process.

Recently, a multi-variable ADT of Gamma process has been proposed to model a damage at high stress-loading levels for performing reliability inferences by Ling et al.[15], Park and Padgett [20, 21], Tsai et al. [25], and Tsai et al. [27] via the maximum likelihood estimates (MLEs). Chiang et al. [3] proposed Markov chain Monte Carlo method to the estimation for the ADT Gamma process. Because of the complexity, the aforementioned studies under multi-variate Gamma accelerated variables were conducted under the independent assumption. In this chapter, the copula will be proposed to describe the dependent complexity of two stress variables. In this investigation, we consider three bivariate Gamma processes utilizing the Clayton, Frank, and Gumbel copulas to describe the dependence of two variables.

The rest of this chapter is organized as follows. More details of the two stress variables ADT of the Gamma process with copulas and the corresponding likelihood functions will be presented in Sect. 2. The Bayesian Markov chain Monte Carlo estimation of model parameters and model fitting will be discussed in Sect. 3. A Monte Carlo simulation study to evaluate the performance of the estimation method and a copula model selection will be provided in Sect. 4. Finally, some discussions and concluding remarks are given in Sect. 5.

2 Gamma Process with Copula

Let the increments of two degradation damages, (Y_1, Y_2), from a highly reliable product under a constant-stress ADT that collects these two degradation observations at the same predetermined time schedules be governed by marginal gamma processes, respectively, with positive shape parameters, ν_1 and ν_2, and scale parameters, β_1 and β_2, where the shape parameters, ν_1 and ν_2, depend upon the stress level L of the ADT. Therefore, the marginal probability density functions of Y_l for $l = 1, 2$ are, respectively, given as

$$f_l(y; \nu_l, \beta_l) = \frac{1}{\Gamma(\nu)\,\beta_l^{\nu}}\, y^{\nu_l} e^{-y/\beta_l}, \quad y > 0,\ l = 1, 2. \tag{1}$$

This chapter focuses on the modeling of these two possibly dependent increments of the degradation damages, (Y_1, Y_2). According to Sklar's Theorem, if $H(y_1, y_2; \nu_1, \beta_1, \nu_2, \beta_2)$ is a joint distribution with marginals $F_1(y; \nu_1, \beta_1)$ and $F_2(y; \nu_2, \beta_2)$, then there exists a copula C such that the following is true: $H(y_1, y_2; \nu_1, \beta_1, \nu_2, \beta_2) = C(F_1(y_1 : \nu_1, \beta_1), F_2(y_2 : \nu_2, \beta_2))$. Practically, a copula has been approved to be a flexible and convenient method to combine two marginal distributions into a bivariate distribution to address the possible dependence of two marginal distributions. Therefore, we would like to use the form of copula to address the dependence of these two random increments at all stress levels. There are many useful copula functions that include elliptical family (such as Gaussian, t, etc.) and Archimedean family (such as Frank, Gumbel, Clayton, etc.). Three aforementioned Archimedean copula functions that include the Clayton, Frank, and Gumbel copula with the parameter θ are introduced briefly as follows.

Clayton copula is a symmetric copula for bivariate random variables. The CDF of Clayton copula is given by

$$C_{\theta_1}(u, v) = \left(u^{-\theta} + v^{-\theta} - 1\right)^{-1/\theta} \tag{2}$$

with the corresponding density as

$$c_{\theta_1}(u, v) = (\theta + 1)(uv)^{-(\theta+1)}(u^{-\theta} + v^{-\theta} - 1)^{-\frac{2\theta+1}{\theta}}. \tag{3}$$

The second copula is Frank copula. Its CDF is given by

$$C_{\theta_2}(u, v) = \frac{-1}{\theta}\log\left\{1 + \frac{[e^{-\theta u} - 1][e^{-\theta v} - 1]}{e^{-\theta} - 1}\right\} \tag{4}$$

with the corresponding density as

$$c_{\theta_2}(u, v) = \frac{\theta[1 - e^{-\theta u}][e^{-\theta(u+v)}]}{1 - e^{-\theta} - [1 - e^{-\theta u}][1 - e^{-\theta v}]}. \tag{5}$$

The third copula is Gumbel copula and its CDF is given by

$$C_{\theta_3}(u, v) = \exp\{-[(-\log u)^{\theta} + (-\log v)^{\theta}]^{1/\theta}\} \tag{6}$$

with the corresponding density as

$$c_{\theta_3}(u, v) = C_{\theta_3}(u, v)(uv)^{-1} \frac{[(\tilde{u})(\tilde{v})]^{\theta-1}}{[\tilde{u}^{\theta} + \tilde{v}^{\theta}]^{2-1/\theta}} \left\{(\tilde{u}^{\theta} + \tilde{v}^{\theta})^{\frac{1}{\theta}} + \theta - 1\right\}, \tag{7}$$

where $\tilde{u} = -\log(u)$ and $\tilde{v} = -\log(v)$.

2.1 *The Likelihood Function*

Let a highly reliable product have two cumulative damage paths, labeled by $W_t = (X_{t_1}, X_{t_2})$, that starts at $w_0 = (0, 0)$ and follows the bivariate GP of Eq. (1) with $C(u, v)$ of Eq.(2), Eq.(4), or Eq.(6). The bivariate GP has marginal GPs, respectively, with positive shape parameters, ν_{L_1} and ν_{L_2}, and scale parameters, β_1 and β_2, where the shape parameters, ν_{L_1} and ν_{L_2}, depend on the stress level L of the ADT. The product is classified as failed when either X_{t_1} passes a given threshold ξ_1 first time or X_{t_2} passes a given threshold ξ_2 first time by the termination of the ADT; otherwise, the product is classified as surviving. Let S_1 be the first passage time of X_{t_1} to ξ_1 and S_2 be the first passage time of X_{t_2} to ξ_2.

The ADT is conducted with the working assumptions (A1) to (A5), which were given by Tsai et al. [27]:

(A1) k treatments are considered for the tested units in the ADT. Treatment i consists of a combination of two stress-loading levels, denoted by $L_i' = (L_{1i}', L_{2i}')$ for $i = 1, 2, \cdots, k$.

(A2) A total of n_i units are allocated to the run i of the ADT, and all units are tested subject to treatment L_i'.

(A3) The two components of stress-loading levels of L_i' are, respectively, standardized as follows:

$$L_{1i} = \frac{1/L_{10}' - 1/L_{1i}'}{1/L_{10}' - 1/L_{1M}'}, \quad \text{for ambient temperature,}$$

$$L_{2i} = \frac{1/L_{20}' - 1/L_{2i}'}{1/L_{20}' - 1/L_{2M}'}, \quad \text{for drive current, } i = 1, 2, \cdots, k,$$

where $1/L_{10}'$ and $1/L_{20}'$ are the respective levels of normal use condition for both treatments; additionally, $1/L_{1M}'$ and $1/L_{2M}'$ are the respective levels of the highest stress loading for both treatments. Obviously, $L_{10} = L_{20} = 0$, $L_{1M} = L_{2M} = 1$, $0 < L_{1i} \leq 1$,$0 < L_{2i} \leq 1$ for $i = 1, 2, \cdots, k$.

Moreover, L_{1i} and L_{2i} are scale-free and increasing functions of $1/L'_{1i}$ and $1/L'_{2i}$, respectively, for $i = 1, 2, \cdots, k$.

(A4) Let the starting time, $t_{ij0} = 0$, of the ADT and the initial damages of two paths for each unit in life test be $x_{ij01} = 0$ and $x_{ij02} = 0$. The damage of first path of each surviving unit at $L_i = (L_{1i}, L_{2i})$ is measured at times, $t_{ij1} < t_{ij2} < \cdots < t_{ijm_1}$, and labeled by $x_{ij11}, x_{ij21}, \cdots, x_{ijm_i1}$, respectively, for $i = 1, 2, \cdots, k$; and the damage of second path of each surviving unit at $L_i = (L_{1i}, L_{2i})$ is measured at times, $t_{ij1} < t_{ij2} < \cdots < t_{ijm_1}$, and labeled by $x_{ij12}, x_{ij22}, \cdots, x_{ijm_i2}$, respectively, for $i = 1, 2, \cdots, k$. The increments of the damages of two processes, $y_{ijh1} = x_{ijh1} - x_{ij(h-1)1}$ and $y_{ijh2} = x_{ijh2} - x_{ij(h-1)2}$, follow a bivariate Gamma distribution of $H(y_{ijh1}, y_{ijh2}; \delta_{ijh1}, \beta_1, \delta_{ijh2}, \beta_2)$ with $C_\theta(u, v)$ of Eq.(3), two shape coefficients $\delta_{ijh1} = \nu_{L_i1}\nu_{ijh}$ and $\delta_{ijh2} = \nu_{L_i2}\nu_{ijh}$, and two scale parameters β_1 and β_2, where $j = 1, 2, \cdots, n_i$, $h = 1, 2, \cdots, m_i$, and $i = 1, 2, \cdots, k$. It should be noticed that the marginal probability density functions of $H(y_{ijh1}, y_{ijh2}; \delta_{ijh1}, \beta_1, \delta_{ijh2}, \beta_2)$ are, respectively, given as follows:

$$f_l(y_{ijhl}; \delta_{ijhl}, \beta_l) = \frac{1}{\Gamma(\delta_{ijhl})\beta_l^{\delta_{ijhl}}} y_{ijhl}^{\delta_{ijhl}-1} e^{-y_{ijhl}/\beta_l}, \quad y_{ijhl} > 0 \text{ for } l = 1, 2. \tag{8}$$

(A5) The two shape parameters of the marginal gamma distribution can be expressed in terms of L_{1i} and L_{2i} through the generalized Eyring model (GEM) as

$$\nu_{L_il} = \exp(\gamma_{0l} + \gamma_{1l} L_{1i} + \gamma_{2l} L_{2i} + \gamma_{3l} L_{1i}L_{2i}), \ i = 1, 2, \cdots, k, \text{ and } l = 1, 2, \tag{9}$$

where $\gamma_{0l} < 0$, $\gamma_{1l}, \gamma_{1l} > 0$ and $\gamma_{3l} \in \mathcal{R}$ for $l = 1, 2$.

The GEM model in Eq. (9) is a generalized function that includes three widely used single-loading acceleration models as special cases: the Arrhenius law model, a power law model, and an exponential law model when only either L_1 or L_2 is used. Using the exact distributions of the first passage times, S_1 and S_2 under Gamma degradation process, to achieve an optimal ADT plan is difficult. For the case of one degradation path, Park and Padgett [19] indicated that the distribution of the first passage time, S_l, can be approximated by the IG distribution if the condition $C_{\beta l}/\sqrt{\nu_{L_l}} \gg C_{\beta l}/\nu_{L_l}$ (i.e., $\sqrt{\nu_{L_l}} \gg 1$) is true, where $C_{\beta l} = (\xi_l - x_{0l})/\beta_l$ for $l = 1, 2$. Let $\mu_{L_l} = C_{\beta l}/\nu_{L_l}$, and $\lambda_{L_l} = C_{\beta l}^2/\nu_{L_l}$ for $l = 1, 2$. Park and Padgett [19] showed that such an approximation is effective even if $\sqrt{\lambda_{L_l}}$ is not excessively greater than μ_{L_l} when μ_{L_l} is high for $l = 1, 2$. The PDF of the IG distribution is defined by

$$g_{S_l}(s; C_l) = g_{S_l}(s; x_{0l} = 0, C_l) = \frac{\frac{C_{\beta l}}{\sqrt{\nu_{L_l}}}}{\sqrt{(2\pi s^3}} \exp\left(\frac{-(\nu_{L_l}(s - \frac{C_{\beta l}}{\sqrt{\nu_{L_l}}})^2}{2s}\right) \text{ for } l = 1, 2. \tag{10}$$

The pdf of the damage increments observed from the marginal gamma process can be presented by Eq. (8), where $\delta_{ijhl} = \nu_{L_i l}\tau_{ijh}$ for $j = 1, 2, \cdots, n_i$, $h = 1, 2, \cdots, m_i$, $i = 1, 2, \cdots, k$, and $l = 1, 2$. Let $D = \{(y_{ijhl}, \tau_{ijh}), i = 1, 2, \cdots, k, j = 1, 2, \cdots, n_i, h = 1, 2, \cdots, m_i, l = 1, 2\}$ denote the data set of join damage increments observed from the bivariate gamma process. The likelihood function and log likelihood function can be presented, respectively, by

$$L(D \mid \Theta) = \prod_{i=1}^{k}\prod_{j=1}^{n_i}\prod_{h=1}^{m_i} C_\theta(F_1(y_{ijh1}; \delta_{ijh1}, \beta_1), F_2(y_{ijh2}; \delta_{ijh2}, \beta_2) \cdot \prod_{l=1}^{2} \frac{y_{ijhl}^{\delta_{ijhl}-1} e^{-y_{ijhl}/\beta_l}}{\Gamma(\delta_{ijhl})\beta_l^{\delta_{ijhl}}} \tag{11}$$

and

$$l(D \mid \Theta) = \sum_{i=1}^{k}\sum_{j=1}^{n_i}\sum_{h=1}^{m_i}\{C_\theta(F_1(y_{ijh1}; \delta_{ijh1}, \beta_1), F_2(y_{ijh2}; \delta_{ijh2}, \beta_2) - \left[\sum_{l=1}^{2} \ln(\Gamma(\delta_{ijhl}) + \delta_{ijhl}\ln(\beta_l) - (\delta_{ijhl} - 1)\ln(\delta_{ijh1} + y_{ijh1}/\beta_l)\right], \tag{12}$$

where C_θ is one of Clayton, Frank, and Gumbel copulas in Eq.(2), Eq.(4), and Eq.(6), θ is the corresponding copula parameter, and $\Theta = (\beta_1, \gamma_{01}, \gamma_{11}, \gamma_{21}, \gamma_{31}, \beta_2, \gamma_{02}, \gamma_{12}, \gamma_{22}, \gamma_{32}, \theta)$.

No close forms of the MLEs $(\hat{\theta})$ can be found due to the complicated log-likelihood function $l(\theta \mid D)$. Numerical computing methods such as the quasi-Newton method can be used to obtain the MLEs of the model parameters to maximize the log-likelihood function $l(\theta \mid D)$. The MCMC approach will be addressed as follows to find the Bayesian estimates of $\hat{\beta}_1, \hat{\gamma}_{01}, \hat{\gamma}_{11}, \hat{\gamma}_{21}, \hat{\gamma}_{31}, \hat{\beta}_2, \hat{\gamma}_{02}, \hat{\gamma}_{12}, \hat{\gamma}_{22}, \hat{\gamma}_{32}$, and $\hat{\theta}$ through using Gibbs sampling algorithm and Metropolis–Hastings algorithm.

3 Markov Chain and Monte Carlo Procedure

Markov Chain and Monte Carlo (MCMC) method is an effective procedure for obtaining information about distributions, especially for estimating posterior distributions in Bayesian inference. It allows one to calculate numerical approximations of multi-dimensional integrals and to sample from the un-normalized posterior distribution over parameters. (See, for example, Cowles and Carlin [5], Chen [2], and Tan et al. [23]). Unlike Monte Carlo sampling methods that draw independent samples from the distribution, MCMC method draws samples from the dependent sample conditionally on the existing sample. This allows the algorithms to approximate the target distribution with the simulated MCMC samplers.

Assume that the model parameter Θ has a joint prior pdf $\pi(\Theta)$. The posterior likelihood function can be represented as

$$\Pr(\Theta \mid D) \propto L(\Theta \mid D)\pi(\Theta), \tag{13}$$

where $\Theta = (\theta_1, \theta_2, \theta_3, \theta_4, \theta_5, \theta_6, \theta_7, \theta_8, \theta_9, \theta_{10}, \theta_{11}) \equiv (\beta_1, \gamma_{01}, \gamma_{11}, \gamma_{21}, \gamma_{31}, \beta_2, \gamma_{02}, \gamma_{12}, \gamma_{22}, \gamma_{32}, \theta)$. In this study, independent priors for parameters will be applied. However, the analytic form of the marginal posterior distribution in Eq.(13) is difficult to be obtained, and it is also infeasible to implement a numerical integration when using the marginal posterior distribution. Hence, in order to derive the Bayesian estimations of the parameters, the MCMC approach through the use of the Metropolis–Hastings algorithm (Hastings [12], Metropolis et al. [17]) to draw the sample of θ_j for $j = 1, 2, 3, \cdots, 11$ via the Gibbs sampling scheme (Geman and Geman [9]) will be applied in this study. When non-informative prior for each parameter (i.e., no prior for each parameter) is used, the MLEs $\hat{\Theta} = (\hat{\beta}_1, \hat{\gamma}_{01}, \hat{\gamma}_{11}, \hat{\gamma}_{21}, \hat{\gamma}_{31}, \hat{\beta}_2, \hat{\gamma}_{02}, \hat{\gamma}_{12}, \hat{\gamma}_{22}, \hat{\gamma}_{32}, \hat{\theta})$ can be derived through the MCMC approach. Readers may refer Chib and Greenberg [4] for more information.

Let the joint prior pdf

$$\pi(\Theta) = \left\{\prod_{l=1}^{2} \pi_{1l}(\beta_l)\pi_{2l}(\gamma_{0l})\pi_{3l}(\gamma_{1l})\pi_{4l}(\gamma_2 l)\pi_{5l}(\gamma_{3l})\right\}\pi_\theta(\theta),$$

where $\pi_{1l}(\beta_l)$ is the pdf of inverse Gamma distribution, $\pi_{jl}(\gamma_{(j-2)l}) \propto 1$ for $j = 2, 3, 4, 5$ and $l = 1, 2$, and $\pi(\theta) \propto 1$. Then, $\pi(\Theta)$ can be represented as

$$\prod_{l=1}^{2} \frac{\eta_l^{\lambda_l}}{\Gamma(\lambda_l)} \beta_l^{-\lambda_l - 1} e^{-\eta_l/\beta_l}, \ \beta_l > 0 \text{ for } l = 1, 2. \tag{14}$$

Then

$$\Pr(\Theta \mid D) \propto \prod_{i=1}^{k}\prod_{j=1}^{n_i}\prod_{h=1}^{m_i} c_{\theta_i}(F_1(y_{ijh1}; \delta_{ijh1}, \beta_1), F_2(y_{ijh2}; \delta_{ijh2}, \beta_2)$$
$$\cdot \prod_{l=1}^{2} \frac{y_{ijhl}^{\delta_{ijhl}-1} e^{-y_{ijhl}/\beta_l}}{\Gamma(\delta_{ijhl})\beta_l^{\delta_{ijhl}}}. \tag{15}$$

The Bayesian estimate of θ_i is close to the MLE for maximizing $l(\theta)$ if the hyper-parameters λ_l and η_l are selected to have a big variance of β_l for $l = 1, 2$ in the pdf (8).

3.1 Blocking

The Metropolis–Hastings is a specific implementation of MCMC. It works well in high-dimensional spaces as opposed to Gibbs sampling and rejection sampling. It uses q to randomly walk in the distribution space, accepting or rejecting jumps to new positions based on how likely the sample is.

It is not necessary to update each of the parameters individually. (see Gelman et al. [8], Chen [2]). Since the marginal distribution of a bivariate Gamma copula is free of the other counterpart parameters and is again Gamma distributed, we consider the following Gibbs sampling scheme that the parameters $B_1 = (\beta_1, \gamma_{01}, \gamma_{11}, \gamma_{21}, \gamma_{31})$, $B_2 = (\beta_2, \gamma_{02}, \gamma_{12}, \gamma_{22}, \gamma_{32})$, and θ are iteratively updated. That is, if $\Theta = (B_1, B_2, \theta)$, the Gibbs sampling scheme consists of three parts:

1. Update $B_1 | D, B_2, \theta$.
2. Update $B_2 | D, B_1, \theta$.
3. Update $\theta | D, B_1, B_2$.

3.2 Updating $B_i | D, B_j, \theta$ $(i \neq j)$

To update $B_1 | D, B_2, \theta$ or equivalently $B_1 | y_{ijh1}, B_2, \theta$, the M–H algorithm that generates the Markov chain $\{B_1^{(i)}\}$ of B_1 is as follows:

1. Set the initial parameter values, $B_1^{(1)}$.
2. At each bth ($b > 1$) Gibbs sampling iteration, simulate the candidates $B_1^{(*)}$ from their transition densities q_1 and $w \overset{iid}{\sim} \mathrm{U}(0, 1)$, then

$$B_1^{(b+1)} = \begin{cases} B_1^{(*)} \text{ if } w \leq \min\left\{1, \dfrac{L(B_1^{(*)} | y_{ijh1}, B_2, \theta)\, q_1(B_1^{(b)} | B_1^{(b)})}{L(B_1^{(b)} | y_{ijh1}, B_2, \theta)\, q_1(B_1^{(*)} | B_1^{(*)})}\right\} \\ B_1^{(b)} \text{ otherwise.} \end{cases}, \quad (16)$$

where $L(B_1 | y_{ijh1}, B_2, \theta)$ is the conditional posterior density proportional to Eq. (15). It is proportional to the product of the marginal likelihood in Eq. (11) times the marginal prior density distributions of B_1 in Eq. (14). Equivalently,

$$L(B_1 | y_{ijh1}, B_2, \theta) = \left\{\prod_{i=1}^{k}\prod_{j=1}^{n_i}\prod_{h=1}^{m_i} \frac{y_{ijh1}^{\delta_{ijhl}-1} e^{-y_{ijh1}/\beta_1}}{\Gamma(\delta_{ijh1})\beta_1^{\delta_{ijh1}}}\right\} \cdot \frac{\eta_l^{\lambda_1}}{\Gamma(\lambda_1)} \beta_l^{-\lambda_1-1} e^{-\eta_1/\beta_1}. \quad (17)$$

Likewise, $B_2 | D, B_1, \theta$ can be updated in a similar way.

1. Set the initial parameter values, $B_2^{(1)}$.

2. At each bth ($b > 1$) Gibbs sampling iteration, simulate the candidates $B_2^{(*)}$ from their transition densities q_2 and $w \overset{iid}{\sim} \text{U}(0, 1)$, then

$$B_1^{(b+1)} = \begin{cases} \theta^{(*)} \text{ if } w \leq \min\left\{1, \dfrac{L(B_2^{(*)} \mid y_{ijh2}, B_1, \theta)\, q_2(B_2^{(b)} | B_2^{(b)})}{L(B_2^{(b)} \mid y_{ijh2}, B_1, \theta)\, q_2(B_2^{(*)} | B_2^{(*)})}\right\} \\ \theta^{(b)} \text{ otherwise.} \end{cases} ,(18)$$

where

$$L(B_1 \mid y_{ijh2}, B_1, \theta) = \left\{ \prod_{i=1}^{k} \prod_{j=1}^{n_i} \prod_{h=1}^{m_i} \frac{y_{ijh2}^{\delta_{ijh2}-1} e^{-y_{ijh2}/\beta_2}}{\Gamma(\delta_{ijh2}) \beta_2^{\delta_{ijh2}}} \right\} \cdot \frac{\eta_2^{\lambda_2}}{\Gamma(\lambda_2)} \beta_2^{-\lambda_2 - 1} e^{-\eta_2/\beta_2}.$$

3.3 Updating Copula Parameter

Copula measures the complex dependence between variables. Although there are lots of ways to estimate the copula parameter θ in the literature, the derivative-based estimation of the copula parameter is ad hoc, especially for high-dimensional data. The MCMC method via M–H algorithm to estimate the copula parameter is an effective alternative. In this case, the M–H algorithm to estimate the parameter $\theta \mid D, B_1, B_2$, is as follows:

1. Set the initial value of θ, say $\theta^{(1)}$.
2. At each bth Gibbs sampling iteration, simulate the candidate $\theta^{(*)}$ from their transition densities q_3 and $w \overset{iid}{\sim} \text{U}(0, 1)$, then

$$\theta^{(b+1)} = \begin{cases} \theta^{(*)} \text{ if } w \leq \min\left\{1, \dfrac{L(\theta^{(*)} \mid D, B_1, B_2)\, q_3(\theta^{(*)} | \theta^{(b)})}{L(\theta^{(b)} \mid D, B_1, B_2)\, q_3(\theta^{(b)} | \theta^{(*)})}\right\} \\ \theta^{(b)} \text{ otherwise.} \end{cases} ,$$

where the posterior likelihood is proportional to Eq.(13) times the non-informative prior of θ, $\pi(\theta) \propto 1$, which is

$$L(\theta | D, B_1, B_2) = \prod_{i=1}^{k} \prod_{j=1}^{n_i} \prod_{h=1}^{m_i} c_\theta(F_1(y_{ijh1}; \delta_{ijh1}^{(b)}, \beta_1^{(b)}), F_2(y_{ijh2}; \delta_{ijh2}^{(b)}, \beta_2^{(b)}) \cdot 1. \tag{19}$$

The sample means of these MCMC samplers, $\{\Theta^{(b)}\}_{b=N_b+1}^{N}$, after some burn-in periods N_b are the Bayes estimates.

3.4 Model Comparison

Once the parameters are estimated, there arises the question of model selection. Bayesian model comparison is a method of model selection based on Bayes factors. See, for example, Gelman et al. [8] and Chen [2]. The Bayes factor is a likelihood ratio of the posterior marginal likelihood of two competing models, which can be written as the posterior probability odds of models M_i and M_j multiplied by the model priors' odds. That is, the Bayes factor in favor of M_i and against M_j is defined as

$$B_{ij} = \frac{\Pr(D|M_i)}{\Pr(D|M_j)} = \frac{\frac{\Pr(M_i|D)\Pr(D)}{\Pr(M_i)}}{\frac{\Pr(M_j|D)\Pr(D)}{\Pr(M_j)}} = \frac{\Pr(M_i|D)}{\Pr(M_j|D)}\frac{\Pr(M_j)}{\Pr(M_i)}, \tag{20}$$

where D is the data, and $\Pr(M_i|D)$ is the posterior probability (likelihood) of model M_i. When the two models are equally probable a priori, i.e., $\Pr(M_i) = \Pr(M_j)$, the Bayes factor is equal to the ratio of the posterior probabilities of M_i and M_j. That $B_{ij} > 1$ indicates that M_i is a better model fitting than M_j. In our case, it is fair to assume $\Pr(M_i) = 1/3$ for $i = 1, 2, 3$ since the underlying three models are equally preferred.

The posterior probability can be approximated by the likelihood function of the MCMC sampler of Θ (see Chen [2]).

$$\Pr(D|M_i) = \int L(D|M_i, \Theta)\pi(\Theta|M_i)\, d\Theta = \mathrm{E}_{\pi(\Theta)}\left(\Pr(D|M_i, \Theta)\right)$$
$$\approx \frac{1}{N - N_b}\sum_{b=N_b}^{N} \Pr(D|M_i, \Theta^{(b)}), \tag{21}$$

where $\{\Theta^{(b)}\}_{b=1}^{N}$ is the MCMC sampler of Θ, N is the number of MCMC iterations, N_b is the burn-in period, and $\Pr(D|M_i, \Theta^{(b)}) = L(D|M_i, \Theta^{(b)})$ is the likelihood function evaluated at $\Theta = \Theta^{(b)}$ in Eq.(11) at each bth Gibbs sampling iteration.

4 Numerical Analysis

4.1 Simulation Study

To show the performance of our proposed approach, an extensive simulation study is conducted to calculate the mean square errors (MSEs) of the Bayes estimates. For the computational simplicity, let us consider the data experiment: let ADT experiment $k = 6$ treatments, 26 weeks (one week = 168 h) for ADT, check the test for every two weeks, the number of measurement times is $m = m_i = 13$ for all treatments, scaled time increment is 14, $[L_{1i}]_{i=1}^{6} = [25, 45, 60, 75, 75, 75]$,

$[L_{2i}]_{i=1}^{6} = [350, 650, 650, 450, 550, 650]$, and the same target parameters (i.e., $B_1 = B_2$) are $r_{01} = -2.902$, $r_{11} = r_{12} = 0.577, r_{21} = r_{22} = 0.533$, and $\beta_1 = \beta_2 = 0.662$, and θ is one of the Clayton, Frank, and Gumbel copula parameters in Eq. (2), (4), and (6). $n_1 = n_2 = n$ pairs of bivariate Gamma variates $\{(y_{ijk1}, y_{ijk2})\}_{i,j,k}$ from the Clayton, Frank, or Gumbel copula with marginal distribution are, respectively, simulated using the R copula package. Our proposed MCMC method in Sect. 3.3 with non-informative parameter prior distributions is then applied to calculate the Bayes estimates.

Using R NIMBLE packages to implement the MCMC estimation computation, see, for example, de Valpine et al. [6, 7], the following tables summarize the approximated MSEs of selected parameters θ, r_{01}, r_{11}, r_{21}, β_1 in 500 times of simulation study. Selected R NIMBLE codes that simulate bivariate Gamma variates with Clayton copula and estimate the corresponding parameters using MCMC method are included in Appendix.

From Table 1, we see, regardless of the Clayton, Frank, or Gumbel copula functions, as the sample size $6 \times n \times 13$ of bivariate data is getting larger, all the MSEs of all parameters get smaller. This demonstrates the effectiveness of our proposed MCMC method.

Table 1 The Bayes estimate of each parameter is the sample mean of its 21,000 MCMC samplers after 1000 burn-in periods at each simulation run. The values at each cell are the MSEs and bias with parenthesis, respectively

Parameter	θ	r_{01}	r_{11}	r_{21}	β_1
Clayton copula $\theta = 3$					
$n_i = 2$	0.15417	0.01619	0.02127	0.01953	0.00489
	(0.05696)	(0.01786)	(−0.01139)	(−0.01141)	(0.00526)
$n_i = 5$	0.11739	0.00776	0.00689	0.00718	0.00158
	(−0.0187)	(0.01544)	(−0.01975)	(−0.00791)	(0.00623)
$n_i = 10$	0.02979	0.00393	0.00352	0.00293	0.00088
	(−0.01236)	(0.00550)	(−0.00168)	(−0.00169)	(−0.00100)
Frank copula $\theta = 3$					
$n_i = 2$	0.37304	0.01539	0.02294	0.02655	0.00388
	(−0.00414)	(0.00972)	(−0.00735)	(−0.02397)	(0.01439)
$n_i = 5$	0.11248	0.00752	0.00844	0.00693	0.00143
	(−0.03808)	(0.01451)	(−0.00969)	(−0.00862)	(0.000695)
$n_i = 10$	0.05625	0.00403	0.00355	0.00295	0.00069
	(0.00559)	(0.00493)	(−0.00756)	(−0.0007)	(0.00237)
Gumbel copula $\theta = 3$					
$n_i = 2$	0.07767	0.02045	0.03455	0.01666	0.00625
	(0.04093)	(0.05120)	(−0.01838)	(−0.06294)	(0.01656)
$n_i = 5$	0.02334	0.01111	0.01115	0.01186	0.00213
	(0.00963)	(0.01589)	(−0.00637)	(−0.01054)	(0.00086)
$n_i = 10$	0.01493	0.00454	0.00413	0.00433	0.00116
	(0.00118)	(0.01660)	(−0.00871)	(−0.01145)	(−0.00140)

4.2 Numerical Example

In this section, three data sets of $\{y_{ijkl}\}$, namely D_1, D_2, and D_3, with sample size 156 (= 6∗2∗13) from the Clayton, Frank, and Gumbel copulas with the same copula parameter $\theta = 3$ are, respectively, simulated. To observe the behavior of bivariate copulas, the scatter plots and contour plots of datasets D_1, D_2, and D_3 along with those for the three copulas with $\theta = 6$ are shown in Figs. 1 and 2, respectively. We see that the two-dimensional density of Frank copula, blue contours in the two figures, is more dense than the Clayton and Gumbel copulas. This shows that the bivariate data from the Frank copula is more highly correlated than the others.

Given the data sets D_1, D_2, and D_3 assuming from Clayton (M_1), Frank (M_2), and Gumbel (M_3) copulas, the Bayes point and interval estimation with non-informative prior distribution is calculated and summarized in Table 2. Look at the estimation of $D_i|M_i$, $i = 1, 2, 3$ in the first, fifth, and ninth rows in Table 2.

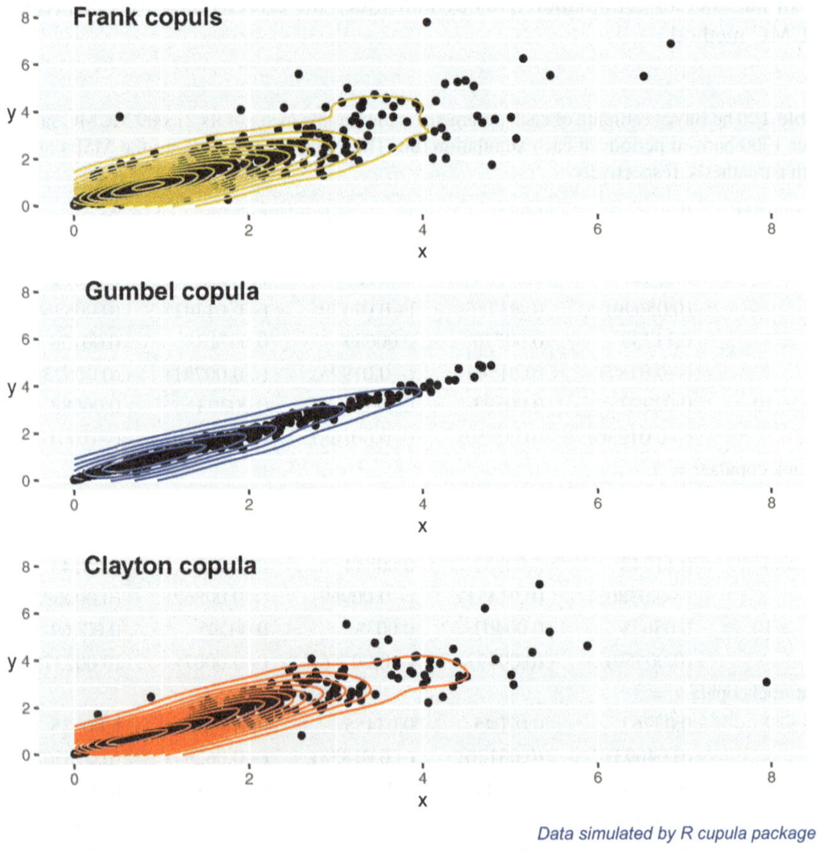

Fig. 1 $\theta = 3$

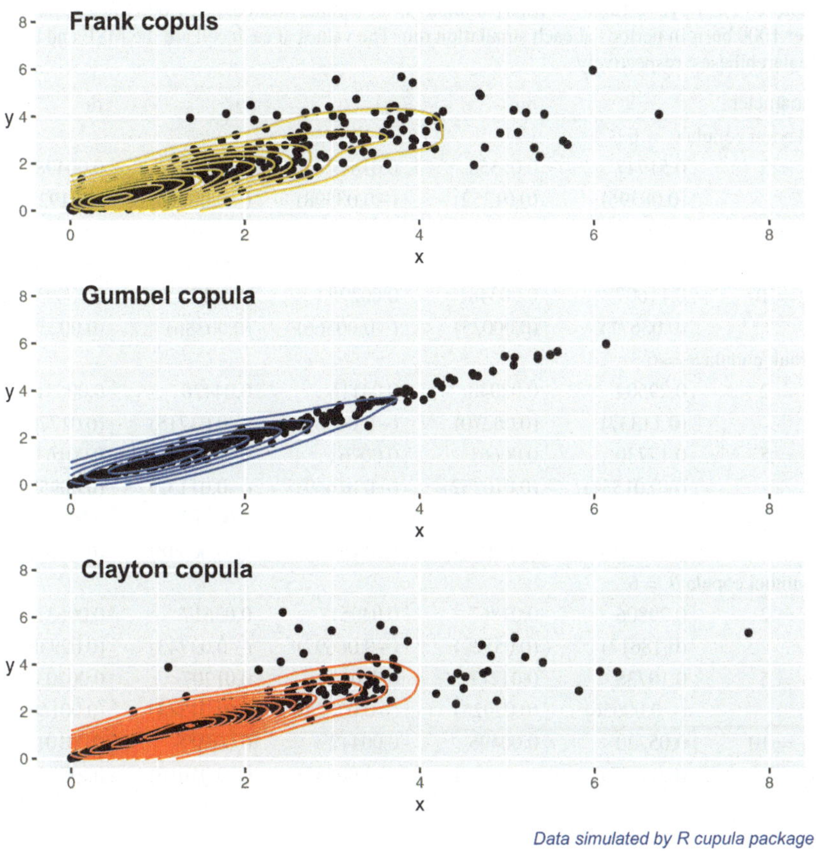

Fig. 2 $\theta = 6$

The point estimates are around the target parameter values, and the corresponding credible sets also cover the true parameters. It is saying that the parameters are correctly estimated if data sets D_1, D_2, or D_3 are from the targeted models M_1, M_2, or M_3, respectively. Otherwise, the estimation is not good since wrong models are analyzed.

Moreover, we see that the marginal likelihood $\Pr(D_1|M_1) = \exp(-267.38)$ by Eq. (21) is greater than $\Pr(D_1|M_2) = \exp(-289.74)$ and $\Pr(D_1|M_3) = \exp(-306.15)$. It indicates that the Bayes factors B_{12} and B_{13} in Eq. (20) with equally likely model preference $\Pr(M_1) = \Pr(M_2) = \Pr(M_2) = \frac{1}{3}$ are much larger than 1. Therefore, given the data set D_1, the model coming from the bivariate Gamma Clayton copula is more likely. Similar conclusions can be drawn that the data sets D_2 and D_3 are from the Frank and Gumbel copulas, respectively, as expected (see, Table 3).

Table 2 The Bayes estimate of each parameter is the sample mean of its 21,000 MCMC samplers after 1000 burn-in periods at each simulation run. The values at each cell are the MSE and bias in the parentheses, respectively

Parameter	θ	r_{01}	r_{11}	r_{21}	β_1
Clayton copula $\theta = 6$					
$n_i = 2$	0.51947	0.01558	0.01844	0.01566	0.00498
	(0.08396)	(0.01352)	(−0.03398)	(−0.00864)	(0.01922)
$n_i = 5$	0.20282	0.00771	0.00555	0.00566	0.00206
	(0.05614)	(0.00911)	(−0.01167)	(0.00349)	(0.00086)
$n_i = 10$	0.11607	0.003481	0.00295	0.00273	0.00093
	(0.03671)	(0.00025)	(−0.00566)	(0.00386)	(0.00231)
Frank copula $\theta = 6$					
$n_i = 2$	0.29509	0.02048	0.04116	0.04420	0.00631
	(0.11337)	(0.06270)	(−0.06062)	(−0.03715)	(0.01770)
$n_i = 5$	0.17730	0.00661	0.00761	0.00737	0.00163
	(−0.01554)	(0.010252)	(−0.01669)	(−0.01132)	(0.00951)
$n_i = 10$	0.07859	0.00351	0.00386	0.00319	0.00067
	(0.02316)	(0.00690)	(−0.01145)	(−0.00048)	(0.00164)
Gumbel copula $\theta = 6$					
$n_i = 2$	0.29806	0.01867	0.04051	0.03617	0.00631
	(0.18612)	(0.05529)	(−0.06697)	(−0.03743)	(0.02938)
$n_i = 5$	0.10738	0.01217	0.01042	0.01207	0.00203
	(−0.00656)	(0.02926)	(−0.02225)	(−0.01314)	(0.00168)
$n_i = 10$	0.05720	0.00496	0.00442	0.00509	0.00101
	(0.00637)	(0.01350)	(−0.00485)	(−0.01015)	(0.00124)

5 Concluding Remarks

The ADT with two stress variables in a GP model has been an important approach to evaluate the reliability of highly reliable products. Following the working assumptions of GEM model, the estimation problem is typically transferred to bivariate Gamma variates. Many researchers had studied the MLEs of the reliability under Gamma process. (See, for example, Ling et al. [15] and Tsai et al. [26]). However, this differentiation-based MLEs of the bivariate Gamma variates are sometimes not steady. The existing estimations are ad hoc.

In this chapter, we proposed three bivariate Gamma processes with the Clayton, Frank, and Gumbel copulas to describe the dependence characteristics of the bivariate ADT variables and apply MCMC method to do Bayesian estimation for the bivariate Gamma variates with copulas and model selection. Intensive simulation studies show that not only the performance of the GP model parameter and copula estimation in terms of the MSEs are as good as the expectation but also for the model selection problem, the Bayes factors given by computing their posterior likelihood identify the correct target model among three possible copulas.

Table 3 The values at each cell are the point estimate and the credible set in the parentheses

$D_1 \sim$ Clayton copula $\theta = 3, r_{01} = -2.9, r_{11} = 0.577, r_{21} = 0.531, \beta_1 = 0.662$						
	$\widehat{\theta}$	$\widehat{r}_{01}$	$\widehat{r}_{11}$	$\widehat{r}_{21}$	$\widehat{\beta}_1$	$\log(\Pr(D_1 \mid M_i))$
M_1	3.2662 (2.47, 4.19)	−2.7214 (−2.99, −2.51)	0.6029 (0.33, 0.88)	0.3066 (0.01, 0.59)	0.6420 (0.53, 0.79)	−267.38
M_2	8.9540 (7.37, 10.6)	−2.9020 (−2.91, −2.90)	0.6776 (0.35, 0.97)	0.3433 (0.01, 0.64)	0.6502 (0.54, 0.78)	−288.74
M_3	2.3442 (1.93, 2.82)	−2.6777 (−2.92, −2.51)	0.5079 (0.10, 0.80)	0.2334 (0.01, 0.57)	0.7276 (0.58, 0.92)	−306.15
$D_2 \sim$ Frank copula $\theta = 3, r_{01} = -2.9, r_{11} = 0.577, r_{21} = 0.531, \beta_1 = 0.662$						
	$\widehat{\theta}$	$\widehat{r}_{01}$	$\widehat{r}_{11}$	$\widehat{r}_{21}$	$\widehat{\beta}_1$	$\log(\Pr(D_2 \mid M_i))$
M_1	0.5831 (0.30, 0.91)	2.7500 (−3.00, −2.53)	0.4135 (0.12, 0.67)	0.5505 (0.29, 0.80)	0.6455 (0.54, 0.77)	−360.93
M_2	3.5226 (2.41, 4.66)	−2.8920 (−2.90, −2.89)	0.5340 (0.27, 0.76)	0.5878 (0.33, 0.84)	0.6544 (0.55, 0.78)	−351.46
M_3	1.4375 (1.25, 1.65)	−2.7292 (−2.98, −2.52)	0.4198 (0.05, 0.68)	0.5037 (0.23, 0.77)	0.6556 (0.54, 0.79)	−357.04
$D_3 \sim$ Frank copula $\theta = 3, r_{01} = -2.9, r_{11} = 0.577, r_{21} = 0.531, \beta_1 = 0.662$						
	$\widehat{\theta}$	$\widehat{r}_{01}$	$\widehat{r}_{11}$	$\widehat{r}_{21}$	$\widehat{\beta}_1$	$\log(\Pr(D_3 \mid M_i))$
M_1	1.8019 (1.27, 2.39)	−2.7872 (−3.07, −2.54)	0.5080 (0.23, 0.75)	0.5368 (0.29, 0.79)	0.6149 (0.50, 0.74)	−290.69
M_2	8.3216 (6.78, 9.94)	−2.9389 (−2.94, −2.93)	0.6407 (0.49, 0.79)	0.5719 (0.42, 0.71)	0.5882 (0.52, 0.66)	−267.81
M_3	2.5861 (2.22, 2.99)	−2.7762 (−2.96, −2.60)	0.5850 (0.41, 0.75)	0.5470 (0.38, 0.70)	0.5493 (0.48, 0.63)	−255.23

Appendix

Below are the R codes via NIMBLE package in Bayesian using Gibbs sampling (BUGS) language to estimate the parameters (s1, r2, s2, r2), including copula parameter (theta).

```
# install.packages("copula")          ## R copula package
                                          (r-nimble.org)
# install.packages("nimble", type="source")
#    NIMBLE needs a C++ compiler and the standard utility 'make'
     to generate and compile C++


library(nimble)                     ## call NIMBLE package
library(copula)                     ## call copula package
                                    ## Generate bivariate Gamma
                                    variates from  Clayton copula
theta =3 # the target copula parameter
n1=n=3                              ## no. of units used for each
                                       treatment

C=50
k=6                                 ## set up k=6 treatments
```

```
tU=168*26                          ## 26 weeks (one week=168
                                      hours) for ADT
t=seq(0,tU,168*2)/24               ## check the test each two weeks
m=length(t)-1                      ## no. of measurement times
dt=t[2:(m+1)]-t[1:m]               ## scaled time increments
LL=L=array(dim=c(6,2))
LL[1,]=c(25, 350)
LL[2,]=c(45, 650)
LL[3,]=c(60, 650)
LL[4,]=c(75, 450)
LL[5,]=c(75, 550)
LL[6,]=c(75, 650)
mL1=max(LL[,1])
mL2=max(LL[,2])
L[,1]=(1/(25+273.15)-1/(LL[,1]+273.15))/(1/(25+273.15)-1/
(mL1+273.15))
L[,2]=(log(LL[,2])-log(350))/(log(mL2)-log(350))
r0=-2.902;  r1=0.577; r2=0.533; r3=0.531; be=0.662
v.r=c(r0,r1,r2,r3,be)

generatedata=function(v,t,be,n1, theta)
 {m=length(t)-1             # no. of measurement times
  y=array(dim=c(2,m,n1,k))
for (i in 1:k)
{for (j in 1:n1){
     cop <- claytonCopula(param = theta, dim = 2)
     U <- rCopula(m, cop)
     y[1,,j,i]= qgamma(U[,1],shape=v[i]*dt[i],scale=be)
     y[2,,j,i]= qgamma(U[,2],shape=v[i]*dt[i],scale=be)
     }
}
return(y) # 4 dimensional data
}

v=rep(0,k)
v0=exp(r0)
for (i in 1:k) {v[i]=v0*exp(r1*L[i,1]+r2*L[i,2]+r3*L[i,1]
                     *L[i,2])} #delta

yy= generatedata (v,t,be,n1, theta)  # generate the bivariate
                                        copula data
y1=yy[1,,,]; y2=yy[2,,,]
zeros=array(0,dim=c(m,n1,k))
mydata=list(xx=y1, yy=y2,  L=L , r3=0.531) # the data set
myinits=function()list(theta=5, r0=-2.8,  r1=0.4, r2=0.4,
                        be=0.5) # initial values

ClaytonCode=nimbleCode({             # likelihood defined below
for (mm in 1:13){
for( nn in 1:n1){
  for (ii in 1:6){
    delta[mm,nn,ii] <- (exp(r0)*exp(r1*L[ii,1]+r2*L[ii,2]+r3
                                 *L[ii,1]*L[ii,2]))* 14
    dummy[mm,nn,ii] ~ dpois(negLogLike[mm,nn,ii]) # zero trick
```

```
    u[mm,nn,ii]<- pgamma(xx[mm,nn,ii], shape=delta[mm,nn,ii],
                       scale=be)      # marginal gamma CDF
    v[mm,nn,ii]<- pgamma(yy[mm,nn,ii], shape=delta[mm,nn,ii],
                                        scale=be)
    negLogLike[mm,nn,ii]<-  100+(-1)*logLike[mm,nn,ii]
    logLike[mm,nn,ii]<- log(theta+1)+(-theta-1)*log(u[mm,nn,ii]
                                                *v[mm,nn,ii])+
         ((-1)*(2*theta+1)/theta)*log(u[mm,nn,ii]^(-theta)+
         v[mm,nn,ii]^(-theta)-1)+
         log(dgamma(xx[mm,nn,ii], delta[mm,nn,ii],scale=be))+
         log(dgamma(yy[mm,nn,ii],delta[mm,nn,ii],scale=be))
  ## negLogLike[mm,nn,ii]= (-1)*log-likelihood, which is
     "the negative value of the log-likelihood function"
  ## logLike[mm,nn,ii] is the log-likelihood of Eq.(3)
}}}
theta~ dgamma(.01,.01)    # parameter's prior distributions
r0  ~ dunif(-3.5,-2.5)
r1  ~ dgamma(.01,.01)
r2  ~ dgamma(.01,.01)
be ~  dgamma(.01,.01)
}) # end of nimbleCode function
                                                 # computing the
                                                 estimation by MCMC
                                                 method
mcmc.out=nimbleMCMC(ClaytonCode,                 # call  "Clayton
                                                 Code" nimbleCode
 monitors=c("theta","r0", "r1", "r2","be"),      # interested param-
                                                     eters
 constants=list(xx=y1, yy=y2, L=L, r3=0.531, n1=n1),
 data=list(dummy=zeros),                         # data and constants
 inits=myinits, thin=1,                          #  initial values
 nchains=2, niter=20000, nburnin=1000,           # 2 chains, 20000
                                                   MCMC iterations,
                                                   1000 burn-in periods
 summary=TRUE)                                   #  summary of the MCMC
                                                   estimation


mcmc.out$summary                                 # the MCMC estimates
## The Bayes estimates:  be=0.6242, r0=-2.8598, r1= 0.4528,
   r2=0.6806, theta= 2.7733
## Below are the sample MCMC outputs.

#$chain1
#             Mean    Median  St. Dev. 95%CI_low 95%CI_upp
#    be      0.6267   0.6231   0.0619    0.5205       0.7647
#    r0     -2.8652  -2.8627   0.1334   -3.1288      -2.6053
#    r1      0.4543   0.4579   0.1364    0.1846       0.7146
#    r2      0.6802   0.6780   0.1255    0.4274       0.9284
#    theta  2.7884   2.7655   0.3917    2.0927       3.6011

#$chain2
#            Mean    Median  St. Dev.  95%CI_low 95%CI_upp
#    be      0.6217   0.6183   0.0629    0.5083       0.7606
```

```
#     r0      -2.8545  -2.8513   0.1357   -3.1315         -2.6027
#     r1       0.4513   0.4509   0.1303    0.1917          0.7012
#     r2       0.6810   0.6815   0.1218    0.4339          0.9195
#     theta  2.7581   2.7353   0.3877    2.0658          3.5689

#$all.chains
#              Mean     Median  St. Dev. 95%CI_low 95%CI_upp
#     be       0.6242   0.6205   0.0625    0.5141          0.7623
#     r0      -2.8598  -2.8568   0.1347   -3.1300         -2.6035
#     r1       0.4528   0.4544   0.1334    0.1886          0.7081
#     r2       0.6806   0.6796   0.1237    0.4306          0.9247
#     theta  2.7733   2.7475   0.3900    2.0775          3.5940
```

References

1. Boulanger, M., Escobar, L. A.: Experimental design for a class of accelerated degradation tests. Technometrics **36**, 260–272 (1994)
2. Chen, M. H.: Computing marginal likelihoods from a single MCMC output. Statistica Neerlandica **59**, 16–29 (2005)
3. Chiang, J.-Y, Zhu, J., Lin, Y.-J., Lio, Y.L., Tsai, T.-R.: Inference from two-variable degradation data using genetic algorithm and Markov Chain Monte Carlo Methods. Int. J. Inform. Manag. Sci. **29**, 235–256 (2018)
4. Chib, S., Greenberg, E.: Understanding the metropolis-hastings algorithm. Am. Stat. **49**, 327–335 (1995)
5. Cowles, M.K., Carlin, B.P.: Markov chain Monte Carlo convergence diagnostics: a comparative review. J. Am. Stat. Assoc. **91**(434), 883–904 (1996)
6. de Valpine, P., Paciorek, C., Turek, D., Michaud, N., Anderson-Bergman, C., Obermeyer, F., Wehrhahn Cortes, C., Rodríguez, A., Temple Lang, D., Paganin, S.: NIMBLE: MCMC, Particle Filtering, and Programmable Hierarchical Modeling (2021). https://cran.r-project.org/package=nimble
7. de Valpine, P., Paciorek, C., Turek, D., Michaud, N., Anderson-Bergman, C., Obermeyer, F., Wehrhahn Cortes, C., Rodríguez, A., Temple Lang, D., Paganin, S.: NIMBLE User Manual (2021). r-nimble.org
8. Gelman, A., Carlin, J.B., Stern, H.S., Dunson, D., Vehtari, A., Rubin, D.B.: Bayesian Data Analysis (3rd edn.) Chapman & Hall, London (2013)
9. Geman, S., Geman, D.: Stochastic relaxation, gibbs distributions, and the bayesian restoration of images. IEEE Trans. Pattern Anal. Math. Intell. **6**, 721–741 (1984)
10. Gertsbackh, I.B., Kordonskiy, K.B.: Models of Failure. Springer, New York (1969)
11. Guan, Q., Tang, Y.-C.: Optimal design of accelerated degradation test based on gamma process models. Chinese J. Appl. Probab. Stat. **29**, 213–224 (2013)
12. Hastings, W.K.: Monte Carlo sampling methods using Markov Chains and their applications. Biometrika **57**, 97–109 (1970)
13. Liao, C.-M., Tseng, S.-T.: Optimal design for step-stress accelerated degradation tests. IEEE Trans. Reliab. **55**, 59–66 (2006)
14. Lim, H., Yum, B.-J.: Optimal design of accelerated degradation tests based on Wiener process models. J. Appl. Stat. **38**, 309–325 (2011)
15. Ling, M.H., Tsui, K.L., Balakrishnan, N.: Accelerated degradation analysis for the quality of a system based on the gamma process. IEEE Trans. Reliab. **64**, 463–472 (2015)
16. Lu, C.J., Meeker, W.Q.: Using degradation measures to estimate a time-to-failure distribution. Technometrics **35**, 161–174 (1993)

17. Metropolis, N., Rosenbluth, A.W., Rosenbluth, M.N., Teller, A.H., Teller, E.: Equations of state calculations by fast computing machines. J. Chem. Phys. **21**, 1087–1092 (1953)
18. Padgett, W.J., Tomlinson, M.A.: Inference from accelerated degradation and failure data based on Gaussian process models. Lifetime Data Anal. **10**, 191–206 (2004)
19. Park, C., Padgett, W.J.: Accelerated degradation models for failure based on geometric Brownian motion and gamma process. Lifetime Data Anal. **11**, 511–527 (2005)
20. Park, C., Padgett, W.J.: Stochastic degradation models with several accelerating variables. IEEE Trans. Reliab. **55**, 379–390 (2006)
21. Park, C., Padgett, W.J.: Cumulative damage models for failure with several accelerating variables. Quality Technol. Quant. Manag. **4**, 17–34 (2007)
22. Peng, J.-Y.: A note on optimal allocations for the second elementary symmetric function with applications for optimal reliability design. Nav. Res. Logist. **59**, 278–284 (2012)
23. Tan, M.T., Tian, G.L., Ng, K.W.: Bayesian Missing Data Problems: EM, Data Augmentation and Noniterative Computation. Chapman & Hall/CRC CRC Press, Florida (2010)
24. Tsai, T.-R., Lin, C.-W., Sung, Y.-L., Chou, P.-T., Chen C.-L., Lio, Y.L.: Inference from lumen degradation data under Wiener diffusion process. IEEE Trans. Reliab. **61**, 710–718 (2012)
25. Tsai, C.-C., Tseng, S.-T., Balakrishnan, N.: Optimal burn-in policy for highly reliable products using gamma degradation process. IEEE Trans. Reliab. **60**, 338–350 (2013)
26. Tsai, T.-R., Lio, Y. L., Jiang, N.: Optimal decision on the accelerated degradation test plan under the Wiener process. Qual. Technol. Quantit. Manag. **11**, 461–470 (2014)
27. Tsai, T.-R., Sung, W-Y, Lio, Y. L., Chang, S., Lu, J.-C.: Optimal two-variable accelerated degradation test plan for gamma degradation processes. IEEE Trans. Reliab. **65**, 459–468 (2016)
28. Tseng, S.-T., Balakrishnan N., Tsai, C.-C.: Optimal step-stress accelerated degradation test plan for gamma degradation process. IEEE Trans. Reliab. **58**, 234–245 (2011)
29. Whitmore, G.A.: Estimating degradation by a Wiener diffusion process subject to measurement error. Lifetime Data Anal. **1**, 307–319 (1995)

Part III
Biomedical Data Analysis

Review of Statistical Treatment for Oncology Dose-Escalation Trial with Prolonged Evaluation Window or Fast Enrollment

Xin Wei and Rong Liu

Abstract In this chapter, we start with the review on three classes of methodologies for oncology dose-escalation trial design: the 3+3, the statistical model-based approach including Continuous Reassessment Method (CRM) and Bayesian Logistic Regression Model (BLRM), and the toxicity interval-based algorithms such as Bayesian Optimal Interval Design (BOIN) and Toxicity Probability Interval method (TPI) and their respective variations. The focus of this chapter is to give a comprehensive outline of the various statistical extensions of these methods to address the statistical challenges caused by the prolonged safety evaluation window, or equivalently, the fast enrollment rate. They include, in CRM and BLRM class, the weighted likelihood function method (TITE-CRM), TITE-CRM aided by suspension rule or Bayesian predictive risk for toxicity to avoid aggressive dose escalation, the TITE-CRM that leverages drug cycle information, adaptive time-to-event toxicity distribution, and three-parameter logistic regression extension on the basis of BLRM. In the toxicity interval-based class, we review R-TPI method for the Toxicity Probability Interval method, TITE-BOIN which imputes the unobserved DLT, and BOIN12 which models the long-term toxicity and efficacy concurrently. The methods under discussion can play a valuable role in improving the accuracy of optimal dose identification without sacrificing patient safety or significantly prolonging the trial duration.

1 Introduction

In the pharmaceutical industry, identifying the proper dose of experimental drugs is a critical mission in early phase development. In the field of oncology, the 1960s–1970s witnessed the advent of chemo/radiotherapy for cancer treatment. In these settings, the correlation between the dose of chemotherapy drugs and efficacy is

---

X. Wei · R. Liu (✉)
Global Biometrics and Data Science, Bristol Myers Squibb, New York, NY, USA
e-mail: Xin.Wei@bms.com

Y. Lio et al. (eds.), *Bayesian Inference and Computation in Reliability and Survival Analysis*, Emerging Topics in Statistics and Biostatistics,
https://doi.org/10.1007/978-3-030-88658-5_9

established within a certain dose range. However, dose is a double-edged sword, that is, when the dose is too low, there is little chance for patients to derive treatment benefit while enduring possible toxicity. On the other hand, the unnecessarily high dose increases the risks of adverse events that might offset the improvement of the quality of life as a result of tumor response. Dose-limiting toxicity, DLT, is defined as the type of adverse events that prohibit further dose escalation in the hope for better efficacy.

In a traditional oncology setting, it is generally accepted that the chances for both DLT and tumor response increase concurrently as the dose escalates. A desirable dose that can be used in the latter development stage, therefore, should be at the level that strikes a proper balance between the possibility of achieving efficacy and the level of toxicity that can be managed. Such a dose level, which is defined as maximumly tolerated dose (MTD) or recommended dose for phase 2 trial (RD2P), typically has a DLT rate ranging from 20 to 30%, depending on the specific disease condition and drugs' mechanism of action [18].

The first-in-human (FIH) oncology trial is typically a dose-escalation study with the primary objective of identifying MTD or RD2P. The oldest yet still the most widely used approach is a rule-based algorithm such as the 3+3 method [17]. Briefly, the patients will be enrolled to a specific dose level in a cohort with a fixed size (typically $N = 3$). If none of them experiences any DLT, the next cohort of three subjects will be enrolled to the next higher level. If one subject has at least one DLT, the current dose will be expanded to another three subjects to further characterize the safety profile with the emphasis on DLT. If two or more subjects have DLT among six subjects, the dose will be declared as a non-tolerated dose (NTD). The dose that is one level below NTD, if already has six subjects tested for DLT, will be declared as MTD.

Apparently, the 3+3 method suffers several shortcomings. In theory, it can only target MTD with a DLT rate between 17 and 33% without adequate precision due to its simple rule-based nature. Secondarily, empirical experience shows that the 3+3 approach tends to prematurely stop a trial by identifying as MTD the dose level that is lower than a potentially efficacious and tolerable level. As a result, this design leads to a majority of the trial participants being treated at the suboptimal level and not getting the clinical benefit they otherwise could.

It has been reported that one of the main reasons for the failures in late-phase clinical development is improper dose selection during early phase trials. The methodology such as the 3+3 design, which lacks statistical rigor, is arguably to blame. In 1990, O'Quigley et al. [14] proposed a statistical model-based dose-finding algorithm called Continual Reassessment Method (CRM), which later adopted the full Bayesian solution. It updates the parametric model for dose-toxicity curves based on prior knowledge and the accumulative data in real time. For a first-in-human trial with sparse data and rapid decision-making, this approach is conceptually appealing and in practice demonstrates ability superior to 3+3 in identifying dose levels that have a better chance to succeed in the later development stage. Within the Bayesian framework inspired by CRM, a more modified version of model-based methods, such as Escalation with Overdose Control (EWOC) and

Bayesian Logistic Regression Model (BLRM), have also been put forward and widely applied in the pharmaceutical industry [13].

On the other hand, it has been debated whether it is either necessary or feasible to characterize the full dose-toxicity model using sparse phase I trial data. Both CRM and BLRM require Bayesian modeling of the toxicity data at all dose levels, increasing the operational complexity. More importantly, they are not as simple and transparent as the 3+3 design which the clinical team can readily understand and deploy.

Therefore, simplified versions of model-based methods, sometimes dubbed as statistical model-assisted methods, have also been proposed, as exemplified by the Bayesian Optimal Interval (BOIN) design and the Modified Toxicity probability Interval (mTPI) design [8, 11]. These models do not attempt to characterize the whole dose-toxicity relationship within the dose range being tested; instead, they base the dose recommendation on the frequentist or Bayesian posterior probability of observed toxicity at individual dose level in relation to a prespecified target DLT interval. By doing away with modeling all the observed toxicity data all at once, these interval-based designs provide transparent decision rules that are uniformly applicable to all the dose levels, which is based on the exhaustive enumeration of foreseeable cohort size and DLT number. Essentially, BOIN and mTPI methods provide nearly as transparent and simple implementation as the 3+3 design, with a performance at least comparable to the more complicated CRM or BLRM model.

Among many challenges Phase I dose-finding trials face, delayed or long-term dose-limiting toxicity (DLT) is the one that greatly increases the trial duration. In the first-in-human trial, subjects are tested at a new drug/dose in a very small cohort size, for the sake of caution, typically not exceeding three, before the next group of subjects can be dosed. In order for experimental drugs to be studied in an affordable sample size ($N = 30 \sim 40$) with a reasonable time span, the current dose level needs to be cleared of DLT quickly before the next dose level can be tested. Fortunately, the traditional concept of DLT, conceived during the early days of chemotherapy, presumes cytotoxicity-related DLT develops shortly after the first dosing within the first cycle (28 days). These features make the phase I dose-escalation trial what they look like today.

As more and more molecularly targeted therapies enter the pipeline and market, however, they demonstrate diverse mechanisms of action (MOA) that could impact the onset of DLT. For example, immuno-oncology therapies such as PD-1 checkpoint pathway inhibitors are known for their delayed immuno-response related toxicities and efficacy [12]. Since all the current patients need to clear the DLT window before any new patients can enter the trial, a long DLT observation window will lead to a prolonged trial duration. As an example, a simulation study showed that it will take 4–8 years to complete a dose-escalation trial with 24–48 patients if the DLT window is as long as 6 months [3]. Similarly, even if the DLT observation period itself is not exceedingly long, a relatively rapid enrollment, in case of the high willingness of patient participation, may cause a backlog and long waiting list of enrollment and eventually turn away patients who urgently need the opportunity coming with the potential new therapies.

In these two scenarios, it is beneficial to allow new patients to start treatment while the ones before them are still in the DLT observation period. For an early phase trial with small sample size, however, it is not efficient nor ethical to disregard even the partial information without the ultimate DLT outcome yet. Currently, there are numerous approaches to allow new patients to be enrolled in trial while taking account into the incomplete information carried by patients who have not yet complete DLT window. In this chapter, we will use three sections to discuss the current algorithms to handle the late-onset DLT problems in dose-escalation trials. This section is the summary of the background for the dose-escalation trial. The second section will summarize the basic types of dose-escalation algorithms, and the third section will review the extensions of these basic methods to the case of late-onset toxicity or fast patient enrollment.

2 Dose-Escalation Algorithm

2.1 *The 3+3 method*

Firstly, escalate the dose from the lowest level to the highest level in cohort size of three subjects.

(1) If no DLT is encountered among the three subjects, escalate to the next higher dose level.
(2) In the case of one DLT, three more subjects will be enrolled to the same dose level.
(3) In the case of two or more DLT, the next cohort of three subjects will be dosed at one level lower.
(4) Eventually, if two or more DLT are observed among six subjects treated at one dose, this dose will be declared as a non-tolerable dose (NTD). The dose that is one level below NTD, if already being tested in six subjects, will be declared as MTD.

2.2 *Model-Based Method*

2.2.1 Continual Reassessment Method

First of all, a guessed DLT probability ($\pi(\theta)^d$) for all the dose levels will be solicited from the consultation with the clinical team based on the best available knowledge, such as clinical data from the similar compound, preclinical PK, and toxicity data, etc. The parametric dose-toxicity relationship is expressed by the following one-parameter power model:

$$\pi_\theta(d) = c_d^\theta, \theta > 0$$

where a suggested prior for log(θ) is a normal distribution with mean 0 and variance 1.342. If the prior median of θ is 1, C_d is the prior median at dose *d*.

With the one-parameter exponential function as likelihood function and log normal as the prior distribution for θ, one can derive the posterior distribution of θ via Bayesian theorem:

$$f(y) = \frac{f(y|\lambda)\, g(\lambda)}{g(\lambda|y)}$$

The next dose level, recommended for the incoming new cohort of patients, will be the one whose posterior point estimate of DLT rate is the closest to the MTD level with prespecified DLT rate [14].

2.2.2 Bayesian Logistic Regression Model

Unlike the one-parameter exponential model for CRM, Neuenschwander et al recommend a two-parameter logistic curve to model the dose-toxicity relationship. This curve has quite a few resemblances in the field of biology and medicine, thus has good acceptance among clinicians and translational scientists.

$$\text{logit}\{\pi_\theta(d)\} = \log(\alpha) + \beta \log\left(\frac{d}{d*}\right), \quad \alpha, \beta > 0$$

The logistic model, coupled with the Bernoulli distribution of DLT status, forms the likelihood function for DLT rate. The prior distribution of alpha and beta is specified by lognormal distribution as follows:

$$\log(\alpha) \sim N\left(\mu, \sigma^2\right); \log(\beta) \sim N\left(\mu, \sigma^2\right),$$

where the mean of the logistic parameter can be derived from historical data of the same or similar compound while the variance can be calibrated based on the level of certainty on this prior knowledge [13].

Another feature of BLRM framework, besides making the parametric inference on the dose-toxicity relationship, is to take into consideration the uncertainty of the point estimate of the posterior distribution, which is updated by the upcoming toxicity data based on the prior distribution. The rationale is that various DLT rates can be considered equivalent if they fall into a probability interval that is close or distant enough from MTD with the prespecified DLT probability. Briefly, the MCMC draws from posterior distribution are tabulated based on their chance of falling into the probability regions such as "too low/under dose", "about right/on target" and "too high/overly toxic". The dose level that maximizes the on-target probability, while maintaining the risk of overdose below a prespecified value such as 25%, will be recommended to the next cohort of patients. This approach has been shown to avoid aggressive escalation encountered in CRM method.

2.3 *Toxicity Interval-Based Method*

2.3.1 Modified Toxicity Probability Interval (mTPI)

"All models are wrong, some are useful."

If the main purpose of a dose-escalation algorithm is to identify the one singular dose level that achieves the proper balance between efficacy and safety, some might argue, the attempt to characterize the whole dose-toxicity curve, which could be complex and parameter-rich, might seem to be an overkill. In this spirit, Ji et al proposed a probability interval-based method which only focuses on the toxicity estimation for the current dose level, without borrowing information from other dose levels such as CRM and BLRM [8].

This simple approach is fundamentally Bayesian. With a flat prior beta (1,1), the posterior distribution of DLT rate for the current dose can be expressed as follows:

$$\mathrm{Beta}\left(1 + r_i, 1 + n_i - r_i\right)$$

where n_i is the number of patients enrolled at dose level I, and r_i is the number of patients who experience DLT.

Like BLRM approach, the rate of DLT can be split into three regions: low/under-dose, medium/on-target and high/overdose, which correspond to three different decisions: escalate, retainment and de-escalate, respectively. The chance of true DLT falling into these regions can be modeled by the posterior distribution of the DLT rate, which is often a bell-shaped beta distribution. The region with the highest Unit Probability Mass (UPM), which is specified in the following formula:

$$\mathrm{UPM}\left(i, d\right) = \frac{\Pr\left(M_i \mid \{x_d, n_d\}\right)}{S\left(M_i\right)}$$

will be the recommended decision for the next cohort of patients.

The implementation of this rule causes some unease in practice. For example, when three out of six patients experience DLT, the escalation region will have the highest UPM, thus becoming the recommended decision of the next dose, when most clinicians would probably agree that this kind of safety profile might warrant de-escalation.

To fine-tune mTPI, mTPI-2, the modified version of the original method has been proposed by the same group [5]. Instead of relying on the overall UPM for the whole decision region (low, medium and overdose), a series of sub-regions are constructed within each decision region using the length for the narrowest interval of the three, which typically is the on-target region. Then the maximum UPM for the resulting sub-intervals from the three regions will be compared, and the region with the highest maximum sub-region UPM will be selected as the recommended action. This change enables dose de-escalation in the case of 3 DLT out of 6 subjects.

2.3.2 Bayesian Optimal Interval Design (BOIN)

BOIN is another popular interval-based method that, similar to mTPI-2, makes dose recommendation based on the local point estimator of the toxicity at an individual dose level [10]. It first specifies three toxicity boundaries: Φ, Φ_1 and Φ_2, where Φ is the target DLT rate for MTD, Φ_1 is the highest DLT considered to be suboptimal, and Φ_2 is the lowest DLT rate deemed too toxic. Conceptually, the implementation of BOIN is even simpler than mTPI-2. It directly compares the observed toxicity rate to Φ_1 and Φ_2 , then makes dose recommendation as follows:

(1) Escalate the dose when DLT rate is lower than Φ_1
(2) De-escalate when DLT rate is higher than Φ_2
(3) Otherwise have the next cohort of patients remain on the sample dose level

Φ, as the target MTD level, is solicited from the clinical team through consultation. The selection of Φ_1 and Φ_2 can be optimized by minimizing the selection error rate through the following formulation:

$$\lambda_{1j} = \frac{\log\left(\frac{1-\phi_1}{1-\phi}\right)+n_j^{-1}\log\left(\frac{\pi_{1j}}{\pi_{0j}}\right)}{\log\left(\frac{\phi(1-\phi_1)}{\phi_1(1-\phi)}\right)}$$

$$\lambda_{2j} = \frac{\log\left(\frac{1-\phi}{1-\phi_2}\right)+n_j^{-1}\log\left(\frac{\pi_{0j}}{\pi_{2j}}\right)}{\log\left(\frac{\phi_2(1-\phi)}{\phi(1-\phi_2)}\right)}$$

where λ_{1j} and λ_{2j} are the joint error rates when it comes to making decision in relation to lower and higher bounds of the target DLT interval. It can be shown that $\Phi_1 = 0.6\Phi$ and $\Phi_2 = 1.4\Phi$ provides satisfactory operating characteristics in most clinical scenarios.

3 Time-to-Event Consideration

As discussed in the previous section, both scenarios including long DLT follow-up window/normal enrollment time and normal DLT window/fast enrollment rate may lead to a significant patient backlog. This could result in excessively long trial duration and ethical issues such as delaying patients with terminal illness the access to potential life-saving experimental drugs. To solve this problem, numerous extensions have been built on the previously described frameworks, allowing for the continuous enrollment of new patients before all the current patients have completed DLT evaluation period. We will summarize these developments in this section.

3.1 The 3+3 Method

The rolling-six method has been proposed by Skolnik et al as an extension to the 3+3 rule to accommodate the need to keep enrollment going while the patients of the current cohort are still under DLT evaluation [16]. Instead of suspending enrollment after every three subjects in the 3+3 method, this rolling-six design allows six patients to be under concurrent evaluation before halting enrollment.

Briefly, if the number of the patients who are at the current dose level reaches three, the fourth patient will

(1) Be escalated to the next higher level of the current dose if all three subjects' DLT window are cleared
(2) Stay at the current dose level if at least one subject among the three has not completed their DLT window or one DLT has been reported from these three subjects
(3) Be de-escalated to the next lower level of the current dose if two or more DLT had been reported.

The dosing decision of the fifth and the sixth subject will be the same as above. Extensive simulations results demonstrate that the expansion of three-patients cohort to the "rolling-six" cohort lowers the duration of the dose-escalation trial without exposing patients to excessive toxicity.

The detailed decision rule is summarized as follows (Table 1):

Table 1 The decision table for rolling-six design

	Observed data at dose *d*			Decision	
#Enrolled	# DLTs	# Non-DLTs	# Pending	MTD not exceeded	MTD exceeded
2	0, 1	any	any	S	–
2	2	0	0	D	–
3	0	0, 1, 2	3, 2, 1	S	–
3	0	3	0	E	–
3	1	0, 1, 2	2, 1, 0	S	–
3	≥ 2	any	any	D	–
4	0	0, 1, 2, 3	4, 3, 2, 1	S	S
4	0	4	0	E	S
4	1	0, 1, 2, 3	3, 2, 1, 0	S	S
4	≥ 2	any	any	D	D
5	0	0, 1, 2, 3, 4	5, 4, 3, 2, 1	S	S
5	0	5	0	E	S
5	1	0, 1, 2, 3, 4	4, 3, 2, 1, 0	S	S
5	≥ 2	any	any	D	D
6	0	0, 1, 2, 3, 4	6, 5, 4, 3, 2	Suspend	Suspend
6	0	5, 6	1, 0	E	MTD
6	1	0, 1, 2, 3, 4	5, 4, 3, 2, 1	Suspend	Suspend
6	1	5	0	E	MTD
6	≥ 2	any	any	D	D

From Skolnik [16]

3.2 *CRM/BLRM*

3.2.1 Weighted Likelihood Function Method (TITE-CRM)

The essence of model-based Bayesian framework is to construct posterior distribution of toxicity profile by combing the prior distribution and observed data. In the case of the CRM, the likelihood function of binary DLT data is shown by the following:

$$L_n(\beta) = \prod_{i=1}^{n} F\left(d_{[i]}, \beta\right)^{y_i} \left\{1 - F\left(d_{[i]}, \beta\right)\right\}^{1-y_i}$$

A natural challenge, therefore, is how to deal with the partial toxicity data when concurrently enrolling new patients, while the current patients have not yet finished the whole DLT evaluation window. Entirely discarding the data points due to the lack of the final toxicity call would be inefficient. Before reaching the end of DLT window, a DLT-free subject with a long follow-up already carries more information than the one who just starts the treatment. This difference should be reflected in the data likelihood function when it comes to model update, which is particularly important to the situation of data scarcity in phase I dose-escalation trial.

One solution, as Cheung et al proposed in 2000, is to have the information of unfinished patients contribute less to the posterior distribution than the patients who have the known DLT outcome [3]. This is achieved by penalizing the contribution of an unfinished patient with a weighted likelihood function as follows:

$$\tilde{L}_n(\beta) = \prod_{i=1}^{n} G\left(d_{[i]}, w_{i,n}, \beta\right)^{y_{i,n}} \left\{1 - G\left(d_{[i]}, w_{i,n}, \beta\right)\right\}^{1-y_{i,n}}$$

Cheung et al. showed that a simple linear form of weight function from 0 to 1, in which the information carried by uncompleted DLT-free subject is proportional to the ratio of his/her follow-up time to the length of DLT window, is adequate to provide the satisfactory estimate of MTD while reducing the whole trial duration. The weight function can be expressed as follows:

$$w(u; T) = \frac{u}{T}$$

This weight function assumes a uniform distribution for time-to-DLT. They had also shown that the more complicated forms of the time-to-DLT distribution, such as logistic and Weibull distribution, have similar performance in improving MTD identification and shortening trial duration.

Cheung et al. 's method is called time-to-event continuous reassessment method (TITE-CRM) because the time-to-DLT event is taken into account in the update of the posterior distribution.

3.2.2 TITE-CRM with Suspension Rule

TITE-CRM, in theory, allows for continuous patient accrual without any suspension, for the model already takes full advantage of data that, even when they are incomplete, are available in real time. The real-world clinical practice, however, shows that TITE-CRM could lead to overly aggressive escalation behavior. In order to mitigate this risk, Polley introduced a principled approach to halting accrual for new subjects when the current ones are not adequately followed up [15].

Two user-defined threshold values, m and c, are solicited from clinicians for this purpose. First of all, m is the maximum waiting time a physician is willing to place a prospective subject on the waiting list. c is a threshold to measure the extent of patient safety being evaluated. If the total follow-up time for the patients on the current dose level, defined as V, exceeds threshold c, then it means that the current safety assessment is adequate and the new subjects can start treatment right away without any delay. Otherwise, the clinical team will assign the prospective patient a waiting time that is proportional to the inadequacy of current safety follow-up, setting a cap at m, the maximum waiting time that the clinician team can tolerate. This rule can be expressed by the following formula:

$$S = \begin{cases} m - \left(\frac{m}{c}\right) V, & \text{if } V < c, \\ 0, & \text{if } V \geq c, \end{cases}$$

where S is the waiting time.

Simulation study shows that this mitigation improves the overall trial safety without scarifying the accuracy of the MTD identification.

3.2.3 TITE-CRM with Predictive Risk

In parallel, a more computationally intensive approach had been proposed by Bekele et al. [1]. Instead of assuming DLT occurs at a constant rate during the entire span of clinical observation, they use sequential ordinal modeling to describe the relationship between the dose and time-to-toxicity with the likelihood function as follows:

$$L\left(\boldsymbol{\beta} | D_n\right) = \prod_{i=1}^{n} \Phi\left(\beta_{Y_i^0,k(i)}\right)^{\delta_i} \prod_{h=1}^{Y_i^0-1} \left\{1 - \Phi\left(\beta_{h,k(i)}\right)\right\}$$

This method is basically Bayesian. It calculates the predictive toxicity probability from the posterior distribution. If the predictive toxicity for the prospective patient is too high, too low, on-target, or on-target with a high level of uncertainty, the decision will be to de-escalate, escalate, stay on the same dose or stop accrual to collect more safety information from the ongoing patients, respectively.

The appeal of this approach is that the decision to suspend accrual can be made quantitatively with the predictive toxicity risk. Due to its complexity in rule-setting and derivation of the posterior distribution, however, this method is not used as widely as TITE-CRM and its other variations.

3.2.4 TITE-CRM with Cycle Information

It can be argued that the uniform distribution may be too simplistic to model the true nature of time-to-toxicity distribution, to which the aggressive dose-escalation behavior of TITE-CRM may attribute. Huang et al. propose to leverage the cyclic nature of cancer drug administration to model the time-to-DLT distribution [6]. Due to the cumulative effect of drug exposure, the patients, even when they are not followed up long enough at the current cycle, may carry a large amount of safety information if they are already at a later cycle without experiencing any DLT in the previous cycles. As result, the weight, which will be used to adjust the contribution of incomplete observation to the posterior DLT distribution, is an adaptive function that combines the DLT probability distribution of the previous cycle with the proportion of local safety follow-up time to cycle length, as follows:

$$\hat{w}\left(t, \hat{\boldsymbol{P}}(m)\right) = \begin{cases} \hat{p}_1(m)G(t) & 0 < t \leq t_0 \\ \hat{p}_1(m) + \hat{p}_2(m)G(t - t_0) & t_0 < t \leq 2t_0 \\ \vdots & \vdots \\ \sum_i^{k-1} \hat{p}_i(m) + \hat{p}_k(m)G(t - (k-1)t_0) & (k-1)t_0 < t \leq kt_0 \end{cases}$$

Then the implantation of the weighted likelihood function, the update of prior distribution will follow in the same manner as the standard TITIE-CRM.

3.2.5 TITE-CRM with Adaptive Time-to-DLT Distribution

Another line of effort recognized that the distribution of time-to-toxicity, similar to the dose-toxicity relationship, can be adaptively learned from the real data. Braun proposed that the probability of DLT, rather than being assumed to have constant rate across the evaluation window, can be modeled by a beta distribution Beta $(1, \theta)$ where θ can vary with the dose and determine whether DLT is early or late-onset event. The objective of this approach is to let the learning of time-to-event distribution follow a data-driven mode without the strong assumption for the constant rate [2].

In Braun's method, the initial uniform distribution of time-to-DLT over DLT assessment window [0, T] is generalized to a beta distribution Beta $(1, \theta)$, which is an adaptive weight function with unknown parameter θ:

$$F_c\left(u|Y_i=1,\theta_i\right)=[u/T]^{\theta_i},\ \ \theta_i>0$$

where T is DLT window and u is the incomplete follow-up time.

This becomes uniform distribution when θ =1, as the initial TITE-CRM paper adopted. To model the DLT kinetics as close to reality as possible, θ is allowed to vary with dose as follows:

$$\theta_i=Z_{[i]}^{\lambda},-\infty<\lambda<\infty$$

The likelihood function involving λ and β is:

$$\mathcal{L}_i\left(\beta,\lambda|X_{[i]},T_i,\delta_i\right)=\left[p\left(X_{[i]};\beta\right)(T_i/T)^{\theta_i}\right]^{\delta_i}\left[1-p\left(X_{[i]};\beta\right)(T_i/T)^{\theta_i}\right]^{1-\delta_i}$$

In the following computation, λ, with the prior N (0, σ^2), can be inferred from the posterior DLT distribution along with β, which characterizes the dose-toxicity relationship in the CRM and the TITE-CRM.

Adaptively training the weight function and time-to-event distribution based on real toxicity data seems to be data-driven and less arbitrary. However, as the author suggested, this approach may not manifest its full potential in a phase I setting with a very small sample size. Furthermore, estimating additional parameters might have a statistical cost that, when the performance gain is arguably marginal, is not justifiable.

3.2.6 BLRM Adaptation

In the early phase dose-escalation trial for oncology, it is often time quite common to consider the first cycle as DLT evaluation window, when DLT is projected to occur rather soon after the first dose. This practice may negate the need to account for the time to toxicity in case of long DLT assessment period. When one has a good rationale to extend the DLT window beyond the first cycle, nonetheless, it turns out not to be trivial to explicitly define the length of DLT window. Zheng et al. proposed a three-parameter logistic regression model, built on BLRM framework advocated by Neuenschwander et al, to model patients' different extent of drug exposure during the whole duration, beyond an arbitrarily determined DLT window [22].

BLRM is based upon the assumption that only the tangible variable that impacts DLT rate is the dose, which can be modeled by two parameters: the DLT rate at reference dose (α) and the slope of dose-toxicity curve (β). The approach of Zheng et al. extends BLRM to an additional parameter, the ratio of treatment time of a patient to a reference time window, which can be adopted from a commonly used DLT window. The joint likelihood function based on three-parameter logistic model is described as follows:

$$p(\boldsymbol{d}, \boldsymbol{T}, \boldsymbol{\delta}|\alpha, \beta, \gamma) = \prod_{i=1}^{N} \left\{ \frac{\exp(\alpha)(1/T_0)^{\beta} T_i^{(h)\beta-1} (d_i/d_0)^{\gamma} \beta}{\left[1+\exp(\alpha)(T_i/T_0)^{\beta}(d_i/d_0)^{\gamma}\right]^2} \right\}^{\boldsymbol{I}_{\{\delta_i=1\}}} \left\{ \frac{1}{1+\exp(\alpha)(T_i/T_0)^{\beta}(d_i/d_0)^{\gamma}} \right\}^{\boldsymbol{I}_{\{\delta_i=0\}}}$$

This function will become identical to BLRM formation when the time-to-DLT is capped at T_0, making it a fixed DLT window design.

The rest of the computation can follow the routine of BLRM, though what Zheng et al. actually used in their paper is to go after the dose level with the posterior DLT mean closest to the target MTD.

3.3 *Model-Assisted Method*

3.3.1 R-TPI

The m-TPI2 version of time-to-DLT adjustment is called R-TPI (Rolling-TPI) [4]. Interestingly, this modification, in order to maintain the simplicity in its original formulation, does not require statistically modeling the partial information carried by the patients who have not completed the full DLT evaluation. Instead, R-TPI operates similarly as the rolling-six design.

It first makes dose recommendations based on the status of completed subjects alone, without considering the pending ones. Then, by assuming the safest case scenario (no DLT for pending patients) and the most toxic scenario (all the pending patients will develop DLT eventually by the end of DLT evaluation period), the algorithm checks whether the initial decision is altered by these hypotheticals. If yes, it means that the pending result for the incomplete patients would be a game-changer for dose decision and cautions must be taken; thus the initial dose recommendation will be moderated in terms of its aggressiveness, or the trial will require more pending patients to complete their DLT observation period before the new patient can start the treatment, in order to garner more safety information.

Specifically, the study statistician will work with the clinical team to determine a trial parameter C, which is the maximum pending patients the team can tolerate before enrolling any new patients from safety perspective. Therefore, if the number of pending patients exceeds parameter C, study team would have no option but to halt the patient accrual. On the other hand, if all patients (n_d) in the current dose level complete the required observation window, the decision rule will follow as a routine m-TPI2 approach.

The situation becomes trickier if the number of incomplete patients is between 0 and C, where the following rule will be followed if that is the case:

(1) If the m-TPI2 decision is de-escalation after excluding the pending patients (m_d), it means that the safety profile for the current level is a bit precarious even solely based on the completed subjects (n_d). Then m-TPI2 calculation will be repeated assuming all the pending patients (m_d) are DLT-free eventually. The following are two possible outcomes:

   (a) If the result remains de-escalation, the final decision will be de-escalation, reflecting the fact that even the safest assumption for the pending subjects (m_d) would not neutralize the overly toxic signal from the patients with known outcomes.
   (b) If the recommended change is staying on the same dose (S), it implies moderate but volatile toxicity signal based on the complete patients (n_d). Then R-TPI will check the number of patients who are enrolled to the current dose (k_d) in the last batch. If it is below a certain threshold (say, three), which should be prespecified by the study team and simulation exercises, the new patient will be enrolled to the current dose, that is, to increase the sample size thus reducing the uncertainty by honoring the recommended action: stay. If k_d is greater than the prespecified threshold, on the other hand, it means that the current dose level already has an adequate sample size; the only way to increase the information content will be to halt new patient accrual, letting more pending patients reach their endpoint.

(2) If the m-TPI2 decision is escalating after excluding the pending patients ($\mathrm{m_d}$), it means that the current dose level is confidently safe even solely based on the completed subjects (n_d). Then m-TPI2 calculation will be repeated assuming all the pending patients (m_d) without unknown outcome will develop DLT eventually.

   (a) If the re-calculated decision remains escalation, then the final decision will be to escalate, reflecting the fact that even the most toxic assumption for the pending subjects (m_d) would not change the conclusion of dose being safe based on the patients with the known outcomes.
   (b) If the recommended change is staying on the same dose, it implies a moderate toxicity signal based on the complete patients (n_d), which has a high degree of uncertainty. Then the R-TPI will check the number of patients who are enrolled to the current dose (k_d) in the last batch. If it is below a certain threshold (say, three), new patients will be added to the current dose, that is, to increase the sample size and reduce the uncertainty, by honoring the recommended action: stay. If k_d is greater than the prespecified threshold, it means that the current dose level already has an adequate sample size; the only way to increase the information content will be to halt the patient accrual, letting more pending patients reach their endpoint.

Similar to m-TPI2, the decision rule for R-TPI can also be pre-calculated in the protocol. Its strength of transparency is not lost (Table 2).

Table 2 R-TPI decision table with target DLT rate = 0.3, width of MTD range = 0.1, and C = 3

Observed data at dose d				Decision	
$n_d + m_d$	y_d	n_d	k_d	R-TPI	RSD
1	0	0	1	S	–
1	0	1	1	E	–
1	1	1	1	D	–
2	0	0, 1	any	S	S
2	0	2	any	E	S
2	>0	any	any	D	S or D
3	0	0, 1, 2	3	Suspend	S
3	0	1, 2	<3	S	S
3	0	3	any	E	E
3	1	any	any	S	S
3	>1	any	any	D	D
4	0	1, 2, 3	3	Suspend	S
4	0	2, 3	<3	S	S
4	0	4	any	E	E
4	1	any	any	S	S
4	>1	any	any	D	D
5	0	2, 3, 4	3	Suspend	S
5	0	3, 4	<3	S	S
5	0, 1	5	any	E	E or S
5	1	3, 4	≥3	Suspend	S
5	1	3, 4	<3	S	S
5	>1	any	any	D	D
6	0	3, 4	3	Suspend	Suspend
6	0	4	<3	S	–
6	0	5	any	E	E
6	1	3, 4, 5	3	Suspend	Suspend
6	1	4, 5	<3	S	–
6	0, 1	6	any	E	E
6	2	any	any	S	D
6	>2	any	any	D	D
7	0	4, 5	3	Suspend	–
7	0	5	<3	S	–
7	0	6	any	E	–
7	1	4, 5, 6	3	Suspend	–
7	1	5, 6	<3	S	–
7	0, 1	7	any	E	–
7	2	6, 7	any	S	–
7	>2	any	any	D	–

RSD rolling-six design
From Guo [4]

3.3.2 TITE-BOIN

The time-to-event version of BOIN method takes a different approach from R-TPI. When the new patients are waiting while some patients on the current dose level are still pending without final DLT results, the algorithm goes ahead to impute the DLT result for these pending patients, so that the waiting patients can enter the study in a timely manner, based on both the observed and imputed DLT results [20].

It can be shown that the point estimator of DLT rate at the current dose level, based on both the observed and unknown data, can be given as follows:

$$\hat{p} = \frac{\sum_{i \in O} y_i + \sum_{i \in M} \hat{y}_i}{n} = \frac{s + \frac{p}{1-p}\,(c - \mathrm{STFT})}{n}$$

where O is the set of patients with known outcome of DLT (observed) and M is the set of patients whose DLT status is still pending. With c being the total number of pending patients, STFT is the sum of total follow-up time for the c patients divided by the length of DLT follow-up window, representing the ratio of information carried by those pending patients up to time t_i. This representation assumes the uniform distribution of DLT rate across the DLT evaluation window, which has been proven robust in previous literatures. The only unknown entity in the right side of the equation is p, which can be estimated from the posterior beta distribution for DLT rate based on a vague prior and the patients who cleared DLT window. The p hat on the left will be compared with the toxicity interval in the regular BOIN to facilitate the dose recommendation.

One common strength of R-TPI and TITE-BOIN is that they both produce a transparent decision table in protocol before the first patient is accrued. For TITIE-BOIN at each dose level, the sample size, the number of DLT, the number of pending patients, and the threshold value of STFT are enumerated with the corresponding four different decision-makings for the incoming patients: de-escalate, stay, suspend accrual, and escalation, as follows (Table 3):

Table 3 Dose-escalation and de-escalation rule for TITE-BOIN with a target DLT rate of 02 and cohort size of 3

No. treated	No. DLTs	No. data pending	STFT			No. treated	No. DLTs	No. data pending	STFT		
			Escalate	Stay	Deescalate				Escalate	Stay	Deescalate
3	0	≤1	Y			12	1	6	≥1.24	<1.24	
3	0	≥2		Suspend accrual		12	1	≥7		Suspend accrual	
3	1	≤2			Y	12	2	≤6		Y	
3	≥2	≤1			Y&Elim	12	2	≥7		Suspend accrual	
6	0	≤3	Y			12	3, 4	≤9			Y
6	0	≥4		Suspend accrual		12	≥5	≤7			Y&Elim
6	1	≤3		Y		15	0	≤7	Y		
6	1	≥4		Suspend accrual		15	0	≥8		Suspend accrual	
6	2	≤4			Y	15	1	≤7	Y		
6	≥3	≤3			Y&Elim	15	1	≥8		Suspend accrual	
9	0	≤4	Y			15	2	≤2	Y		
9	0	≥5		Suspend accrual		15	2	3	≥1.14	<1.14	
9	1	≤2	Y			15	2	4	≥2.31	<2.31	
9	1	3	≥0.77	<0.77		15	2	5	≥3.48	<3.48	
9	1	4	≥2.15	<2.15		15	2	6	≥4.65	<4.65	
9	1	≥5		Suspend accrual		15	2	7	≥5.82	<5.82	
9	2	0		Y		15	2	≥8		Suspend accrual	
9	2	1		>0.52	≤0.52	15	3	≤2		Y	
9	2	2		>1.59	≤1.59	15	3	3		>1.16	≤1.16
9	2	3		>2.66	≤2.66	15	3	4		>2.34	≤2.34
9	2	4		>3.73	≤3.73	15	3	5		>3.53	≤3.53
9	2	≥5		Suspend accrual		15	3	6		>4.72	≤4.72
9	3	≤6			Y	15	3	7		>5.90	≤5.90
9	≥4	≤5			Y&Elim	15	3	≥8		Suspend accrual	
12	0	≤6	Y			15	4, 5	≤11			Y
12	0	≥7		Suspend accrual		15	≥6	≤9			Y&Elim
12	1	≤5	Y								

From Yuan et al. [20]

3.3.3 BOIN12

During a long DLT period, which we have discussed so far, it is possible for efficacy signal to emerge alongside with toxicity. An efficient design, therefore, is called for to select the dose with optimal risk-benefit trade-off. Sometimes, it is desirable to model both efficacy and toxicity simultaneously even when DLT window is not very long. For example, CAR-T cell therapy can induce quick and robust efficacy response and potentially severe toxicity at the same time.

Lin et al. proposed that the efficacy/toxicity balance can be quantitated by the following 2 × 2 table [9].

Toxicity \ Efficacy	Yes	No
No	u_1	u_2
Yes	u_3	u_4

where $u_1 - u_4$ represent the utility scores which can be solicited from consultation with the clinical team. Typically, the optimal situation, in which tumor response is achieved in absence of toxicity, can be rewarded 100 (u_1) points with magnitude of 0–100, while toxicity without efficacy, the most undesirable scenario, has score of 0. Different scores between 0 and 100 can be assigned to u_2 and u_3 based on medical consideration, such as value of tumor response, the clinical sequelae of DLT, etc.

Corresponding to the four scenarios laid out above, the number of patients who have clinical outcomes (efficacy/toxicity) can be denoted as $Y(d) = (y_1(d), y_2(d), y_3(d), y_4(4))$, which can be modeled by multinomial distribution. In order to simplify the computation, however, the authors proposed an "quasi-beta distribution" method to solve this complex situation with binomial approximation.

In a regular binomial setting for toxicity alone, the number of DLT at dose d follows a binomial distribution $B(p, n)$. Similarly, the equivalent of the binomial DLT count in "quasi-likelihood" theory here is $x(d)$, the weighted utility score which can be normalized as follows:

$$x(d) = \frac{u_1 y_1(d) + u_2 y_2(d) + u_3 y_3(d) + u_4 y_4(d)}{100}$$

$x(d)$ follows a "quasi-binomial" distribution $Bq\ (u(d), n(d))$ where the expected $u(d)$ is as follows:

$$u(d) = u_1 p_1(d) + u_2 p_2(d) + u_3 p_3(d) + u_4 p_4(d)$$

and $n(d)$ is the total patients treated at dose level d.

The likelihood function, as shown below, has a similar form as binomial probability:

$$L\left(D(d)|u^*(d)\right) \propto \left(u^*(d)\right)^{x(d)}\left(1 - u^*(d)\right)^{n(d)-x(d)}$$

In Bayesian framework, if we assign probability of the utility, $u(d)$, to a beta distribution Beta (α, β) ($\alpha = 1$ and $\beta = 1$ renders a flat prior), its posterior distribution can be formulated as follows:

$$u^*(d) \mid D(d) \sim Beta\,(\alpha + x(d), \beta + n(d) - x(d))$$

In BOIN12 algorithm, the dose recommendation is based on the posterior inference on the probability of the utility, as opposed to DLT rate used in standard BOIN method. Its step-by-step guideline can be laid out as follows:

1. Define the DLT rate boundary for de-escalation and escalation (λ_e, λ_d) in the same fashion as regular BOIN method and start to treat patients at the lowest dose level.
2. Upon observing the DLT rate at dose level d, follow the rules below:
   a. If the observed DLT rate is greater than the upper boundary λ_d, de-escalate to the next lower level $d - 1$.
   b. If DLT rate is on the target range (between λ_e and λ_d), and there are adequate number of patients at the current level (no less than a prespecified number, say, 6 or 9, etc), the dose level d or $(d - 1)$ will be recommended for the new patients, depending on which level has the higher posterior probability of the drug utility, $Pr(u(d) > u_b|D(d))$. Here dose level $d+1$ is not considered for potential better utility because of relatively strong confidence that the current level is not underdose.
   c. If the observed DLT rate is below the lower bound λ_e, or within the target range (between λ_e and λ_d) but with a high degree of uncertainty (the number of treated patients at the current dose is less than a prespecified threshold value), even the dose level $d+1$ which is one level higher than the current dose, in addition to the current level d and its adjacent lower level $d-1$, can be explored for their posterior probability of the utility score. Among these three levels, the one with the highest posterior probability of functional utility will be recommended to the new patients.
3. Once the maximum sample size is reached, DLT level at each dose level will be estimated isotonically and the one whose DLT rate is closest to the target DLT

rate will be declared as MTD. The final recommended dose for phase 2 (RDP2) should be the dose level with highest estimated utility score while not exceeding MTD level.

BOIN12 method retains the strength of BOIN and mTPI-2 that is the transparency to pre-tabulate all the decision-making points prior to the start of a trial. The following is example of decision table (Table 4).

Table 4 Rank-based desirablity score (RDS) table for the BOIN12 design with the upper toxicity limit = 0.35, the lower efficacy limit = 0.25

No. Pts.	No. Tox.	No. Eff.	Desirability Score	No. Pts.	No. Tox.	No. Eff.	Desirability Score	No. Pts.	No. Tox.	No. Eff.	Desirability Score
0	0	0	60	6	3	2	22	9	2	4	45
3	0	0	35	6	3	3	38	9	2	5	58
3	0	1	55	6	3	4	51	9	2	6	70
3	0	2	76	6	3	5	67	9	2	7	83
3	0	3	91	6	3	6	81	9	2	8	92
3	1	0	24	6	4	0	1	9	2	9	98
3	1	1	44	6	4	1	6	9	3	0	E
3	1	2	63	6	4	2	15	9	3	1	7
3	1	3	80	6	4	3	27	9	3	2	14
3	2	0	13	6	4	4	42	9	3	3	25
3	2	1	31	6	4	5	56	9	3	4	36
3	2	2	48	6	4	6	72	9	3	5	49
3	2	3	69	6	≥ 5	≥ 0	E	9	3	6	61
3	3	≥ 0	E	9	0	0	E	9	3	7	74
6	0	0	22	9	0	1	25	9	3	8	85
6	0	1	38	9	0	2	36	9	3	9	94
6	0	2	51	9	0	3	49	9	4	0	E
6	0	3	67	9	0	4	61	9	4	1	3
6	0	4	81	9	0	5	74	9	4	2	9
6	0	5	93	9	0	6	85	9	4	3	17
6	0	6	100	9	0	7	94	9	4	4	29
6	1	0	15	9	0	8	99	9	4	5	40
6	1	1	27	9	0	9	102	9	4	6	53
6	1	2	42	9	1	0	E	9	4	7	65
6	1	3	56	9	1	1	17	9	4	8	78
6	1	4	72	9	1	2	29	9	4	9	88
6	1	5	87	9	1	3	40	9	5	0	E
6	1	6	96	9	1	4	53	9	5	1	2
6	2	0	8	9	1	5	65	9	5	2	5
6	2	1	19	9	1	6	78	9	5	3	10
6	2	2	34	9	1	7	88	9	5	4	20
6	2	3	47	9	1	8	97	9	5	5	32
6	2	4	64	9	1	9	101	9	5	6	45
6	2	5	77	9	2	0	E	9	5	7	58
6	2	6	90	9	2	1	10	9	5	8	70
6	3	0	4	9	2	2	20	9	5	9	83
6	3	1	12	9	2	3	32	9	≥ 6	≥ 0	E

Lin et al., personal communication

3.3.4 Imputation of Unobserved DLT Data

The idea of using imputed DLT outcome from the pending subjects to guide dose recommendation, as has been done in TITE-BOIN method, has seen its application in other literatures [7, 11, 21]. We will have two examples as follows.

Liu et al. showed that the imputed DLT status from pending patients, along with the observed DLT count, can be fit into regular CRM model, leading to the update of the posterior DLT rate and dose recommendation for the incoming patients based on the posterior mean [11]. This process is an iterative process consisting two fundamental steps: (1) imputation of missing DLT value, (2) posterior estimation of the CRM parameter, as summarized below:

1. The time to DLT for subject i is modeled by a piece-wise exponential model as follows:

$$L\left(\mathcal{Y}|\boldsymbol{\lambda}\right) = \prod_{i=1}^{n}\prod_{k=1}^{K} \lambda_k^{\delta_{i,k}} \exp\left\{-\mathcal{Y}_i \lambda_k s_{ik}\right\}$$

where y is DLT status, s_{ik} is the length of k sub-interval of DLT evaluation window, λ_k is the constant hazard rate for kth time interval. In Bayesian framework, λ_k is assumed to follow a prior Gamma distribution:

$$f\left(\lambda_k\right) = G_a\left(\widetilde{\lambda_k}/C, 1/C\right)$$

where the value C can be calibrated to render the prior vague ($C = 2$).

This leads to the posterior distribution, which is conditional on the observed data and model parameters including the power parameter α of the CRM and the DLT hazard rate λ, as follows:

$$\mathcal{Y}_i \mid \left(\mathcal{D}_{\text{obs}}, \boldsymbol{\alpha}, \daleth\right) \sim \text{Bernoulli}\left(\frac{\alpha_{d_i}^{\exp(a)} \exp\left(-\sum_{k=1}^{K} \lambda_k s_{ik}\right)}{1 - \alpha_{d_i}^{\exp(a)} + \alpha_{d_i}^{\exp(a)} \exp\left(-\sum_{k=1}^{K} \lambda_k s_{ik}\right)}\right)$$

The missing DLT data can be imputed by drawing posterior samples from the distribution above.

2. The observed and imputed DLT data can be used to update the posterior distribution of the CRM model, from which α can be sampled. The DLT hazard rate λ_k can be sampled from the conjugate Gamma posterior distribution as follows:

$$\lambda_k \mid \mathcal{Y} \sim \boldsymbol{G_a}\left(\frac{\widetilde{\lambda_k}}{C} + \sum_{i=1}^{n} \delta_{ik}, \frac{1}{C} + \sum_{i=1}^{n} y_i s_{ik}\right)$$

3. The drawn samples of α and λ_k will be fed back into step 1, updating imputation of the missing DLT data. Then α and λ_k will be sampled again from the posterior distribution of the CRM model based on the renewed imputed data. This iterative process, which is also called Bayesian data augmentation method, will go on until Markov chain sampling achieves convergence.
4. The final posterior sampling of α will determine the point estimator of the posterior DLT rate, which will determine the dose recommendation.

This approach is evidently complex. So far there is no definite evidence showing it outperforms other simpler approaches such as R-TPI.

In a related paper published by the same group, this iterative data augmentation process is implemented by EM (Estimation-Maximization) algorithm [21]. In the Estimation step, the missing DLT outcome of y_i can be substituted with its expectation in the form of

$$E\left(\boldsymbol{Y}_i|\boldsymbol{t}_i > \boldsymbol{u}_i, \alpha^{(r)}, \gimel^{(r)}\right) = \frac{p_{di}^{\exp(\alpha^r)} \prod_{k:\tau_k < u_i} \left(1 - \lambda_k^{(r)}\right)}{1 - p_{di}^{\exp(\alpha^r)} + p_{di}^{\exp(\alpha^r)} \prod_{k:\tau_k < u_i} \left(1 - \lambda_k^{(r)}\right)}$$

Then in the M step, the MLE of the CRM power parameter α and the DLT hazard rate λ_k by the following likelihood function:

$$\lambda_k^{(r+1)} = m_k / \sum_{j=k}^{K} \left(m_j + \sum_{i \in C_j} \hat{y}_i\right)$$

$K = 1, \ldots, K$, an estimate analogous to Kaplan-Meier's estimator and

$$\boldsymbol{L}\left(\mathbf{y}|\boldsymbol{\alpha}\right) = \prod_{\boldsymbol{i}=1}^{\boldsymbol{n}} \left\{p_{di}^{\exp(\alpha)}\right\}^{y_i} \left\{1 - p_{di}^{\exp(\alpha)}\right\}^{1-\boldsymbol{y}_{\boldsymbol{i}}}$$

respectively.

Furthermore, this EM-CRM framework also allows multiple dose-toxicity "skeletons" to be selected, and the Bayesian model selection and averaging will be employed to give the best estimate for the CRM power parameter α, which is the basis for DLT rate estimation and subsequent dose recommendation.

3.4 *Use Kaplan-Meier Method to Derive Fractional DLT for Pending Subjects*

Finally, the missing DLT status of pending patients can be replaced by fraction of 1, depending on the proportion of follow-up time to the full DLT observation window. This fractional value can be used in either rule-based method such as the 3+3 after rounding, or model-based method such as CRM/BLRM , given that the specification of likelihood function can take fraction as the input value [19].

When a subject completes the DLT window, his DLT status y_i will be either 0 or 1, depending on whether they experience DLT. When a patient's final DLT status is still pending upon a new patient enters, however, their fractional DLT values can be computed as follows:

$$\hat{y}_i = \frac{\hat{S}(u_i) - \hat{S}(\tau)}{\hat{S}(u_i)}$$

where S is Kaplan-Meier estimator of survival function at u_i or τ. The KM survival estimator is expressed as:

$$\hat{S}(t_i) = \prod_{j=1}^{i} \left(1 - d_j/Y_j\right)$$

With the missing DLT data replaced by a fractional DLT, they can serve as input for any dose-escalation method mentioned above.

4 Summary

In this chapter, we started with the review on three classes of methodologies for oncology dose-escalation trial design: the 3+3, the statistical model-based approach including Continuous Reassessment Method (CRM) and Bayesian Logistic Regression Model (BLRM), and the toxicity interval-based algorithms such as Bayesian Optimal Interval Design (BOIN) and Toxicity Probability Interval method (TPI) and their respective variations. The focus of this chapter is to give a comprehensive outline of the various statistical extensions of these methods to address the statistical challenges caused by the prolonged safety evaluation window, or equivalently, the fast enrollment rate. They include, in CRM and BLRM class, the weighted likelihood function method (TITE-CRM), TITE-CRM aided by suspension rule or Bayesian predictive risk for toxicity to avoid aggressive dose escalation, the TITE-CRM that leverages drug cycle information, adaptive time-to-event toxicity distribution, and three-parameter logistic regression extension on the basis of BLRM. In the toxicity interval-based class, we review R-TPI method for Toxicity Probability Interval method, TITE-BOIN which imputes the unobserved DLT and BOIN12 which models the long-term toxicity and efficacy concurrently. The methods under discussion can play a valuable role in improving the accuracy of optimal dose identification without sacrificing patient safety or significantly prolonging the trial duration.

References

1. Bekele, B., Ji, Y., Shen, Y., Thall, P.: Monitoring late-onset toxicities in phase I trials using predicted risks. *Biostatistics*. **9**(3), 442–457 (2008)
2. Braun, T.: Generalizing the TITE-CRM to adapt for early- and late-onset toxicities. *Stat Med*. **25**(12), 2071–2083 (2006)
3. Cheung, Y., Chappell, R.: Sequential designs for phase I clinical trials with late-onset toxicities. *Biometrics*. **56**(4), 1177–1182 (2000)
4. Guo, W., Ji, Y., Li, D.: R-TPI: rolling toxicity probability interval design to shorten the duration and maintain safety of phase I trials. *J Biopharm Stat*. **29**(3), 411–424 (2019)
5. Guo, W., Wang, S.J., Yang, S., Lynn, H., Ji, Y.: A Bayesian interval dose-finding design addressing Ockham's razor: mTPI-2. *Contemp Clin Trials*. **58**, 23–33 (2017)
6. Huang, B., Kuan, P.: Time-to-event continual reassessment method incorporating treatment cycle information with application to an oncology phase I trial. *Biom J*. **56**(6), 933–946 (2014)
7. Jin, I., Liu, S., Thall, P., Yuan, Y.: Using data augmentation to facilitate conduct of phase I-II clinical trials with delayed outcomes. *J Am Stat Assoc*. **109**(506), 525–536 (2014)
8. Ji, Y., Liu, P., Li, Y., Bekele, B.N.: A modified toxicity probability interval method for dose-finding trials. *Clin Trials*. **7**(6), 653–663 (2010)
9. Lin, R., Zhou, Y., Yan, F., Li, D., Yuan, Y.: Personal communication (2020)
10. Liu, S., Yuan, Y.: Bayesian optimal interval designs for phase I clinical trials. J. R. Stat. Soc. Ser. C. **64**, 507–523 (2015)
11. Liu, S., Yin, G., Yuan, Y.: Bayesian data augmentation dose finding with continual reassessment method and delayed toxicity. *Ann Appl Stat*. **7**(4), 1837–2457 (2013)
12. Shah, N.J., et al.: Delayed toxicities with anti-PD-1 and anti-PDL-1 immune checkpoint inhibitors (ICIs). *J. Clin. Oncol*. **36**(15 suppl) (2018)
13. Neuenschwander, B., Branson, M., Gsponer, T.: Critical aspects of the Bayesian approach to phase I cancer trials. *Stat Med*.**27**(13), 2420–2439 (2008)
14. O'Quigley, J., Pepe, M., Fisher, L.: Continual reassessment method: a practical design for phase 1 clinical trials in cancer. *Biometrics*. **46**(1), 33–48 (1990)
15. Polley, M.: Practical modifications to the time-to-event continual reassessment method for phase I cancer trials with fast patient accrual and late-onset toxicities. *Stat Med*. **30**(17), 2130–2143 (2011)
16. Skolnik, J., Barrett, J., Jayaraman, B., Patel, D., Adamson, P.: Shortening the timeline of pediatric phase I trials: the rolling six design. *J Clin Oncol*. **26**(2), 190–195 (2008)
17. Storer, B.E.: Design and analysis of phase I clinical trials. *Biometrics*. **45**(3), 925–937 (1989)
18. Ting, N., Chen, D.G., Ho, S., Cappelleri, J.C.: Phase II Clinical Development of New Drugs. Springer, Cham (2017)
19. Yin, G., Zheng, S., Xu, J.: Fractional dose-finding methods with late-onset toxicity in phase I clinical trials. *J Biopharm Stat*. **23**(4), 856–870 (2013)
20. Yuan, Y., Lin, R., Li, D., Nie, L., Warren, K.: Time-to-event bayesian optimal interval design to accelerate phase I trials. *Clin Cancer Res*. **24**(20), 4921–4930 (2018)
21. Yuan, Y., Yin, G.: Robust EM continual reassessment method in oncology dose finding. *J Am Stat Assoc*. **106**(495), 818–831 (2011)
22. Zheng, W., Zhao, Y., Lu, Y., Miao, H., Liu, H.: A Bayesian three-parameter logistic model for early- and late-onset DLTs in oncology phase I studies. *J Biopharm Stat*. **26**(2), 339–351 (2016)

A Bayesian Approach for the Analysis of Tumorigenicity Data from Sacrificial Experiments Under Weibull Lifetimes

Man Ho Ling, Hon Yiu So, and Narayanaswamy Balakrishnan

Abstract This chapter details a Bayesian approach for inference on onset time of tumors based on tumorigenicity data from sacrificial experiments under Weibull lifetimes. We assume that both shape and scale parameters are related to various covariates in log-linear forms. Metropolis–Hastings sampling method is then used for the estimation of posterior means of quantities of interest. A simulation study and a sensitivity analysis are carried out to assess the performance of the developed Bayesian approach with different priors. A comparison is also made with the likelihood estimates determined from an EM algorithm. Finally, a known mice tumor toxicology dataset is analyzed to illustrate the developed Bayesian approach.

1 Introduction

In sacrificial experiments that examine tumor occurrence in different organ sites, each animal under study is sacrificed at a pre-specified time and is examined to determine the presence of tumors [11]. The data consist of a single sacrifice time for each animal, and indicators of whether tumors are present at the time of sacrifice. If a specific type of tumor is found in the animal at the time of sacrifice, it indicates that the tumor onset time is before the sacrifice time, thus resulting in left-censoring. On the other hand, if the tumor type is not found in the animal at the time of sacrifice, it

M. Ho Ling (✉)
Department of Mathematics and Information Technology, The Education University of Hong Kong, Hong Kong, China
e-mail: amhling@eduhk.hk

H. Y. So
Department of Mathematics and Statistics, Oakland University, Rochester, MI, USA
e-mail: hso@oakland.edu

N. Balakrishnan
Department of Mathematics and Statistics, McMaster University, Hamilton, ON, Canada
e-mail: bala@mcmaster.ca

Y. Lio et al. (eds.), *Bayesian Inference and Computation in Reliability and Survival Analysis*, Emerging Topics in Statistics and Biostatistics,
https://doi.org/10.1007/978-3-030-88658-5_10

indicates that the tumor onset time is after the sacrifice time, thus resulting in right-censoring. Consequently, all tumor onset times are therefore either left- or right-censored, and the exact tumor onset times can never be observed in this experiment. This is a special case of current status data [19, 22, 24].

Numerous studies on current status data analysis have been carried out in the literature. Dinse [10] and Lindsey and Ryan [17] analyzed data on bladder tumor, liver tumor, lung tumor, lymphoma tumor, and reticulum cell sarcomas in sacrificial experiments. Subsequently, Dunson and Dinse [12] studied bivariate current status data on adrenal and lung tumors for male mice from the control and high-dose groups and found that there is a moderate level of dependence between the onset times of adrenal and lung tumors. Wang and Ding [23] presented a procedure to estimate the dependence between the onset times of hypertension, diabetes mellitus, and hypercholesterolemia under Clayton copula models, and Ding and Wang [9] further developed an independence test for bivariate current status data. In addition, current status data may consist of some covariates that may have influence on the tumor onset times, such as gender, dose level of a chemical, type of strain, radiation level, etc. [8, 16, 18].

Balakrishnan and Ling [3, 4] developed EM algorithms for estimating the model parameters under Weibull and gamma lifetime distributions, respectively, to measure the effects of each covariate on the tumor onset times based on mice tumor toxicology data [16]. In this chapter, we extend the work of Fan et al. [13] by assuming tumor onset times to have Weibull distributions and develop a Bayesian estimation method for tumorigenicity data from sacrificial experiments. In their work [13], three priors were used in the Bayesian estimation: Exponential, Normal, and Beta. Their simulation results showed that all the priors performed similarly when the data possess enough information, while normal performed better when the data possess zero-failure cases. Here, we adopt Laplace distribution, normal distribution with non-informative prior for the variance, and beta distribution for the prior. A simulation study and a sensitivity analysis are then carried out to evaluate the performance of the developed Bayesian approach under these three priors. A comparison is also made with the maximum likelihood estimation determined from the EM algorithm. Finally, an example of a mice tumor toxicology dataset in [16] is used to illustrate all the inferential results developed here.

2 Model Specification

Tumorigenicity experiments with serial sacrifice are set up as follows:

1. There are I groups of J covariates $\mathbf{x}_i$, for $i = 1, 2, \ldots, I$.
2. The number of mice in the i-th group is K_i.
3. The mice in the i-th group are sacrificed at time τ_i, for $i = 1, \ldots, I$.
4. The number of mice having tumors, n_i, are collected from the i-th group.

As in the work of Balakrishnan and Ling [3], we assume that the tumor onset time of the k-th mice in the i-th group, t_{ik}, has a Weibull distribution with scale parameter $\alpha_i > 0$ and shape parameter $\eta_i > 0$, for $i = 1, \ldots, I$ and $k = 1, \ldots, K_i$. The corresponding pdf and cdf are

$$f_T(t, \alpha_i, \eta_i) = \frac{\eta_i t^{\eta_i - 1}}{\alpha_i^{\eta_i}} \exp\left(-\left(\frac{t}{\alpha_i}\right)^{\eta_i}\right), \quad t > 0,$$

and

$$F_T(t, \alpha_i, \eta_i) = 1 - \exp\left(-\left(\frac{t}{\alpha_i}\right)^{\eta_i}\right), \quad t > 0,$$

respectively. We now assume that the scale and shape parameters are linked to the covariates in the following log-linear forms:

$$\alpha_i = \exp\left(\sum_{j=0}^{J} a_j x_{ij}\right) = \exp(\mathbf{a} \cdot \mathbf{x}_i) \text{ and } \eta_i = \exp\left(\sum_{j=0}^{J} b_j x_{ij}\right) = \exp(\mathbf{b} \cdot \mathbf{x}_i).$$

If the tumor onset times of all the mice are independent, then n_i is a binomial random variable with the number of mice K_i and probability of having tumors

$$1 - p_i = F_T(\tau_i; \alpha_i, \eta_i), \tag{1}$$

and so the joint likelihood function of $\mathbf{a}$ and $\mathbf{b}$ is

$$L(\mathbf{a}, \mathbf{b}) = \prod_{i=1}^{I} L_i(\mathbf{a}, \mathbf{b} | \mathbf{x}_i, \tau_i, n_i) \tag{2}$$

$$\propto \prod_{i=1}^{I} (1 - p_i)^{n_i} \, p_i^{K_i - n_i}. \tag{3}$$

For example, survival and sacrifice data taken from the National Center for Toxicological Research involved 1816 mice, of which 553 mice had tumors. These data have been considered earlier by Kodell and Nelson [16], Finkelstein and Ryan [14], and Lindsey and Ryan [17]. The original data were classified into 5 groups and were reported by Kodell and Nelson [16]. Note that not all mice were sacrificed at pre-specified times because some died of tumors naturally before the sacrifice time. So, the time of natural death would also be treated as the sacrifice time. We considered the mice sacrificed with tumors, died of tumors, and died of competing risks with liver tumors as those having tumors, while the mice sacrificed without tumors and died of competing risk without liver tumors as those not having tumors. Part of these data is presented in Table 1.

Table 1 A partial data from the tumorigenicity experiments of benzidine dihydrochloride in mice, giving the number of mice tested, K_i, number of mice having tumors, n_i, time to being sacrificed or natural death, τ_i, strain of offspring ($F1 = 0$, $F2 = 1$), x_{i1}, gender ($F = 0$, $M = 1$), x_{i2}, and concentration of the chemical (in ppm), x_{i3}

K_i	n_i	τ_i	x_{i1}	x_{i2}	x_{i3}	K_i	n_i	τ_i	x_{i1}	x_{i2}	x_{i3}	K_i	n_i	τ_i	x_{i1}	x_{i2}	x_{i3}
24	0	9.37	0	0	60	1	1	16.57	0	0	120	1	1	14.03	0	0	200
24	1	13.97	0	0	60	1	1	16.90	0	0	120	1	1	14.23	0	0	200
24	0	9.37	0	0	120	1	1	15.13	0	0	120	1	1	18.67	0	0	200
24	5	13.97	0	0	120	1	1	15.40	0	0	120	24	16	9.33	0	0	400
23	9	14.03	0	0	120	47	4	9.33	0	0	200	10	9	14.00	0	0	400
26	25	18.67	0	0	120	45	38	14.00	0	0	200	1	1	9.87	0	0	400
48	0	9.27	0	1	120	22	11	14.00	0	1	400	1	0	17.13	1	0	60
44	7	14.00	0	1	120	15	11	18.70	0	1	400	24	2	9.27	1	0	120
22	7	18.73	0	1	120	1	1	7.87	0	1	400	22	0	9.37	1	0	120
20	4	19.30	0	1	120	1	1	14.73	0	1	400	41	15	14.00	1	0	120
24	0	9.27	1	1	60	18	5	18.70	1	1	120	1	1	15.43	1	1	200
23	0	9.30	1	1	60	1	1	9.57	1	1	120	24	1	9.30	1	1	400
21	0	9.37	1	1	60	1	1	14.43	1	1	120	21	4	14.00	1	1	400
44	3	14.00	1	1	60	1	1	17.87	1	1	120	12	6	18.67	1	1	400

3 Bayesian Approach

For analyzing tumorigenicity data as presented in Table 1, the classical approach will be based on maximum likelihood estimation method. In this regard, Balakrishnan and Ling [3] developed an EM algorithm for determining the MLEs of the model parameters under Weibull lifetimes. These authors observed that the method yields accurate estimates when the sample size is large, but the estimation is not satisfactory for small sample sizes, especially when cases of zero failure are present. By incorporating prior information, Bayesian estimation can provide more accurate inference in the case of small sample sizes; see, for example, Fan et al. [13] and Berger [7]. For this reason, it is of great interest to develop a Bayesian estimation method for the model parameters based on tumorigenicity data.

Fan et al. [13] developed a Bayesian approach for estimating the model parameters under exponential lifetimes. Here, we develop results for the Weibull case along their lines, but for this purpose, several modifications are needed in their algorithm as described below. Let $\pi(\mathbf{a}, \mathbf{b})$ be the joint prior density of $(\mathbf{a}, \mathbf{b})$. Then, the joint posterior density of $\mathbf{a}$ and $\mathbf{b}$ is

$$\pi(\mathbf{a}, \mathbf{b}|\mathbf{x}, \boldsymbol{\tau}, \mathbf{n}) = \frac{L(\mathbf{a}, \mathbf{b}|\mathbf{x}, \boldsymbol{\tau}, \mathbf{n})\pi(\mathbf{a}, \mathbf{b})}{\int\int L(\mathbf{a}, \mathbf{b}|\mathbf{x}, \boldsymbol{\tau}, \mathbf{n})\pi(\mathbf{a}, \mathbf{b})d\mathbf{a}d\mathbf{b}}. \tag{4}$$

Due to the presence of non-linear link functions, the denominator in (4) is usually not in a closed form, and consequently the posterior distribution and the Bayesian estimates of different lifetime characteristics are not in analytical form. So, we apply the Metropolis–Hastings algorithm [15] to generate samples and approximate the posterior distribution.

Following the method of Fan et al. [13], the Bayesian point estimates of $\mathbf{a}$ and $\mathbf{b}$ are $\hat{\mathbf{a}} = \frac{1}{M}\sum_{m=1}^{M} \mathbf{a}^{(m)}$ and $\hat{\mathbf{b}} = \frac{1}{M}\sum_{m=1}^{M} \mathbf{b}^{(m)}$, where $\mathbf{a}^{(m)}$ and $\mathbf{b}^{(m)}$ are the m-th values out of M samples generated from the posterior distribution. We may be interested in estimating some characteristics of interest for mice with covariate $\mathbf{x}_0$, such as the probability of mice without tumors at time t, $S(t, \mathbf{x}_0) = 1 - F_T(t)$, and the mean of tumor onset time $\mu(\mathbf{x}_0)$. They can then be readily estimated as follows:

$$\hat{S}(t, \mathbf{x}_0; \hat{\mathbf{a}}, \hat{\mathbf{b}}) = \frac{1}{M}\sum_{m=1}^{M} \exp\left(-\left(\frac{t}{\alpha_0^{(m)}}\right)^{\eta_0^{(m)}}\right), \tag{5}$$

$$\hat{\mu}\left(\mathbf{x}_0, \hat{\mathbf{a}}, \hat{\mathbf{b}}\right) = \frac{1}{M}\sum_{m=1}^{M} \alpha_0^{(m)}\Gamma\left(1 + \frac{1}{\eta_0^{(m)}}\right), \tag{6}$$

where $\alpha_0^{(m)} = \exp(\mathbf{x}_0 \cdot \mathbf{a}^{(m)})$ and $\eta_0^{(m)} = \exp(\mathbf{x}_0 \cdot \mathbf{b}^{(m)})$.

Several prior distributions are considered in this study and the corresponding hyperparameters based on experts' information are discussed below.

3.1 Laplace Prior

The parameters a_j and b_j, $j = 0, \cdots, J$, may not always be positive. In analogy to the exponential prior in Fan et al. [13], the Laplace distribution is chosen as one of the prior distributions. The parameters are assumed to be independent, and the joint prior density function is

$$\pi_1(\mathbf{a}, \mathbf{b}) = \prod_{j=0}^{J} \exp\left(-\left|\frac{a_j}{a_j^*}\right|\right) \prod_{j=0}^{J} \exp\left(-\left|\frac{b_j}{b_j^*}\right|\right), \tag{7}$$

where $-\infty < a_j < \infty$ and $-\infty < b_j < \infty$ for $j = 0, \cdots, J$.

$|a_j^*|$ and $|b_j^*|$ are the unknown hyperparameters with $\mathrm{E}(|a_j|) = |a_j^*|$ and $\mathrm{E}(|b_j|) = |b_j^*|$. Fan et al. [13] assumed that p_i are around $\hat{p}_i$, for $i = 1, \cdots, I$, and so $\hat{p}_i$ can be empirically estimated as $1 - \frac{n_i}{K_i}$. If one of these estimates is zero, then it will be hard to determine the initial value. Zero-frequency problem has long been discussed in the literature, and Agresti [1] suggested adding a constant, say 0.5, to both failure and success cases, that is,

$$\tilde{p}_i = 1 - \frac{n_i + 0.5}{K_i + 1}. \tag{8}$$

We try to obtain the hyperparameters, a_j^* and b_j^*, by the least-squares method:

$$\{\mathbf{a}^*, \mathbf{b}^*\} = \mathrm{argmin}_{\mathbf{a},\mathbf{b}} \sum_{i=0}^{I} \left(\exp\left(-\left(\frac{\tau_i}{e^{\mathbf{a}\cdot\mathbf{x}_i}}\right)^{e^{\mathbf{b}\cdot\mathbf{x}_i}}\right) - \tilde{p}_i\right)^2, \tag{9}$$

where $\mathbf{a}^* = (a_j^*)_{j=0,\cdots,J}$ and $\mathbf{b}^* = (b_j^*)_{j=0,\cdots,J}$. With the presence of $\eta_i = \exp(\mathbf{b} \cdot \mathbf{x}_i)$, the LSEs are not in closed form. We can minimize the summation in (9) by some standard routines such as `optim` in R or `fminsearch` in MATLAB.

3.2 Normal Prior

Since differences exist between the prior belief and the true values of the unknown parameters, we may assume

$$\tilde{p}_i = p_i + \epsilon_i, \tag{10}$$

where the error terms ϵ_i are assumed to be i.i.d. $N(0, \sigma^2)$ variables. Then, the conditional likelihood function of **a** and **b**, given σ^2, is

$$L(\mathbf{a}, \mathbf{b}|\boldsymbol{\tau}, \mathbf{x}, \tilde{p}_i, \sigma^2) \propto \prod_{i=1}^{I} \frac{1}{\sqrt{2\pi\sigma^2}} \exp\left\{-\frac{1}{2\sigma^2}(p_i - \tilde{p}_i)^2\right\},$$

where p_i and $\tilde{p}_i$ are as specified in Eqs. (1) and (8), respectively. We will now adopt the likelihood function as the prior distribution of **a** and **b**:

$$\pi_2(\mathbf{a}, \mathbf{b}|\boldsymbol{\tau}, \mathbf{x}, \sigma^2) \propto \prod_{i=1}^{I} \frac{1}{\sqrt{2\pi\sigma^2}} \exp\left\{-\frac{1}{2\sigma^2}(p_i - \tilde{p}_i)^2\right\}. \tag{11}$$

Since σ^2 is unknown, we adopt Jeffrey's non-informative prior

$$\pi(\sigma^2) \propto \frac{1}{\sigma^2}, \quad \sigma^2 > 0,$$

which yields the joint prior density of **a** and **b** as

$$\begin{aligned}\pi_2(\mathbf{a}, \mathbf{b}|\boldsymbol{\tau}, \mathbf{x}) &\propto \int_0^\infty \pi_2(\mathbf{a}, \mathbf{b}|\boldsymbol{\tau}, \mathbf{x}, \sigma^2)\pi(\sigma^2)d\sigma^2 \\ &\propto \int_0^\infty (\sigma^2)^{-\frac{I+2}{2}} \exp\left\{-\frac{1}{2\sigma^2}\sum_{i=1}^{I}(p_i - \tilde{p}_i)^2\right\} d\sigma^2 \\ &\propto \left\{\sum_{i=1}^{I}(p_i - \tilde{p}_i)^2\right\}^{-I}. \end{aligned} \tag{12}$$

Then, by Eq. (4), the joint posterior density of **a** and **b** becomes

$$\pi_2(\mathbf{a}, \mathbf{b}|\mathbf{n}, \boldsymbol{\tau}, \mathbf{x}) \propto \prod_{i=1}^{I} (1 - p_i)^{n_i} p_i^{K_i - n_i} \times \left\{\sum_{i=1}^{I}(p_i - \tilde{p}_i)^2\right\}^{-I}. \tag{13}$$

3.3 Beta Prior

Fan et al. [13] considered a beta conjugate prior, beta(α_i, β_i), for p_i of the form

$$\pi_3(\mathbf{a}, \mathbf{b}) = \prod_{i=1}^{I} p_i^{\alpha_i - 1}(1 - p_i)^{\beta_i - 1}, \tag{14}$$

where the hyperparameters α_i and β_i are chosen such that $\mathrm{E}(p_i) = \alpha_i/(\alpha_i + \beta_i) \approx \tilde{p}_i$ and $\mathrm{var}(p_i) = \alpha_i\beta_i/\{(\alpha_i + \beta_i)^2(\alpha_i + \beta_i + 1)\} = c_i^2$, for a given prior belief on

$\tilde{p}_i$ and the uncertainty of the prior belief, c_i^2. If the uncertainty is constant for all groups, $c^2 = c_i^2$, the hyperparameters then become

$$\alpha_i = \tilde{p}_i \left(\frac{\tilde{p}_i(1-\tilde{p}_i)}{c^2} - 1 \right) \text{ and } \beta_i = (1-\tilde{p}_i) \left(\frac{\tilde{p}_i(1-\tilde{p}_i)}{c^2} - 1 \right).$$

Note that the uncertainty has to be small in order for the prior belief to be useful and $\alpha_i > 0$ and $\beta_i > 0$, for $i = 1, \cdots, I$. Then, the posterior distribution becomes

$$\pi_3(\mathbf{a}, \mathbf{b}|\mathbf{n}, \boldsymbol{\tau}, \mathbf{x}) \propto \prod_{i=1}^{I} \prod_{j=1}^{J} p_i^{K_i - n_i + \alpha_i - 1} (1-p_i)^{n_i + \beta_i - 1}; \qquad (15)$$

here, p_i is as specified in (1), and $\tilde{p}_i$ is as specified in (8).

3.4 Prior Belief on p_i

Normally, the prior belief on p_i is the estimates of the probabilities based on previous experiments or experts' judgments. When the prior information is not available, the estimate based on the data, $\tilde{p}_i = 1 - n_i/K_i$, is used as if we have the prior information. It is an approximation in the Bayesian method, and it may be regarded as an empirical Bayes method.

In the study of Fan et al. [13], they supposed that $\hat{p}_i$ is very reliable with regard to the true unknown parameter p_i. So, they generated p_i from a beta distribution with specific choice of parameters. Now, we suppose that $\hat{p}_i$ is also very reliable in the sense that the variance of prior belief on the survival probability, $\text{var}(\hat{p}_i) = c^2$, is small, with c^2 being a small constant. We also assume that $E(\hat{p}_i) = p_i$. Then, with the choice of parameters being similar to the one in Eq. (14), we have

$$f(\hat{p}_i) \propto \hat{p}_i^{\alpha_i^* - 1} (1-\hat{p}_i)^{\beta_i^* - 1}, \qquad (16)$$

where $0 < \hat{p}_i < 1$. The parameters α_i^* are chosen to be

$$\alpha_i^* = p_i \left(\frac{p_i(1-p_i)}{c^2} - 1 \right) \text{ and } \beta_i^* = (1-p_i) \left(\frac{p_i(1-p_i)}{c^2} - 1 \right),$$

for the underlying true value $p_i, i = 1, \cdots, I$.

The prior belief on the parameter can be used to replace $\tilde{p}_i$ in Eqs. (9), (13), and (15), and the corresponding posterior distribution will then result. Note that $\alpha_i^* > 0$ and $\beta_i^* > 0$, and so there is a restriction on the uncertainty of prior belief that $c^2 < p_i(1-p_i)$.

4 Simulation Study

In this section, we will compare the performance of the Bayesian estimation with the three prior distributions and two prior beliefs, $\tilde{p}_i$ and $\hat{p}_i$, with that of the MLEs determined by the EM algorithm developed in [3]. We consider $9K$ mice receiving 3 dose levels of a chemical in their drinking water. At each level, $3K$ mice are equally divided into 3 groups and sacrificed at various times. The detailed parameter settings used in this simulation study are summarized in Table 2. We repeated this experiment with different sample sizes of K mice allocated to each condition.

In this Monte Carlo simulation study, 1000 sets of data were simulated under each specified setting. For the EM algorithm, the iteration was terminated when the sum of squares of the differences in the model parameter estimates was less than 10^{-5}. For the Bayesian estimates, we used Metropolis–Hastings algorithm to simulate the posterior distributions. We generated a vector of four normal random variables with mean parameters equal to the previous estimates and different variance, which gave an acceptance rate of about 0.25, approximately; this is considered to be optimal in practice as stated in Roberts et al. [20] and Roberts and Rosenthal [21]. We generated a sequence of 111,000 vectors of random variables from the algorithm, and the first 10,000 data points were dropped as burn-in. We then chose one sample for every 100 random variables simulated to avoid correlation between the iterated samples and, thus, a sample of size 1000 was finally obtained. For each simulation setting, the MLEs of the model parameters from the EM algorithm, which are often close to the true parameters, were used as the initial guess for the model parameters in the Bayesian framework. This ensures the Metropolis–Hastings algorithm to converge to the posterior distribution in a reasonable amount of time. To evaluate the relative performance of the estimators, we will compare their bias $\frac{1}{N}\sum_{i=1}^{N}\theta^{(i)}-\theta$ and the MSE $\frac{1}{N}\sum_{i=1}^{N}(\theta^{(i)}-\theta)^2$, where $\theta^{(i)}$ is the estimate of a quantity of interest from the i-th sample out of $N = 1000$ simulations and θ is the true parameter.

Table 2 Parameter values used in the simulation study for tumorigenicity experiments with serial sacrifice

Parameters	Symbols	Reaction rates	Values
		Quick	(4.9, −0.05)
Scale link function	a_0, a_1	Moderate	(5.3, −0.05)
		Slow	(5.7, −0.05)
Shape link function	b_0, b_1		(−0.6, 0.03)
Dose level	x_{11}, x_{21}, x_{31}		(30, 40, 50)
		Quick	(5, 10, 15)
Sacrifice time (days)	$\boldsymbol{\tau}$	Moderate	(8, 16, 24)
		Slow	(12, 24, 36)
Sample size	K_1, K_2, K_3		(30, 50, 100)
Prior belief variance	c^2		0.001

Table 3 Bias and MSE of the estimates of parameters for chemical with quick reaction rate under different estimation methods

	Bias			MSE		
$a_{L0} = 4.9$	$K = 30$	$K = 50$	$K = 100$	$K = 30$	$K = 50$	$K = 100$
EM	**1.199e-01**	**6.159e-02**	2.968e-02	**6.744e-01**	**3.65e-01**	**1.555e-01**
Laplace($\tilde{p}$)	**4.498e-02**	**9.514e-03**	**2.832e-03**	8.363e-01	4.601e-01	1.872e-01
Norm($\tilde{p}$)	1.314e-01	6.818e-02	**2.872e-02**	6.988e-01	3.875e-01	1.708e-01
Beta($\tilde{p}$)	1.257e-01	6.167e-02	3.332e-02	6.938e-01	3.74e-01	1.625e-01
Laplace($\hat{p}$)	**2.79e-02**	**6.907e-03**	**1.29e-02**	8.109e-01	4.385e-01	2.109e-01
Norm($\hat{p}$)	1.412e-01	7.271e-02	4.051e-02	**6.01e-01**	**3.266e-01**	**1.422e-01**
Beta($\hat{p}$)	1.316e-01	7.027e-02	3.601e-02	**5.093e-01**	**2.886e-01**	**1.336e-01**
$a_1 = -0.05$	$K = 30$	$K = 50$	$K = 100$	$K = 30$	$K = 50$	$K = 100$
EM	−2.441e-03	−1.231e-03	−6.336e-04	**2.852e-04**	**1.552e-04**	**6.697e-05**
Laplace($\tilde{p}$)	**2.24e-04**	**9.754e-04**	**8.733e-05**	6.492e-04	7.076e-04	8.608e-05
Norm($\tilde{p}$)	−2.544e-03	−1.287e-03	**−5.683e-04**	2.954e-04	1.654e-04	7.356e-05
Beta($\tilde{p}$)	**−2.394e-03**	**−1.156e-03**	−6.826e-04	2.923e-04	1.594e-04	7.016e-05
Laplace($\hat{p}$)	**1.154e-03**	**6.17e-04**	**3.34e-04**	7.95e-04	2.967e-04	4.155e-04
Norm($\hat{p}$)	−2.793e-03	−1.423e-03	−8.125e-04	**2.529e-04**	**1.383e-04**	**6.095e-05**
Beta($\hat{p}$)	−2.59e-03	−1.368e-03	−7.21e-04	**2.149e-04**	**1.227e-04**	**5.751e-05**
$b_0 = -0.6$	$K = 30$	$K = 50$	$K = 100$	$K = 30$	$K = 50$	$K = 100$
EM	**−1.785e-03**	1.869e-02	**−1.592e-03**	**7.008e-01**	**4.068e-01**	**1.928e-01**
Laplace($\tilde{p}$)	9.959e-02	6.43e-02	2.913e-02	7.356e-01	4.623e-01	2.154e-01
Norm($\tilde{p}$)	**−5.591e-03**	**1.457e-02**	**−1.514e-03**	7.502e-01	4.428e-01	2.078e-01
Beta($\tilde{p}$)	−1.932e-02	1.796e-02	−3.606e-03	7.277e-01	4.134e-01	2.09e-01
Laplace($\hat{p}$)	9.829e-02	8.348e-02	2.329e-02	7.96e-01	4.776e-01	2.334e-01
Norm($\hat{p}$)	**−1.697e-05**	**1.318e-02**	−4.351e-03	**6.667e-01**	**3.904e-01**	**1.977e-01**
Beta($\hat{p}$)	−1.513e-02	**1.529e-02**	**−1.107e-03**	**6.033e-01**	**3.623e-01**	**1.846e-01**
$b_1 = 0.03$	$K = 30$	$K = 50$	$K = 100$	$K = 30$	$K = 50$	$K = 100$
EM	**2.532e-04**	**−4.409e-04**	1.647e-04	**3.347e-04**	**1.943e-04**	**9.284e-05**
Laplace($\tilde{p}$)	−3.376e-03	−2.173e-03	−8.215e-04	4.046e-04	2.389e-04	1.116e-04
Norm($\tilde{p}$)	−5.626e-04	−8.815e-04	**−7.63e-05**	3.642e-04	2.145e-04	1.009e-04
Beta($\tilde{p}$)	−9.677e-04	−1.166e-03	**3.556e-05**	3.524e-04	2.012e-04	1.022e-04
Laplace($\hat{p}$)	−3.501e-03	−2.75e-03	−8.182e-04	4.5e-04	2.65e-04	1.287e-04
Norm($\hat{p}$)	**−3.6e-04**	**−5.128e-04**	**3.595e-06**	**3.057e-04**	**1.792e-04**	**9.201e-05**
Beta($\hat{p}$)	**−2.287e-04**	**−7.283e-04**	−1.162e-04	**2.734e-04**	**1.646e-04**	**8.564e-05**

Also, it is of interest to compare the estimation methods for the probability of mice receiving $\mathbf{x}_0 = 25$ dose level of the chemical and without tumors. For this purpose, we simulated data sets for different a_0 values, with other parameters being kept constant. We assumed that the accuracy of the prior belief is high and the variance was set to be $c^2 = 0.001$. The corresponding results obtained for the estimates of the parameters for various rates of chemical reaction are presented in Tables 3, 4, and 5. The estimates of the mean of tumor onset time and the probability

Table 4 Bias and MSE of the estimates of parameters for chemical with moderate reaction rate under different estimation methods

	Bias			MSE		
$a_{M0} = 5.3$	$K = 30$	$K = 50$	$K = 100$	$K = 30$	$K = 50$	$K = 100$
EM	**6.68e-02**	**3.045e-02**	2.852e-02	**4.923e-01**	**2.445e-01**	**1.5e-01**
Laplace($\tilde{p}$)	**5.003e-03**	**−8.739e-03**	**7.035e-03**	5.96e-01	3.159e-01	1.994e-01
Norm($\tilde{p}$)	8.219e-02	4.225e-02	3.712e-02	5.177e-01	2.652e-01	1.626e-01
Beta($\tilde{p}$)	7.708e-02	3.405e-02	3.139e-02	5.16e-01	2.513e-01	1.613e-01
Laplace($\hat{p}$)	**2.42e-02**	**−1.021e-02**	**−7.28e-03**	6.248e-01	3.111e-01	2.273e-01
Norm($\hat{p}$)	8.836e-02	3.96e-02	3.708e-02	**4.058e-01**	**2.077e-01**	**1.296e-01**
Beta($\hat{p}$)	9.282e-02	4.631e-02	**2.842e-02**	**3.55e-01**	**1.827e-01**	**1.183e-01**
$a_1 = -0.05$	$K = 30$	$K = 50$	$K = 100$	$K = 30$	$K = 50$	$K = 100$
EM	**−1.357e-03**	**−6.837e-04**	**−5.982e-04**	**2.11e-04**	**1.051e-04**	**6.48e-05**
Laplace($\tilde{p}$)	**8.255e-04**	1.186e-03	**1.253e-04**	4.235e-04	1.083e-03	1.383e-04
Norm($\tilde{p}$)	−1.549e-03	−8.564e-04	−7.434e-04	2.214e-04	1.142e-04	7.034e-05
Beta($\tilde{p}$)	−1.444e-03	**−6.81e-04**	−6.489e-04	2.221e-04	1.081e-04	6.98e-05
Laplace($\hat{p}$)	**7.262e-04**	**5.687e-04**	7.109e-04	7.124e-04	2.015e-04	3.1e-04
Norm($\hat{p}$)	−1.732e-03	−7.849e-04	−7.37e-04	**1.73e-04**	**8.921e-05**	**5.598e-05**
Beta($\hat{p}$)	−1.802e-03	−9.146e-04	**−5.388e-04**	**1.52e-04**	**7.843e-05**	**5.146e-05**
$b_0 = -0.6$	$K = 30$	$K = 50$	$K = 100$	$K = 30$	$K = 50$	$K = 100$
EM	**−1.313e-02**	**−3.635e-03**	1.189e-02	**6.952e-01**	**3.291e-01**	**1.939e-01**
Laplace($\tilde{p}$)	8.349e-02	4.282e-02	3.941e-02	7.755e-01	3.779e-01	2.312e-01
Norm($\tilde{p}$)	**−1.887e-02**	**4.422e-04**	**9.795e-03**	7.334e-01	3.521e-01	2.14e-01
Beta($\tilde{p}$)	−3.308e-02	−1.385e-02	**1.134e-02**	7.234e-01	3.439e-01	2.093e-01
Laplace($\hat{p}$)	8.249e-02	5.532e-02	5.522e-02	8.024e-01	3.755e-01	2.282e-01
Norm($\hat{p}$)	**−1.293e-02**	**−7.044e-04**	1.592e-02	**5.975e-01**	**3.24e-01**	**1.944e-01**
Beta($\hat{p}$)	−2.949e-02	−4.146e-03	**7.319e-03**	**5.708e-01**	**2.931e-01**	**1.82e-01**
$b_1 = 0.03$	$K = 30$	$K = 50$	$K = 100$	$K = 30$	$K = 50$	$K = 100$
EM	6.192e-04	2.7e-04	**−2.344e-04**	**3.458e-04**	**1.593e-04**	**9.177e-05**
Laplace($\tilde{p}$)	−2.8e-03	−1.423e-03	−1.158e-03	4.323e-04	2.076e-04	1.161e-04
Norm($\tilde{p}$)	**−1.617e-04**	−3.873e-04	−4.716e-04	3.691e-04	1.714e-04	1.03e-04
Beta($\tilde{p}$)	−4.394e-04	**−2.106e-04**	**−3.879e-04**	3.751e-04	1.68e-04	1.004e-04
Laplace($\hat{p}$)	−2.855e-03	−1.691e-03	−1.582e-03	4.404e-04	1.969e-04	1.254e-04
Norm($\hat{p}$)	**1.575e-04**	**−6.625e-06**	−5.375e-04	**2.861e-04**	**1.529e-04**	**9.151e-05**
Beta($\hat{p}$)	**2.738e-04**	**−7.88e-05**	**−3.516e-04**	**2.681e-04**	**1.367e-04**	**8.622e-05**

of mice without tumors at some time points of interest are presented in Tables 6, 7, and 8. The values in bold indicate the three smallest absolute values of bias and MSEs in each simulation setting. Also, the values within borders indicate which method is the best under a particular simulation setting.

From all these results, the method with the best performance in terms of the least absolute values of bias and MSE is summarized in Tables 9 and 10, respectively.

Table 5 Bias and MSE of the estimates of parameters for chemical with slow reaction rate under different estimation methods

	Bias			MSE		
$a_{H0} = 5.7$	$K = 30$	$K = 50$	$K = 100$	$K = 30$	$K = 50$	$K = 100$
EM	**6.069e-02**	**6.06e-02**	**1.614e-02**	**4.977e-01**	**2.884e-01**	**1.306e-01**
Laplace($\tilde{p}$)	**−4.148e-02**	**1.58e-02**	**−1.451e-02**	6.863e-01	3.853e-01	1.886e-01
Norm($\tilde{p}$)	6.985e-02	7.985e-02	1.829e-02	5.282e-01	3.06e-01	1.41e-01
Beta($\tilde{p}$)	7.53e-02	6.08e-02	2.138e-02	5.213e-01	2.957e-01	1.372e-01
Laplace($\hat{p}$)	**−1.982e-02**	**−2.828e-02**	**−1.325e-02**	6.784e-01	4.886e-01	1.961e-01
Norm($\hat{p}$)	6.844e-02	7.574e-02	2.256e-02	**4.178e-01**	**2.468e-01**	**1.203e-01**
Beta($\hat{p}$)	7.858e-02	8.176e-02	2.837e-02	**3.658e-01**	**2.281e-01**	**1.046e-01**
$a_1 = -0.05$	$K = 30$	$K = 50$	$K = 100$	$K = 30$	$K = 50$	$K = 100$
EM	**−1.299e-03**	**−1.268e-03**	**−3.663e-04**	**2.149e-04**	**1.245e-04**	**5.686e-05**
Laplace($\tilde{p}$)	4.466e-03	**5.124e-04**	9.349e-04	2.703e-03	6.266e-04	4.816e-04
Norm($\tilde{p}$)	**−1.39e-03**	−1.596e-03	**−3.767e-04**	2.286e-04	1.322e-04	6.158e-05
Beta($\tilde{p}$)	−1.505e-03	**−1.194e-03**	−4.729e-04	2.265e-04	1.283e-04	5.996e-05
Laplace($\hat{p}$)	2.364e-03	2.808e-03	7.463e-04	1.219e-03	1.488e-03	2.318e-04
Norm($\hat{p}$)	**−1.342e-03**	−1.505e-03	**−4.628e-04**	**1.789e-04**	**1.061e-04**	**5.238e-05**
Beta($\hat{p}$)	−1.529e-03	−1.618e-03	−5.803e-04	**1.565e-04**	**9.804e-05**	**4.568e-05**
$b_0 = -0.6$	$K = 30$	$K = 50$	$K = 100$	$K = 30$	$K = 50$	$K = 100$
EM	**3.967e-02**	**−2.853e-02**	**−1.157e-03**	**6.186e-01**	**3.658e-01**	**1.838e-01**
Laplace($\tilde{p}$)	1.337e-01	**2.89e-02**	2.446e-02	7.161e-01	4.034e-01	2.105e-01
Norm($\tilde{p}$)	4.368e-02	−4.078e-02	−3.5e-03	6.653e-01	4.022e-01	1.956e-01
Beta($\tilde{p}$)	**1.919e-02**	−4.306e-02	−3.991e-03	6.425e-01	3.833e-01	2.014e-01
Laplace($\hat{p}$)	1.067e-01	**2.446e-02**	2.706e-02	7.106e-01	4.236e-01	2.116e-01
Norm($\hat{p}$)	4.708e-02	−3.633e-02	**−3.072e-03**	**5.821e-01**	**3.376e-01**	**1.804e-01**
Beta($\hat{p}$)	**1.702e-02**	−3.361e-02	**−2.581e-03**	**5.371e-01**	**3.276e-01**	**1.703e-01**
$b_1 = 0.03$	$K = 30$	$K = 50$	$K = 100$	$K = 30$	$K = 50$	$K = 100$
EM	**−5.368e-04**	6.938e-04	1.095e-04	**2.938e-04**	**1.748e-04**	**8.943e-05**
Laplace($\tilde{p}$)	−4.233e-03	−1.279e-03	−8.436e-04	4.176e-04	2.169e-04	1.174e-04
Norm($\tilde{p}$)	−1.478e-03	**4.027e-04**	**−7.712e-05**	3.226e-04	1.946e-04	9.579e-05
Beta($\tilde{p}$)	−1.531e-03	**3.027e-04**	**2.386e-05**	3.241e-04	1.868e-04	9.981e-05
Laplace($\hat{p}$)	−3.394e-03	−1.431e-03	−9.157e-04	3.845e-04	2.634e-04	1.215e-04
Norm($\hat{p}$)	**−1.203e-03**	6.023e-04	**2.777e-05**	**2.705e-04**	**1.563e-04**	**8.652e-05**
Beta($\hat{p}$)	**−7.506e-04**	**3.842e-04**	−7.85e-05	**2.484e-04**	**1.509e-04**	**8.162e-05**

It should be mentioned that corresponding to quick, moderate, and slow rates of chemical reaction, we used sacrifice times $(\tau_1, \tau_2, \tau_3) = (10, 20, 30)$, $(30, 40, 50)$, and $(60, 70, 80)$, respectively. From Table 9, we observe that the Laplace prior is good for estimating a_0 and a_1. As expected, Laplace($\hat{p}$) is good for chemicals with quick reaction rate and Laplace($\tilde{p}$) performs better in the cases of slow reaction rate. There is no single dominant method for estimating b_0, b_1, but Norm($\hat{p}$) seems to outperform others in general. For estimating the mean of tumor onset time,

Table 6 Bias and MSE of the estimates of mean of tumor onset time at normal level, $\mu(\mathbf{x_0})$, and the probability of mice without tumors, $S(\cdot, \mathbf{x}_0)$, for chemical with quick reaction rate under different estimation methods

	Bias			MSE		
$\mu(\mathbf{x}_0) = 36.51$	$K = 30$	$K = 50$	$K = 100$	$K = 30$	$K = 50$	$K = 100$
EM	**1.832e+01**	**6.52e+00**	**2.44e+00**	**1.048e+04**	**6.328e+02**	**1.278e+02**
Laplace($\tilde{p}$)	1.267e+19	3.548e+29	**2.733e+00**	1.605e+41	1.259e+62	2.301e+02
Norm($\tilde{p}$)	2.322e+01	7.598e+00	2.841e+00	2.019e+04	7.456e+02	1.527e+02
Beta($\tilde{p}$)	2.193e+01	7.314e+00	2.795e+00	**1.21e+04**	7.455e+02	1.392e+02
Laplace($\hat{p}$)	9.753e+14	9.146e+06	4.995e+08	9.51e+32	8.364e+16	2.495e+20
Norm($\hat{p}$)	**2.133e+01**	**7.09e+00**	2.857e+00	1.939e+04	**7.025e+02**	**1.322e+02**
Beta($\hat{p}$)	**1.633e+01**	**6.473e+00**	**2.629e+00**	**4.844e+03**	**5.948e+02**	**1.193e+02**
$S(10, \mathbf{x}_0) = 0.8114$	$K = 30$	$K = 50$	$K = 100$	$K = 30$	$K = 50$	$K = 100$
EM	**8.725e-04**	**1.226e-03**	**3.447e-04**	**3.315e-03**	**2.02e-03**	**9.869e-04**
Laplace($\tilde{p}$)	−2.433e-03	−2.437e-03	−8.904e-04	3.941e-03	2.622e-03	1.221e-03
Norm($\tilde{p}$)	−4.638e-03	−2.39e-03	−1.53e-03	3.671e-03	2.285e-03	1.101e-03
Beta($\tilde{p}$)	−1.072e-02	−3.661e-03	−8.962e-04	3.713e-03	2.164e-03	1.13e-03
Laplace($\hat{p}$)	−3.953e-03	**−1.188e-03**	−6.577e-04	4.213e-03	2.541e-03	1.321e-03
Norm($\hat{p}$)	**1.158e-03**	1.229e-03	**−1.468e-04**	**2.561e-03**	**1.624e-03**	**9.668e-04**
Beta($\hat{p}$)	**−1.033e-03**	**9.504e-04**	**−2.666e-04**	**2.259e-03**	**1.505e-03**	**8.73e-04**
$S(20, \mathbf{x}_0) = 0.6265$	$K = 30$	$K = 50$	$K = 100$	$K = 30$	$K = 50$	$K = 100$
EM	**−8.383e-03**	**−4.479e-03**	**−2.272e-03**	**5.604e-03**	**3.1e-03**	**1.365e-03**
Laplace($\tilde{p}$)	−1.633e-02	−1.178e-02	−5.784e-03	8.722e-03	4.854e-03	2.019e-03
Norm($\tilde{p}$)	−1.18e-02	−6.981e-03	−4.114e-03	6.148e-03	3.456e-03	1.59e-03
Beta($\tilde{p}$)	−1.672e-02	−8.226e-03	−2.957e-03	5.748e-03	3.353e-03	1.518e-03
Laplace($\hat{p}$)	−1.873e-02	−1.066e-02	−4.349e-03	8.813e-03	4.437e-03	2.051e-03
Norm($\hat{p}$)	**−4.265e-03**	**−2.796e-03**	**−1.241e-03**	**2.921e-03**	**1.822e-03**	**9.507e-04**
Beta($\hat{p}$)	**−4.441e-03**	**−2.129e-03**	**−1.548e-03**	**1.671e-03**	**1.317e-03**	**8.345e-04**
$S(30, \mathbf{x}_0) = 0.4729$	$K = 30$	$K = 50$	$K = 100$	$K = 30$	$K = 50$	$K = 100$
EM	−2.088e-02	**−1.337e-02**	**−6.506e-03**	1.57e-02	**9.072e-03**	**4.008e-03**
Laplace($\tilde{p}$)	−2.881e-02	−2.222e-02	−1.18e-02	1.976e-02	1.207e-02	5.259e-03
Norm($\tilde{p}$)	**−2.041e-02**	−1.406e-02	−7.845e-03	1.576e-02	9.463e-03	4.408e-03
Beta($\tilde{p}$)	−2.297e-02	−1.453e-02	−6.594e-03	**1.497e-02**	9.176e-03	4.182e-03
Laplace($\hat{p}$)	−3.26e-02	−2.196e-02	−9.582e-03	2.048e-02	1.162e-02	5.306e-03
Norm($\hat{p}$)	**−1.489e-02**	**−1.06e-02**	**−4.523e-03**	**1.133e-02**	**6.871e-03**	**3.203e-03**
Beta($\hat{p}$)	**−1.315e-02**	**−9.141e-03**	**−4.761e-03**	**8.426e-03**	**5.562e-03**	**2.98e-03**

Table 7 Bias and MSE of the estimates of mean of tumor onset time at normal level, $\mu(\mathbf{x_0})$, and the probability of mice without tumors, $S(\cdot, \mathbf{x}_0)$, for chemical with moderate reaction rate under different estimation methods

	Bias			MSE		
$\mu(\mathbf{x}_0) = 54.46$	$K = 30$	$K = 50$	$K = 100$	$K = 30$	$K = 50$	$K = 100$
EM	**2.237e+01**	**6.346e+00**	**3.573e+00**	**2.196e+04**	**9.372e+02**	**2.843e+02**
Laplace($\tilde{p}$)	2.93e+10	3.212e+27	4.925e+05	8.582e+23	1.031e+58	2.422e+14
Norm($\tilde{p}$)	3.206e+01	7.944e+00	4.395e+00	6.513e+04	1.171e+03	3.22e+02
Beta($\tilde{p}$)	2.807e+01	7.514e+00	4.121e+00	2.833e+04	9.855e+02	3.309e+02
Laplace($\hat{p}$)	6.034e+10	9.051e+07	4.167e+10	3.64e+24	8.191e+18	1.736e+24
Norm($\hat{p}$)	**2.093e+01**	**6.701e+00**	**3.887e+00**	**1.68e+04**	**9.061e+02**	**2.674e+02**
Beta($\hat{p}$)	**2.073e+01**	**6.559e+00**	**3.565e+00**	**1.733e+04**	**7.963e+02**	**2.481e+02**
$S(30, \mathbf{x}_0) = 0.6246$	$K = 30$	$K = 50$	$K = 100$	$K = 30$	$K = 50$	$K = 100$
EM	**−1.072e-02**	**−6.11e-03**	**−1.053e-03**	**4.664e-03**	**2.486e-03**	**1.224e-03**
Laplace($\tilde{p}$)	−1.792e-02	−1.117e-02	−4.093e-03	6.932e-03	3.58e-03	1.936e-03
Norm($\tilde{p}$)	−1.373e-02	−7.271e-03	−1.772e-03	4.961e-03	2.76e-03	1.379e-03
Beta($\tilde{p}$)	−1.93e-02	−9.987e-03	−1.93e-03	5.159e-03	2.691e-03	1.403e-03
Laplace($\hat{p}$)	−1.466e-02	−1.108e-02	−4.331e-03	7.051e-03	4.02e-03	2.147e-03
Norm($\hat{p}$)	**−5.201e-03**	**−3.567e-03**	**4.105e-04**	**2.232e-03**	**1.607e-03**	**7.872e-04**
Beta($\hat{p}$)	**−5.112e-03**	**−2.244e-03**	**−1.114e-03**	**1.234e-03**	**1.002e-03**	**6.626e-04**
$S(40, \mathbf{x}_0) = 0.5182$	$K = 30$	$K = 50$	$K = 100$	$K = 30$	$K = 50$	$K = 100$
EM	**−2.025e-02**	**−1.132e-02**	**−4.376e-03**	**9.778e-03**	**4.906e-03**	**2.523e-03**
Laplace($\tilde{p}$)	−2.96e-02	−1.803e-02	−8.644e-03	1.331e-02	6.76e-03	3.66e-03
Norm($\tilde{p}$)	−2.071e-02	−1.14e-02	−4.475e-03	9.943e-03	5.266e-03	2.754e-03
Beta($\tilde{p}$)	−2.436e-02	−1.325e-02	−5.002e-03	9.796e-03	4.968e-03	2.743e-03
Laplace($\hat{p}$)	−2.573e-02	−1.815e-02	−9.536e-03	1.316e-02	7.15e-03	4.057e-03
Norm($\hat{p}$)	**−1.237e-02**	**−8.059e-03**	**−2.379e-03**	**5.641e-03**	**3.516e-03**	**1.831e-03**
Beta($\hat{p}$)	**−1.064e-02**	**−5.719e-03**	**−3.509e-03**	**3.766e-03**	**2.397e-03**	**1.553e-03**
$S(50, \mathbf{x}_0) = 0.4266$	$K = 30$	$K = 50$	$K = 100$	$K = 30$	$K = 50$	$K = 100$
EM	−2.428e-02	−1.426e-02	−6.763e-03	1.518e-02	8.057e-03	**4.498e-03**
Laplace($\tilde{p}$)	−3.336e-02	−2.145e-02	−1.157e-02	1.877e-02	1.037e-02	5.955e-03
Norm($\tilde{p}$)	**−2.22e-02**	**−1.322e-02**	**−6.215e-03**	1.488e-02	8.453e-03	4.826e-03
Beta($\tilde{p}$)	−2.411e-02	−1.433e-02	−7.09e-03	**1.46e-02**	**7.918e-03**	4.769e-03
Laplace($\hat{p}$)	−2.961e-02	−2.174e-02	−1.292e-02	1.854e-02	1.059e-02	6.503e-03
Norm($\hat{p}$)	**−1.607e-02**	**−1.081e-02**	**−4.487e-03**	**1.049e-02**	**6.375e-03**	**3.623e-03**
Beta($\hat{p}$)	**−1.371e-02**	**−8.033e-03**	**−5.245e-03**	**8.147e-03**	**4.862e-03**	**3.137e-03**

Table 8 Bias and MSE of the estimates of mean of tumor onset time at normal level, $\mu(\mathbf{x_0})$, and the probability of mice without tumors, $S(\cdot, \mathbf{x}_0)$, for chemical with slow reaction rate under different estimation methods

	Bias			MSE		
$\mu(\mathbf{x}_0) = 81.25$	$K = 30$	$K = 50$	$K = 100$	$K = 30$	$K = 50$	$K = 100$
EM	**3.69e+01**	**1.333e+01**	**4.543e+00**	**1.781e+05**	**2.904e+03**	**6.295e+02**
Laplace($\tilde{p}$)	7.185e+38	8.346e+18	5.678e+12	5.061e+80	6.965e+40	3.224e+28
Norm($\tilde{p}$)	5.6e+01	1.73e+01	5.43e+00	8.481e+05	4.743e+03	7.456e+02
Beta($\tilde{p}$)	5.423e+01	1.558e+01	5.259e+00	**5.797e+05**	4.192e+03	**6.421e+02**
Laplace($\hat{p}$)	2.527e+38	5.261e+20	1.523e+09	6.386e+79	2.767e+44	2.318e+21
Norm($\hat{p}$)	**5.255e+01**	**1.406e+01**	**5.149e+00**	7.985e+05	**2.688e+03**	6.971e+02
Beta($\hat{p}$)	**3.162e+01**	**1.389e+01**	**4.913e+00**	**7.85e+04**	**2.562e+03**	**5.045e+02**
$S(60, \mathbf{x}_0) = 0.5161$	$K = 30$	$K = 50$	$K = 100$	$K = 30$	$K = 50$	$K = 100$
EM	**−1.779e-02**	−9.626e-03	**−6.362e-03**	**1.028e-02**	**5.022e-03**	**2.556e-03**
Laplace($\tilde{p}$)	−2.974e-02	−1.68e-02	−1.073e-02	1.407e-02	7.479e-03	3.497e-03
Norm($\tilde{p}$)	−1.925e-02	**−9.19e-03**	−7.194e-03	1.066e-02	5.211e-03	2.836e-03
Beta($\tilde{p}$)	−2.117e-02	−1.212e-02	−6.4e-03	1.029e-02	5.059e-03	2.707e-03
Laplace($\hat{p}$)	−3.169e-02	−2.059e-02	−9.945e-03	1.492e-02	7.885e-03	3.426e-03
Norm($\hat{p}$)	**−1.323e-02**	**−5.603e-03**	**−5.056e-03**	**6.166e-03**	**3.346e-03**	**2.012e-03**
Beta($\hat{p}$)	**−1.06e-02**	**−3.668e-03**	**−3.225e-03**	**4.292e-03**	**2.614e-03**	**1.574e-03**
$S(70, \mathbf{x}_0) = 0.4533$	$K = 30$	$K = 50$	$K = 100$	$K = 30$	$K = 50$	$K = 100$
EM	**−2.223e-02**	−1.122e-02	−7.72e-03	1.399e-02	7.352e-03	**3.725e-03**
Laplace($\tilde{p}$)	−3.417e-02	−1.881e-02	−1.249e-02	1.816e-02	1.012e-02	4.85e-03
Norm($\tilde{p}$)	−2.244e-02	**−9.636e-03**	−8.145e-03	1.426e-02	7.536e-03	4.031e-03
Beta($\tilde{p}$)	−2.268e-02	−1.229e-02	**−7.517e-03**	**1.365e-02**	**7.22e-03**	3.879e-03
Laplace($\hat{p}$)	−3.53e-02	−2.253e-02	−1.164e-02	1.893e-02	1.066e-02	4.709e-03
Norm($\hat{p}$)	**−1.765e-02**	**−6.475e-03**	**−6.174e-03**	**9.408e-03**	**5.271e-03**	**3.075e-03**
Beta($\hat{p}$)	**−1.402e-02**	**−4.419e-03**	**−4.156e-03**	**7.164e-03**	**4.41e-03**	**2.495e-03**
$S(80, \mathbf{x}_0) = 0.3969$	$K = 30$	$K = 50$	$K = 100$	$K = 30$	$K = 50$	$K = 100$
EM	−2.365e-02	−1.138e-02	−8.332e-03	1.684e-02	9.511e-03	**4.872e-03**
Laplace($\tilde{p}$)	−3.45e-02	−1.879e-02	−1.324e-02	2.071e-02	1.228e-02	6.105e-03
Norm($\tilde{p}$)	−2.266e-02	**−8.73e-03**	−8.329e-03	1.7e-02	9.685e-03	5.176e-03
Beta($\tilde{p}$)	**−2.155e-02**	−1.117e-02	**−7.893e-03**	**1.622e-02**	**9.223e-03**	5.033e-03
Laplace($\hat{p}$)	−3.487e-02	−2.229e-02	−1.238e-02	2.137e-02	1.288e-02	5.907e-03
Norm($\hat{p}$)	**−1.955e-02**	**−6.283e-03**	**−6.63e-03**	**1.231e-02**	**7.191e-03**	**4.151e-03**
Beta($\hat{p}$)	**−1.544e-02**	**−4.268e-03**	**−4.571e-03**	**9.96e-03**	**6.301e-03**	**3.496e-03**

Table 9 The method of estimation with the least bias

Reaction rate	Quick		
Size	$K = 30$	$K = 50$	$K = 100$
a_0	Laplace($\hat{p}$)	Laplace($\tilde{p}$)	Laplace($\hat{p}$)
a_1	Laplace($\tilde{p}$)	Laplace($\hat{p}$)	EM
b_0	Norm($\hat{p}$)	Norm($\hat{p}$)	Beta($\hat{p}$)
b_1	Beta($\hat{p}$)	Norm($\hat{p}$)	EM
$\mu(x_0)$	Beta($\hat{p}$)	Beta($\hat{p}$)	Beta($\hat{p}$)
$S(\tau_1, x_0)$	EM	Beta($\hat{p}$)	Beta($\hat{p}$)
$S(\tau_2, x_0)$	Norm($\hat{p}$)	Beta($\hat{p}$)	Beta($\hat{p}$)
$S(\tau_3, x_0)$	Beta($\hat{p}$)	Beta($\hat{p}$)	Beta($\hat{p}$)
Reaction rate	Moderate		
Size	$K = 30$	$K = 50$	$K = 100$
a_0	Laplace($\hat{p}$)	Laplace($\tilde{p}$)	Laplace($\tilde{p}$)
a_1	Laplace($\hat{p}$)	Laplace($\hat{p}$)	Laplace($\tilde{p}$)
b_0	Norm($\hat{p}$)	Norm($\tilde{p}$)	Laplace($\hat{p}$)
b_1	EM	Norm($\hat{p}$)	Beta($\tilde{p}$)
$\mu(x_0)$	Beta($\hat{p}$)	EM	EM
$S(\tau_1, x_0)$	Beta($\hat{p}$)	Beta($\hat{p}$)	Beta($\hat{p}$)
$S(\tau_2, x_0)$	Beta($\hat{p}$)	Beta($\hat{p}$)	Beta($\hat{p}$)
$S(\tau_3, x_0)$	Beta($\hat{p}$)	Beta($\hat{p}$)	Beta($\hat{p}$)
Reaction rate	Slow		
Size	$K = 30$	$K = 50$	$K = 100$
a_0	Laplace($\tilde{p}$)	Laplace($\tilde{p}$)	Laplace($\hat{p}$)
a_1	Laplace($\tilde{p}$)	Laplace($\tilde{p}$)	EM
b_0	Beta($\hat{p}$)	Beta($\hat{p}$)	EM
b_1	Norm($\hat{p}$)	EM	Beta($\tilde{p}$)
$\mu(x_0)$	EM	Beta($\hat{p}$)	EM
$S(\tau_1, x_0)$	Norm($\hat{p}$)	Norm($\hat{p}$)	Beta($\hat{p}$)
$S(\tau_2, x_0)$	Norm($\hat{p}$)	Norm($\hat{p}$)	Beta($\hat{p}$)
$S(\tau_3, x_0)$	Norm($\hat{p}$)	Norm($\hat{p}$)	Beta($\hat{p}$)

both Beta($\hat{p}$) and EM perform well. For estimating the probability of mice without tumors, Beta($\hat{p}$) seems to be the best method. However, when the chemical reaction rate is slow, Norm($\hat{p}$) seems better for small and moderate sample sizes. The EM algorithm generally works very well when the sample size is large, and this agrees with the finding of Balakrishnan and Ling [2]. From Table 10, we see that Beta($\hat{p}$) appears to be the best method in terms of minimum MSE in general.

In some cases, the prior belief $\hat{p}$ is not always available. The methods with prior based only on observed data that provide the least bias and MSE in this case are listed in Tables 11 and 12, respectively. From Table 11, we can see that Laplace($\tilde{p}$) estimates the parameters a_0 and a_1 very well. For the parameters b_0 and b_1, there is no particular method that turns out to be best overall. For other quantities, EM

Table 10 The method of estimation with the least MSE

Reaction rate	Quick		
Size	$K = 30$	$K = 50$	$K = 100$
a_0	Beta($\hat{p}$)	Beta($\hat{p}$)	Beta($\hat{p}$)
a_1	Beta($\hat{p}$)	Beta($\hat{p}$)	Beta($\hat{p}$)
b_0	Beta($\hat{p}$)	Beta($\hat{p}$)	Beta($\hat{p}$)
b_1	Beta($\hat{p}$)	Beta($\hat{p}$)	Beta($\hat{p}$)
$\mu(x_0)$	Beta($\hat{p}$)	Norm($\hat{p}$)	Beta($\hat{p}$)
$S(\tau_1, x_0)$	Beta($\hat{p}$)	Beta($\hat{p}$)	Beta($\hat{p}$)
$S(\tau_2, x_0)$	Beta($\hat{p}$)	Beta($\hat{p}$)	Beta($\hat{p}$)
$S(\tau_3, x_0)$	Beta($\hat{p}$)	Beta($\hat{p}$)	Beta($\hat{p}$)
Reaction rate	Moderate		
Size	$K = 30$	$K = 50$	$K = 100$
a_0	Beta($\hat{p}$)	Beta($\hat{p}$)	Beta($\hat{p}$)
a_1	Beta($\hat{p}$)	Beta($\hat{p}$)	Beta($\hat{p}$)
b_0	Beta($\hat{p}$)	Beta($\hat{p}$)	Beta($\hat{p}$)
b_1	Beta($\hat{p}$)	Beta($\hat{p}$)	Beta($\hat{p}$)
$\mu(x_0)$	Beta($\hat{p}$)	Beta($\hat{p}$)	Beta($\hat{p}$)
$S(\tau_1, x_0)$	Beta($\hat{p}$)	Beta($\hat{p}$)	Beta($\hat{p}$)
$S(\tau_2, x_0)$	Beta($\hat{p}$)	Beta($\hat{p}$)	Beta($\hat{p}$)
$S(\tau_3, x_0)$	Beta($\hat{p}$)	Beta($\hat{p}$)	Beta($\hat{p}$)
Reaction rate	Slow		
Size	$K = 30$	$K = 50$	$K = 100$
a_0	Beta($\hat{p}$)	Beta($\hat{p}$)	Beta($\hat{p}$)
a_1	Beta($\hat{p}$)	Beta($\hat{p}$)	Beta($\hat{p}$)
b_0	Beta($\hat{p}$)	Beta($\hat{p}$)	Beta($\hat{p}$)
b_1	Beta($\hat{p}$)	Beta($\hat{p}$)	Beta($\hat{p}$)
$\mu(x_0)$	Beta($\hat{p}$)	Beta($\hat{p}$)	Beta($\hat{p}$)
$S(\tau_1, x_0)$	Beta($\hat{p}$)	Beta($\hat{p}$)	Beta($\hat{p}$)
$S(\tau_2, x_0)$	Beta($\hat{p}$)	Beta($\hat{p}$)	Beta($\hat{p}$)
$S(\tau_3, x_0)$	Beta($\hat{p}$)	Beta($\hat{p}$)	Beta($\hat{p}$)

algorithm seems to be the best method of estimation. From Table 12, EM seems to perform well for estimating the parameters and all the quantities of interest. We also observe that Beta($\tilde{p}$) estimates the probability of mice without tumors quite well in the case of quick reaction rate, large sample size, and long sacrifice time. Also, Beta($\tilde{p}$) is good at predicting the probability of mice without tumors of a long sacrifice time when the number of mice having tumors is large.

Table 11 The method of estimation with the least bias among the methods with prior based only on observed data

Reaction rate	Quick		
Size	$K = 30$	$K = 50$	$K = 100$
a_0	Laplace($\tilde{p}$)	Laplace($\tilde{p}$)	Laplace($\tilde{p}$)
a_1	Laplace($\tilde{p}$)	Laplace($\tilde{p}$)	EM
b_0	EM	EM	Beta($\tilde{p}$)
b_1	EM	Norm($\tilde{p}$)	EM
$\mu(x_0)$	EM	EM	EM
$S(\tau_1, x_0)$	EM	EM	EM
$S(\tau_2, x_0)$	EM	EM	EM
$S(\tau_3, x_0)$	Norm($\tilde{p}$)	Norm($\tilde{p}$)	Beta($\tilde{p}$)
Reaction rate	Moderate		
Size	$K = 30$	$K = 50$	$K = 100$
a_0	Laplace($\tilde{p}$)	Laplace($\tilde{p}$)	Laplace($\tilde{p}$)
a_1	Laplace($\tilde{p}$)	Beta($\tilde{p}$)	Laplace($\tilde{p}$)
b_0	Norm($\tilde{p}$)	Norm($\tilde{p}$)	EM
b_1	EM	Beta($\tilde{p}$)	Beta($\tilde{p}$)
$\mu(x_0)$	EM	EM	EM
$S(\tau_1, x_0)$	EM	EM	Norm($\tilde{p}$)
$S(\tau_2, x_0)$	EM	EM	Norm($\tilde{p}$)
$S(\tau_3, x_0)$	EM	Norm($\tilde{p}$)	Norm($\tilde{p}$)
Reaction rate		Slow	
Size	$K = 30$	$K = 50$	$K = 100$
a_0	Laplace($\tilde{p}$)	Laplace($\tilde{p}$)	Laplace($\tilde{p}$)
a_1	Laplace($\tilde{p}$)	Laplace($\tilde{p}$)	EM
b_0	Norm($\tilde{p}$)	Norm($\tilde{p}$)	EM
b_1	Beta($\tilde{p}$)	EM	Beta($\tilde{p}$)
$\mu(x_0)$	EM	EM	EM
$S(\tau_1, x_0)$	EM	EM	EM
$S(\tau_2, x_0)$	EM	EM	Beta($\tilde{p}$)
$S(\tau_3, x_0)$	EM	Norm($\tilde{p}$)	Beta($\tilde{p}$)

Table 12 The method of estimation with the least MSE among the methods with prior based only on observed data

Reaction rate	Quick			Moderate			Slow		
Size	$K = 30$	$K = 50$	$K = 100$	$K = 30$	$K = 50$	$K = 100$	$K = 30$	$K = 50$	$K = 100$
a_0	EM	EM	EM	EM	EM	EM	EM	EM	EM
a_1	EM	EM	EM	EM	EM	EM	EM	EM	EM
b_0	EM	EM	EM	EM	EM	EM	EM	EM	EM
b_1	EM	EM	EM	EM	EM	EM	EM	EM	EM
$\mu(x_0)$	EM	EM	EM	EM	EM	EM	EM	EM	EM
$S(\tau_1, x_0)$	EM	EM	EM	EM	EM	EM	EM	EM	EM
$S(\tau_2, x_0)$	EM	EM	Beta($\tilde{p}$)	EM	EM	Beta($\tilde{p}$)	EM	EM	EM
$S(\tau_3, x_0)$	Beta($\tilde{p}$)	Beta($\tilde{p}$)	Beta($\tilde{p}$)	EM	Beta($\tilde{p}$)	Beta($\tilde{p}$)	EM	EM	EM

5 Sensitivity Analysis on Prior Accuracy

The prior information with different variances, c^2, may affect the estimation of model parameters. For this reason, we examine the sensitivity of the estimation for varying c^2. It is common in practice to have good prior information in case of most Bayesian analyses. So, we set values of c as $c^2 = 0.005, 0.001$, and 0.0005 in our simulation study, in order to reflect different levels of accuracy with respect to prior information. For different c^2, the bias and MSE of the estimate of a_1 with normal prior distribution using prior information $\hat{p}$ are presented in Table 13. From Table 13, we observe that when c^2 decreases, the MSE also decreases because the prior information becomes more accurate in this case. Of course, decreasing c^2 will not necessarily reduce the bias when the sample size is small or moderate. The reason for this is that the prior information has smaller variance, and so the estimation will depend more on the accurate prior information instead of the imprecise information from the sample. In this case, the estimation will put more weight on the prior information. A decrease in c^2 may not necessarily result in a reduction in the size of bias of the estimates since the samples may be significantly different from the prior information.

6 Application to Tumorigenicity Data from Sacrificial Experiments

In this section, a real data from a study of benzidine dihydrochloride to tumor in mice is analyzed, in which strain of offspring, gender, and concentration of benzidine dihydrochloride used are involved as the covariates. In addition, in each group, the time to being sacrificed, the numbers of mice tested, and the numbers of mice having tumors are all recorded. These data were originally reported by Kodell and Nelson [16] and analyzed by Balakrishnan and Ling [3] under the Weibull distribution. One may also refer to Finkelstein and Ryan [14] and Lindsey and Ryan [17] for some other models in this regard.

Here, let a_1, a_2, and a_3 denote the parameters corresponding to the covariates of strain of offspring, gender, and square root of concentration of the chemical benzidine dihydrochloride in the scale parameter of the Weibull distribution, while b_1, b_2, and b_3 denote similarly for the shape parameter. The estimates of the model parameters and the mean of onset time of tumors for each group are computed by means of the Bayesian approach, along with the corresponding standard errors for all the model parameters. These results are all presented in Tables 14 and 15.

Table 14 presents the Bayesian estimates of the model parameters, along with the corresponding standard errors, based on various priors. The estimates obtained from different priors are not similar for some model parameters, especially a_1 and a_2. However, from the Norm prior and Beta prior, it is evident that both the shape and scale parameters vary with all the covariates. Also, under the Weibull distribution,

Table 13 Comparison of different prior variances c^2 in the estimate of α_1 under Norm($\hat{p}$)

$a_1 = -0.05$		Bias			MSE		
Reaction rate	c^2	$K = 30$	$K = 50$	$K = 100$	$K = 30$	$K = 50$	$K = 100$
Slow	0.005	−1.431e-03	−1.447e-03	−5.004e-04	2.022e-04	1.236e-04	5.964e-05
	0.001	−1.342e-03	−1.505e-03	−4.628e-04	1.789e-04	1.061e-04	5.238e-05
	0.0005	−1.633e-03	−1.468e-03	−3.757e-04	1.751e-04	1.01e-04	4.448e-05
Moderate	0.005	−1.557e-03	−9.033e-04	−8.835e-04	2.009e-04	1.112e-04	6.75e-05
	0.001	−1.732e-03	−7.849e-04	−7.37e-04	1.73e-04	8.921e-05	5.598e-05
	0.0005	−1.79e-03	−1.018e-03	−6.439e-04	1.701e-04	8.629e-05	5.339e-05
Quick	0.005	−2.964e-03	−1.29e-03	−9.535e-04	2.832e-04	1.567e-04	7.179e-05
	0.001	−2.793e-03	−1.423e-03	−8.125e-04	2.529e-04	1.383e-04	6.095e-05
	0.0005	−2.936e-03	−1.473e-03	−7.448e-04	2.45e-04	1.33e-04	5.669e-05

Table 14 Bayesian estimates of the model parameters along with standard errors (within brackets)

	Scale parameter α			
	a_0	a_1	a_2	a_3
Laplace($\tilde{p}$)	3.2877 (0.0347)	0.0143 (0.0113)	0.4786 (0.0422)	−0.0483 (0.0028)
Norm($\tilde{p}$)	3.3828 (0.0671)	0.0311 (0.0007)	0.6997 (0.0617)	−0.0597 (0.0042)
Beta($\tilde{p}$)	3.3178 (0.0185)	0.0774 (0.0129)	0.7423 (0.0403)	−0.0522 (0.0014)
	Shape parameter β			
	b_0	b_1	b_2	b_3
Laplace($\tilde{p}$)	2.0348 (0.1712)	−0.0820 (0.0753)	−0.3566 (0.0873)	−0.0288 (0.0103)
Norm($\tilde{p}$)	1.7357 (0.0391)	−0.2170 (0.0050)	−0.5008 (0.0160)	−0.0706 (0.0014)
Beta($\tilde{p}$)	1.1313 (0.0649)	−0.3215 (0.0284)	−0.6216 (0.0530)	−0.0463 (0.0041)

Table 15 Bayesian estimates of the mean of onset time of tumors along with standard errors (within brackets)

Concentration			$\hat{\mu}$ in months		
Strain	Gender	in ppm	Laplace($\tilde{p}$)	Norm($\tilde{p}$)	Beta($\tilde{p}$)
F1	F	60	17.1094 (0.2679)	16.6401 (0.5491)	16.3120 (0.1404)
F1	F	120	14.5777 (0.1695)	13.6061 (0.2801)	13.8306 (0.0854)
F1	F	200	12.4328 (0.1780)	11.2130 (0.1043)	11.8167 (0.0716)
F1	F	400	9.2810 (0.2623)	8.1532 (0.1102)	9.0860 (0.1056)
F2	F	60	17.2780 (0.2885)	17.0114 (0.5610)	17.8809 (0.3032)
F2	F	120	14.7192 (0.1827)	13.9948 (0.2961)	15.4301 (0.2481)
F2	F	200	12.5524 (0.1820)	11.6632 (0.1272)	13.5046 (0.2090)
F2	F	400	9.3712 (0.2607)	8.8570 (0.1294)	11.1138 (0.2038)
F1	M	60	27.0806 (1.1906)	33.1142 (1.0992)	36.7752 (1.9424)
F1	M	120	23.0676 (0.9134)	27.6913 (1.1414)	32.7747 (1.9602)
F1	M	200	19.6751 (0.7336)	23.7067 (1.1867)	29.9440 (2.1498)
F1	M	400	14.7080 (0.5747)	19.8003 (1.3312)	27.7470 (3.2192)
F2	M	60	27.3419 (1.1785)	34.5574 (1.1557)	45.8196 (2.6647)
F2	M	120	23.2938 (0.8977)	29.5177 (1.2073)	43.3843 (3.0099)
F2	M	200	19.8744 (0.7158)	26.1322 (1.2879)	42.8696 (3.8101)
F2	M	400	14.8749 (0.5553)	24.4588 (1.7216)	48.9678 (7.9914)

the mean of onset time of tumors can be determined. It helps us understand how much the covariates influence the mean of the onset time of tumors. For example, females get tumor earlier than males. Tumors are induced by the increase in dose of benzidine dihydrochloride. F1 strain mice get tumor earlier than F2 strain mice. It is worth noting that the estimate of the mean of the onset time tumors obtained from the Beta prior may not be reasonable because it is observed that the mean is not decreasing when the dose of the chemical is increased.

7 Concluding Remarks

In this work, a Bayesian approach has been developed for tumorigenicity data from sacrificial experiments under Weibull lifetime. Three different prior distributions have been considered, and their corresponding posterior distributions have been derived by the use of Metropolis–Hastings algorithm. The performance of the Bayesian approach has been compared with the maximum likelihood estimation obtained by the use of the EM algorithm by means of Monte Carlo simulations. If accurate prior information is available, the Bayesian approach turns out to be the best. If such prior information is not available, the EM-based likelihood method turns out to be a good method of estimation.

For further study, we can extend the work to the case of gamma lifetimes for which the likelihood approach has been developed by Balakrishnan and Ling [4]. It will also be of interest to generalize the present work to incorporate competing risks along the lines of Balakrishnan et al. [5, 6] who discussed it for the exponential and Weibull cases. We are currently looking into these problems and hope to report the findings in a future research.

Acknowledgments This work was made possible by the facilities of the Shared Hierarchical Academic Research Computing Network (SHARCNET: www.sharcnet.ca) and Compute/Calcul Canada. This work was supported by grants from the Natural Sciences and Engineering Research Council of Canada, the Research Grants Council of the Hong Kong Special Administrative Region, China (Project No. [T32-101/15-R]), and the Education University of Hong Kong (Ref. IDS-2 2019, MIT/SGA05/19-20).

References

1. Agresti, A.: Categorical Data Analysis. Wiley, Hoboken, New Jersey (2013)
2. Balakrishnan, N., Ling, M.H.: EM algorithm for one-shot device testing under the exponential distribution. Comput. Stat. Data Anal. **56**, 502–509 (2012)
3. Balakrishnan, N., Ling, M.H.: Expectation maximization algorithm for one shot device accelerated life testing with Weibull lifetimes, and variable parameters over stress. IEEE Trans. Reliab. **62**, 537–551 (2013)
4. Balakrishnan, N., Ling, M.H.: Gamma lifetimes and one-shot device testing analysis. Reliab. Eng. Syst. Saf. **126**, 54–64 (2014)
5. Balakrishnan, N., So, H.Y., Ling, M.H.: EM algorithm for one-shot device testing with competing risks under exponential distribution. Reliab. Eng. Syst. Saf. **137**, 129–140 (2015)
6. Balakrishnan, N., So, H.Y., Ling, M.H.: EM algorithm for one-shot device testing with competing risks under Weibull distribution. IEEE Trans. Reliab. **65**, 973–991 (2016)
7. Berger, J.: Statistical Decision Theory and Bayesian Analysis. Springer, New York (1985)
8. Berlin, B., Brodsky, J., Clifford, P.: Testing disease dependence in survival experiments with serial sacrifice. J. Am. Stat. Assoc. **74**, 5–14 (1979)
9. Ding, A.A., Wang, W.: Testing independence for bivariate current status data. J. Am. Stat. Assoc. **99**, 145–155 (2004)
10. Dinse, G.E.: Constant risk differences in the analysis of animal tumorigenicity data. Biometrics **47**, 681–700 (1991)

11. Dinse, G.E.: Evaluating constraints that allow survival-adjusted incidence analyses in single-sacrifice studies. Biometrics **49**, 399–407 (1993)
12. Dunson, D.B., Dinse, G.E.: Bayesian models for multivariate current status data with informative censoring. Biometrics **58**, 79–88 (2002)
13. Fan, T.H., Balakrishnan, N., Chang, C.C.: The Bayesian approach for highly reliable electro-explosive devices using one-shot device testing. J. Stat. Comput. Simul. **79**, 1143–1154 (2009)
14. Finkelstein, D.M., Ryan, L.M.: Estimating carcinogenic potency from a rodent tumorigenicity experiment. J. R. Stat. Soc. Ser. C **36**, 121–133 (1987)
15. Hastings, W.K.: Monte Carlo sampling methods using Markov chains and their applications. Biometrika **57**, 97–109 (1970)
16. Kodell, R.L., Nelson, C.J.: An illness-death model for the study of the carcinogenic process using survival/sacrifice data. Biometrics **36**, 267–277 (1980)
17. Lindsey, J.C., Ryan, L.M.: A three-state multiplicative model for rodent tumorigenicity experiments. J. R. Stat. Soc. Ser. C **42**, 283–300 (1993)
18. Ling, M.H., So, H.Y., Balakrishnan, N.: Likelihood inference under proportional hazards model for one-shot device testing. IEEE Trans. Reliab. **65**, 446–458 (2016)
19. Ma, L., Hu, T., Sun, J.: Sieve maximum likelihood regression analysis of dependent current status data. Biometrika **102**, 731–738 (2015)
20. Roberts, G.O., Gelman, A., Gilks, W.R.: Weak convergence and optimal scaling of random walk Metropolis algorithms. Ann. App. Probab. **7**, 110–120 (1997)
21. Roberts, G.O., Rosenthal, J.S.: Optimal scaling for various Metropolis-Hastings algorithms. Stat. Sci. **16**, 351–367 (2001)
22. Rossini, A.J., Tsiatis, A.A.: A semiparametric proportional odds regression model for the analysis of current status data. J. Am Stat. Assoc. **91**, 713–721 (1996)
23. Wang, W., Ding, A.A.: On assessing the association for bivariate current status data. Biometrika **87**, 879–893 (2000)
24. Zhao, S., Hu, T., Ma, L., Wang, P., Sun, J.: Regression analysis of informative current status data with the additive hazards model. Lifetime Data Anal. **21**, 241–258 (2015)

Bayesian Sensitivity Analysis in Survival and Longitudinal Trials with Missing Data

G. Frank Liu and Fang Chen

Abstract Survival and longitudinal clinical trials are commonly conducted to evaluate experimental drug, biologic, and vaccine products. Conventional methods such as the log-rank test and the Cox proportional hazards model assume non-informative censoring for time-to-event data, and mixed model analysis assumes missing-at-random (MAR) in longitudinal trials. Although such assumptions play a critical role in influencing the outcome of the analysis, there are no formal methods to validate such assumptions from the data at hand. Sensitivity analyses are often recommended to test the robustness of an analysis that depends on such assumptions. In this chapter, we discuss how to perform practical sensitivity analysis, in a Bayesian modeling setting, to handle missing and censored data in clinical trials. Specifically, we focus on the delta-adjusted and control-based imputation strategies under informative censoring or missing-not-at-random (MNAR) mechanisms. Applications to real clinical trials are presented to demonstrate these methods.

1 Introduction

In most survival and longitudinal clinical trials, it is inevitable that some patients prematurely withdraw from trials for various reasons, such as adverse events and lack of treatment efficacy. Patients who withdraw from trials can follow different treatment trajectories. For example, they might stop treatment, switch to a different treatment, or receive additional treatment. Discontinuation of treatment often leads to patients dropping out of the study, so no data are collected afterward. Even

G. Frank Liu (✉)
Merck & Co., Inc., North Wales, PA, USA
e-mail: guanghan_frank_liu@merck.com

F. Chen
SAS Institute Inc., Cary, NC, USA
e-mail: fangk.chen@sas.com

Y. Lio et al. (eds.), *Bayesian Inference and Computation in Reliability and Survival Analysis*, Emerging Topics in Statistics and Biostatistics,
https://doi.org/10.1007/978-3-030-88658-5_11

if those patients agree to stay in the study, the outcomes that are collected after treatment is completed can be systematically different from the outcomes if the patients were to continue with the assigned treatment in the trial. Such missing data and potential discrepancies can seriously undermine the validity of the analysis and hinder our ability to assess the effectiveness of the treatment. The recent International Council for Harmonization (ICH) E9 (R1) addendum [1] requires clear definition of the estimands that describe the quantity to be estimated in study protocols. The estimand framework includes how to handle intercurrent events (IEs) such as premature discontinuation that can affect the collection and interpretation of the data for trials. Analyzing trials with appropriate methods to handle IEs and missing data is critical when we want to evaluate the between-group treatment effect.

To investigate the treatment effect of a testing product and avoid potential confounding from other rescue medications, sponsors are often interested in hypothetical estimands. One of the hypothetical estimands is to envision what the outcome would be if a dropout patient had not experienced any IEs and had continued with the assigned treatment. Clearly, data cannot be collected after dropout under this hypothetical scenario. Rather, assumptions are made in analysis models to estimate what treatment effect would be. In survival trials, conventional methods, such as the log-rank test and the Cox proportional hazards model, treat premature discontinuation as non-informative or random censoring [2]. As a result, the hazard ratio from those analyses evaluates the treatment difference with the assumption that all patients would complete the assigned treatment without IEs. This random censoring is similar to the missing-at-random (MAR) assumption commonly used in the analysis of longitudinal trials [3], where the repeated measures after IEs are treated as missing.

Assumptions of random censoring or MAR are not verifiable from observed study data, meaning we cannot rule out that probabilities of missing data can depend on the unobserved outcomes (missing not at random). Sensitivity analysis is recommended by regulatory guidance documents in order to assess the robustness of the analysis results under various deviations from the random censoring or MAR assumptions [1, 4]. In the area of survival analysis, control-based multiple imputation and delta-adjusted methods were put forth as effective and practical approaches in conducting sensitivity analysis [5–8]. The idea is to impute the censored event time, many times over, using estimated survival functions from data in a reference group (e.g., control group) or using adjusted survival functions. For longitudinal trials, similar approaches of control-based and delta-adjusted imputation methods have been proposed [11–16].

In this chapter, we review sensitivity analysis approaches in both survival analysis and longitudinal trials, with a focus on the Bayesian approach using control-based and delta-adjusted imputation methods. The Bayesian paradigm offers an effective modeling approach in this area, largely because of its ability to conduct *proper* multiple imputation and to model uncertainty of outcome trajectories with prior distributions. Because of their dependency on heavy computation and the shortage of user-friendly software packages, Bayesian methods have not been widely used in practice. With modern computers and rapid maturing of Bayesian software packages such as PROC MCMC in SAS, WinBUGS, NIMBLE, and Stan, Bayesian approaches have become a practical solution to address complex missing data problems faced in clinical trials.

The chapter is organized as follows. Sensitivity analysis methods based on multiple imputation (MI) under different assumptions for survival analysis are presented in Sect. 2. Section 3 discusses sensitivity analysis of missing data in longitudinal studies, where a Bayesian approach is introduced to incorporate additional variation for the trajectory responses. Applications to two clinical trial examples are presented in Sect. 4. A summary and discussion are provided in Sect. 5.

2 Sensitivity Analysis for Censoring in Survival Trials

Suppose that T_i is the time to event of interest and C_i is the censoring time for patient i. We observe $Y_i = \min(T_i, C_i)$ and denote the censoring indicator $d_i = I(T_i > C_i)$. Under the proportional hazards assumption, the hazard function is

$$h_i(t) = \lambda_0(t)\exp(\beta Z_i + \boldsymbol{\gamma}'\boldsymbol{X}_i) \tag{1}$$

where $Z_i = 0$ (control) or 1 (test drug) is a treatment indicator and $\boldsymbol{X}_i$ is a vector of baseline covariates. The function $\lambda_0(t)$ is an unspecified baseline hazard that corresponds to the hazards of a patient in the control group at $\boldsymbol{X}_i = 0$. The parameters $\{\beta, \boldsymbol{\gamma}\}$ can be estimated using a partial-likelihood approach that has been widely implemented in many software packages (e.g., PROC PHREG in SAS and the coxph library in R).

In a clinical trial, two types of censoring can occur: administrative and non-administrative censoring. Administrative censoring is an operationally inserted cutoff time point when a patient reaches the end of the study. This type of censoring is often independent of study outcomes and non-informative; thus it is random censoring. For this type of censoring, conventional methods, such as the log-rank test or Cox proportional hazards model, are adequate. Non-administrative censoring is due to premature discontinuation, which often occurs when patients have safety or efficacy concerns. This type of censoring can depend on treatment and potentially the time to event, and therefore it is informative. Sensitivity analysis, under various scenarios, should be applied to non-administrative censoring data.

One way to handle censoring is to impute the missing event times. Suppose that the survival function is

$$S(t) = \exp\left(-\int_0^t h(s)ds\right) \tag{2}$$

Under random censoring, the conditional survival function after censoring time at c is

$$S(t|t > c) = S(t)/S(c) = \exp\left(-\int_c^t h(s)ds\right) \tag{3}$$

Assume that we are able to estimate the survival function, such as by using a parametric model or Kaplan–Meier (KM) estimation, and we denote the estimate to be $\hat{S}(t)$. The following steps provide a recipe to impute survival time for a patient who is censored at c_i:

1. Draw a random number u_i from a uniform distribution: $U[0, \hat{S}(c_i)]$.
2. Use the solution to $u_i = \hat{S}(t|Z_i, \boldsymbol{X}_i)$ as the imputed event time.

Repeat these steps for all censored observations to obtain one copy of a complete dataset. Repeat the process M times. Then use a Cox regression model on each of the complete datasets, and obtain M estimates of the log-hazard ratio. The results can be combined using Rubin's method of inference. The point estimate is the average of the log-hazard ratio estimates from the M imputed datasets, and its variance is a weighted combination of the within and between variances.

2.1 Delta-Adjusted Imputation and Jump-to-Reference

The purpose of sensitivity analysis is to determine how various assumptions, when incorporated into an imputation model, can alter the outcome of an analysis. Suppose that the hazard at time $t > c_i$ for a non-administratively censored patient is $\delta h_i(t)$. Then the estimated survival function for this patient is

$$\hat{S}_i^*(t) = \begin{cases} \hat{S}(t|Z_i, \boldsymbol{X}_i), & \text{if } t \le c_i \\ \hat{S}(c_i|Z_i, \boldsymbol{X}_i)\hat{S}(t|t > c_i, Z_i, \boldsymbol{X}_i)^{\delta}, & \text{if } t > c_i \end{cases} \tag{4}$$

We describe two approaches to assess deviations from the random censoring assumption: use different δ parameter values or modify the hazard function $h_i(t)$ for censored patients in the test drug group.

(1) Delta-Adjusted Imputation

In the delta-adjusted imputation method [8], the hazard function $h_i(t)$ remains identical to that in Cox PH models, but the δ value is set to be greater than 1 for patients in the test drug group (i.e., when $Z_i = 1$). Non-administrative censored observations for patients in the treatment group are imputed using the hazard function $\delta h_i(t)$. No adjustments are made for censored patients in the control group (i.e., assuming random censoring). The conditional survival function is

$$\hat{S}(t|t > c_i, Z_i, \boldsymbol{X}_i) = \begin{cases} \hat{S}(t|t > c_i, Z_i, \boldsymbol{X}_i), & \text{if } Z_i = 0, \\ \hat{S}(t|t > c_i, Z_i, \boldsymbol{X}_i)^{\delta}, & \text{if } Z_i = 1 \end{cases} \tag{5}$$

Sensitivity analysis using the delta-adjusted method is a way to assess modeling robustness under potential departure from non-informative censoring. The δ value, when set to be greater than 1, reflects a less favorable scenario for the test drug group. In practice, we often gradually move the δ value from small to large, until we reach a tipping point where the significant p-value of testing treatment difference becomes insignificant. A larger $\delta(> 1)$ value implies more penalty being applied to the treatment effect. Therefore, a larger tipping point would make us feel more confident in the primary analysis results; i.e., we need to apply a big penalty to the treatment group to turn the results from significant to insignificant.

(2) Jump-to-Reference (J2R)

We assume that censoring is random for all patients in the control group. That is, the hazards for patients who withdraw from a placebo-controlled group should be similar to the hazards of patients who continue with the placebo, because we do not anticipate any biologic differences to be introduced by the placebo. For patients in the test drug group, we set $\delta = 1$ and $h_i(t) = \lambda_0(t)\exp(\boldsymbol{\gamma}'\boldsymbol{X}_i)$ for $t > c_i$; that is, after discontinuation, a patient in the test drug group has the same hazard as a patient in the control group (jump-to-reference, J2R). The conditional survival function used in imputation for discontinued treatment patients is

$$\hat{S}(t|t > c_i, Z_i, \boldsymbol{X}_i) = \exp\left(-\int_{c_i}^{t} \lambda_0(s)\exp(\boldsymbol{\gamma}'\boldsymbol{X}_i)ds\right) \tag{6}$$

The J2R approach is one of the control-based imputation methods. It hypothesizes a situation where patients in the test drug group stop receiving the test drug and switch to a treatment that is similar to the one received by the control group. By replacing the hazard function for patients after the dropout dates, J2R aims to negate the model-implied hazard on the potential treatment effects after censoring.

2.2 *Estimation of Survival Functions*

In both the delta-adjusted and J2R imputation methods, one challenge is to estimate survival functions that can be used to impute censored event times. Instead of using a piecewise exponential model as recommended by Lu et al. [7] and Lipkovich et al. [8], we consider a mixture Weibull model to estimate survival functions and use a Bayesian approach to MI to implement control-based and delta-adjusted sensitivity analysis.

We first briefly describe a piecewise exponential model. As the name indicates, the model fits an exponential survival function to each of the time intervals over the time domain. Let there be $p + 1$ intervals that are defined by p change points: $0 < \tau_1 < \tau_2 < \cdots < \tau_p$. Within each interval, the hazard rate is a constant with respect to t,

$$h_i(t) = \lambda_j \exp(\beta Z_i + \boldsymbol{\gamma}'\boldsymbol{X}_i), \text{ if } \tau_{j-1} < t < \tau_j \tag{7}$$

for $j = 1, \ldots, p+1$, where $\tau_0 = 0$ and $\tau_{p+1} = \infty$. Its survival function is

$$S(t|Z_i, \boldsymbol{X}_i) = \exp\left(-\left[\sum_{l=1}^{j-1}(\tau_l - \tau_{l-1})\lambda_l + (t - \tau_{j-1})\lambda_j\right]\exp(\beta Z_i + \boldsymbol{\gamma}'\boldsymbol{X}_i)\right), \quad \text{if } \tau_{j-1} < t < \tau_j$$

Dedicated Bayesian routines that fit piecewise exponential survival models are readily available in standard software packages (e.g., PROC PHREG in SAS). Posterior samples of $(\lambda_1, \ldots, \lambda_p)$, β, and $\boldsymbol{\gamma}$ are used to impute non-administratively censored data, based on the conditional survival function of Eq. (5) or (6) in either the delta-adjusted or J2R method.

The biggest challenge of using piecewise exponential models to estimate the baseline survival function is how to specify the time intervals. A moderately large value of p is often used. For example, the PHREG procedure uses $p = 8$ by default, and places an approximately equal number of events in each interval. Methods of estimating the change points can be complicated [9, 10]. A fairly large value of p may be needed to fit survival data that have abrupt drops in the cure effect, which often occur in studies such as immuno-oncology trials [17]. In order to fit the model well, each interval must also contain sufficient events. These challenges make it difficult to prespecify the method, a step that is often required in clinical trials for regulatory submission.

To overcome shortcomings of the piecewise exponential model, we consider an alternative approach using a mixture Weibull model. A two- or three-component mixture model can approximate well to the survival curves of a Cox PH model that are based on the non-parametric KM baseline survival estimator [17, 18]. This mixture Weibull model can be prespecified for the sensitivity analysis. In addition, estimated survival curves from the mixture Weibull model are monotonically decreasing and smooth, as opposed to zigzagged estimated step functions from Cox models. The smoothness and monotonicity enable us to efficiently solve the inverse function $u_i = \hat{S}(t|z_i, \boldsymbol{X}_i)$ for imputation.

In general, a q-component mixture Weibull model has a survival function

$$S(t|\boldsymbol{X}_i) = \sum_{j=1}^{q} w_j \exp\left[-\left(\frac{t}{\lambda_j(\boldsymbol{X}_i)}\right)^{\tau_j}\right] \tag{8}$$

where $w_j \geq 0$ are the mixture weights and $\sum w_j = 1$. The scale and shape parameters of a Weibull distribution (for component j) are $\lambda_j(\boldsymbol{X}_i) = \exp(\alpha_j + \boldsymbol{\gamma}'\boldsymbol{X}_i)$ and τ_j, respectively. Based on the research of Liu and Liao [18], a q value of 2 or 3 would provide a good fit for many oncology trials in applications.

A Cox PH model with a q-component mixture Weibull as the baseline survival function has the form [18]

$$S(t|Z_i, \boldsymbol{X}_i) = [S(t|\boldsymbol{X}_i)]^{\exp(\beta Z_i)}$$

where $S(t|\boldsymbol{X}_i)$ is the q-component mixture Weibull defined in Eq. (8). For this fully parametric model, the likelihood function is known. This makes it possible to specify the model in a general Bayesian sampling tool, such as PROC MCMC or Stan, to obtain posterior samples for the parameters of $(\alpha_1, \ldots, \alpha_q, \tau_1, \ldots, \tau_q, \beta, \boldsymbol{\gamma})$ in the model.

2.3 Inference Using the Bootstrap Method

In both the delta-adjusted and J2R imputation methods, we use a modified hazard function in the imputation model to generate missing times to event for patients who withdraw from the test drug group. These imputation models are different from the analysis model for the complete dataset; the latter model fits the same hazard function for both observed and imputed times to event in the treatment group. Disagreement between the two models, in a sensitivity analysis, can result in an uncongenial imputation condition [19]. For this reason, Rubin's combination rule could lead to an inconsistent estimate of the variance, often overestimating it. As is typical in situations where analytical methods or asymptotic theory does not provide adequate estimations of standard errors, the bootstrap method can be called on as a practical, albeit computationally intensive, alternative. The same consideration can be applied here, and a solution is to combine the bootstrap with MI to obtain an unbiased variance estimate, as suggested by Lu et al. [7]. The following steps show how to combine the bootstrap method with MI and perform Bayesian sensitivity analysis:

Step 1 Draw B bootstrap samples from the original dataset with replacement, stratified by treatment group.

Step 2 For each of the B bootstrap samples, fit a Bayesian q-component Weibull PH model and draw M posterior samples for all the parameters in the model.

Step 3 Use each posterior sample from Step 2 to perform δ-adjusted imputation or control-based imputation (J2R) on the bootstrap sample in Step 2 to get one imputed dataset. Repeat this across the M posterior samples to create M imputed datasets.

Step 4 Fit a Cox PH regression to each of the M imputed datasets to obtain M log-HR estimates.

Step 5 Take the average of the M log-HR estimates as the MI estimate of log-HR for the bootstrap sample.

Step 6 Repeat Steps 2–5 to complete the analysis for all B bootstrap samples, and use the sample mean and standard deviation from the B log-HR estimates to estimate the final log-HR and its standard error for statistical inference.

The p-value and 95% confidence interval for the log-HR can be obtained from the final log-HR, and its standard error can be obtained from the bootstrap process using normal approximation. Simulation studies have shown that the bootstrap standard error estimate is generally unbiased and represents the sampling variability of the control-based and delta-adjusted imputation methods [7]. However, adding the bootstrap steps on top of MI can significantly increase the computational run time. From a practical perspective, $B \approx 200$–500 and $M \approx 50$ should be adequate in many situations [7, 20]. When computationally feasible, we can consider using larger values of B and M in order to further reduce random variability in analysis of clinical trials.

3 Sensitivity Analysis in Longitudinal Trials

Missing data due to premature discontinuation in longitudinal trials share similarities to non-administrative censoring in survival trials. In both situations, assumptions must be made about missing data mechanisms. Much of the research on missing data analysis in clinical trials was motivated by longitudinal studies with repeated measures. For a comprehensive review of missing data methods in longitudinal studies and extensive literature citations, see Ibrahim and Molenberghs [21]. The National Research Council report [4] also provides a comprehensive overview, makes recommendations for the prevention of missing data through study design, and suggests common methods of handling missing data in analyses.

Consider a clinical trial with continuous endpoints collected over time. Let Y_{ijk} be an outcome (e.g., change from baseline score) for patient i in treatment group j at time k, where $i = 1, \ldots, N_j$, $j = 0$ (control) or 1 (test drug), and $k = 1, \ldots, T$. A common endpoint to assess the treatment effect is the mean difference at the last time point T.

When there are no missing data, a standard mixed model for repeated measures (MMRM) analysis is often used to evaluate the treatment difference between the test drug and the control [22]. MMRM assumes that the vector of outcomes, $bf Y_{ij} = (Y_{ij1}, \ldots, Y_{ijT})'$, follows a multivariate normal distribution with mean

$$E(Y_{ijk}) = \mu_{jk} + \boldsymbol{X}_{ij}\boldsymbol{\beta}_k \tag{9}$$

and covariance matrix Σ, usually taken to be unstructured. In this model, $\boldsymbol{X}_{ij}$ is a vector of patient baseline covariates. For simplicity, in this section we assume that $\boldsymbol{X}_{ij}$ are centralized, with the overall average $\bar{\boldsymbol{X}}_{..} = 0$. The treatment difference is evaluated at the center of the covariates $\bar{\boldsymbol{X}}_{..}$ and at the primary time point T. It follows that the treatment difference is

$$\theta_T = \mu_{1T} - \mu_{0T} \tag{10}$$

Following the ICH E9 (R1) addendum, we focus our discussions on two hypothetical estimands for a treatment effect that is not confounded by rescue medications: (1) the estimand under the MAR assumption and (2) the estimand using the control-based imputation strategy. We illustrate how to conduct Bayesian sensitivity analysis for these two estimands.

3.1 Models under the MAR

When there are missing data in repeated measures, MAR is the assumption most frequently used to handle the missing values. Its wide usage underscores the importance of the assumption, primarily for the fact that under the MAR assumption, parameters in the MMRM model are identifiable and can be estimated using likelihood-based or MI-based methods [22]. This model evaluates a hypothetical estimand of the "theoretical" treatment difference under the assumed treatment condition; that is, the dropout patients have continued in the study with the assigned therapy, assuming that the reason for dropout is not related to future unobserved data. Analysis on such a model is not difficult in either the frequentist or Bayesian paradigm because of widely available software packages. We can use, for example, PROC MIXED for frequentist inference or PROC BGLIMM for Bayesian estimation, both in SAS [23].

In clinical trials, there are often two types of missing data: intermittent missing data, in which the missing data occur between some observed data; and monotone missing data, in which once a missing observation occurs, all subsequent observations are missing. Intermittent missing data can be caused by missed visits or data collection errors, reasons typically unrelated to treatment; therefore, the MAR assumption is reasonable. In practice, intermittent missing data can be imputed under MAR to create monotone missing data. More details can be found in the chapter "A Competing Risk Model Based on a Two-Parameter Exponential Family Distribution under Progressive Type II Censoring" in O'Kelly and Ratitch [24]. Monotone missing data that are most likely to be attributed to dropouts can be linked to the treatment because of a lack of efficacy or safety issue. This type of missing data presents a more complex scenario because of treatment discontinuation. Here we focus on modeling monotone missing data under different potential assumptions to assess the sensitivity of the analysis under MAR and a control-based imputation assumption.

To model monotone missingness, patients can be classified into T patterns, where T is the total number of repeated time points in the study. Patients in pattern k ($1 \leq k < T$) are those who dropped out after time k and have outcomes that are observed up to time k; patients in pattern T are those who completed the trial. For patients in pattern k, the response vector $\boldsymbol{Y}_{ij}^{(k)}$ can be partitioned into an observed part $\boldsymbol{Y}_{ij}^{\mathrm{o}(k)}$ (of length k) and a missing part $\boldsymbol{Y}_{ij}^{\mathrm{m}(k)}$ (of length $T-k$). The mean and covariance matrix can be partitioned correspondingly as

$$E(\boldsymbol{Y}_{ij}^{(k)}) = \begin{pmatrix} \boldsymbol{\mu}_j^{\mathrm{o}(k)} \\ \boldsymbol{\mu}_j^{\mathrm{m}(k)} \end{pmatrix}, \boldsymbol{\Sigma} = \begin{pmatrix} \boldsymbol{\Sigma}^{\mathrm{oo}(k)}, & \boldsymbol{\Sigma}^{\mathrm{om}(k)} \\ \boldsymbol{\Sigma}^{\mathrm{mo}(k)}, & \boldsymbol{\Sigma}^{\mathrm{mm}(k)} \end{pmatrix}$$

In general, the treatment difference at the last time point can be expressed as a weighted average:

$$\theta_T = \sum_{k=1}^{T} \pi_{1k}\mu_{1T}^{(k)} - \sum_{k=1}^{T} \pi_{0k}\mu_{0T}^{(k)} \tag{11}$$

where $\mu_{jT}^{(k)} = \mu_{jT}^{\mathrm{m}(k)}$ are means of unobserved outcomes in pattern $k, k < T$, and $\mu_{jT}^{(\mathrm{T})} = \mu_{jT}^{\mathrm{o}(\mathrm{T})}, j = 0, 1$.

However, the parameters $\{\mu_{jl}^{\mathrm{o}(k)}, \mu_{jl}^{\mathrm{m}(k)}; k, l = 1, \ldots, T, j = 0, 1\}$ are not identifiable without certain assumptions. The conventional assumptions for a pattern mixture model, such as CCMV (complete-case missing values) or NCMV (neighboring-case missing values), are not interesting or practical for clinical trials (chapter "Bayesian Analysis of a New Bivariate Wiener Degradation Process" [24]).

One of the most commonly used assumptions is MAR, which is an ACMV (all-case missing values) approach. Under MAR, the missing data are ignorable, so the parameters in the MMRM (9) can be estimated from the likelihood of the observed data without the need to model the missing-data mechanism. An MMRM analysis does not estimate the mean parameters $\{\mu_{jl}^{\mathrm{o}(k)}, \mu_{jl}^{\mathrm{m}(k)}; k, l = 1, \ldots, T, j = 0, 1\}$ for all patterns; instead it estimates the $\{\mu_{jl}; l = 1, \ldots, T, j = 0, 1\}$ parameters in (9) for the whole study population.

Alternatively, the parameters $\{\mu_{jl}; l = 1, \ldots, T, j = 0, 1\}$ can be estimated using MI, which provides insights into how the missing data are handled in an MMRM analysis. For missing data in pattern k, imputation is based on the conditional distribution of $\boldsymbol{Y}_{ij}^{\mathrm{m}(k)} | \boldsymbol{Y}_{ij}^{\mathrm{o}(k)}$, a multivariate normal with the following mean and covariance:

$$E(\boldsymbol{Y}_{ij}^{\mathrm{m}(k)} | \boldsymbol{Y}_{ij}^{\mathrm{o}}) = \boldsymbol{\mu}_j^{\mathrm{m}} + \boldsymbol{\Sigma}^{\mathrm{mo}}(\boldsymbol{\Sigma}^{\mathrm{oo}})^{-1}(\boldsymbol{Y}_{ij}^{\mathrm{o}} - \boldsymbol{\mu}_j^{\mathrm{o}}) \tag{12}$$

$$V(\boldsymbol{Y}_{ij}^{\mathrm{m}(k)} | \boldsymbol{Y}_{ij}^{\mathrm{o}(k)}) = \boldsymbol{\Sigma}^{\mathrm{mm}} - \boldsymbol{\Sigma}^{\mathrm{mo}}(\boldsymbol{\Sigma}^{\mathrm{oo}})^{-1}\boldsymbol{\Sigma}^{\mathrm{om}}$$

where $\boldsymbol{\mu}_j' = (\boldsymbol{\mu}_j^{\mathrm{o}\prime}, \boldsymbol{\mu}_j^{\mathrm{m}\prime})'$, $\boldsymbol{\Sigma}^{\mathrm{mm}}$, $\boldsymbol{\Sigma}^{\mathrm{mo}}$, $\boldsymbol{\Sigma}^{\mathrm{oo}}$, and $\boldsymbol{\Sigma}^{\mathrm{om}}$ are sub-vectors or sub-matrices corresponding to the observed and missing data. Imputation uses the population-level parameters $\boldsymbol{\mu}_j$, $j = 0, 1$, and $\boldsymbol{\Sigma}$ that do not depend on the missing data pattern. Under MAR, MI estimates are asymptotically unbiased ([11, 25] supplemental document). The mean of treatment group j at the last time point can be represented as

$$\begin{aligned}\mu_{jT} &= \sum_{k=1}^{T-1} \pi_{jk} E\left[E(\boldsymbol{Y}_{ij}^{\mathrm{m}(k)} | \boldsymbol{Y}_{ij}^{\mathrm{o}(k)})\right]_T + \pi_{jT}\mu_{\mathrm{jT}}^{(\mathrm{T})} \\ &= \sum_{k=1}^{T-1} \pi_{jk}\left[\boldsymbol{\mu}_j^{\mathrm{m}} + \boldsymbol{\Sigma}^{\mathrm{mo}}(\boldsymbol{\Sigma}^{\mathrm{oo}})^{-1}(\boldsymbol{\mu}_j^{\mathrm{o}(k)} - \boldsymbol{\mu}_j^{\mathrm{o}})\right]_T + \pi_{jT}\mu_{jT}^{(\mathrm{T})}\end{aligned} \tag{13}$$

where $[\boldsymbol{X}]_T$ is the Tth element of the vector $\boldsymbol{X}$. It follows that the treatment difference under MAR is

$$\theta_T^{\mathrm{MAR}} = \mu_{1T} - \mu_{0T}. \tag{14}$$

In the imputation model, MMRM under MAR assumes that post-dropout responses are similar to those from patients who continue the treatment, conditioned on their having identical covariates and observed outcomes before dropout. In other words, MMRM analysis addresses a hypothetical estimand for outcomes in the "what if" situation in which the dropout patients continue the assigned treatment. However, this assumption poses challenges in practice for being overly optimistic: Patients who drop out might not be able to continue the assigned treatment, because of concerns about safety or lack of efficacy, for example. If we want to assess treatment effects under a more realistic assumption that patients who drop out cannot continue test treatment, we cannot use MAR analysis, because it leads to a biased estimate that often favors test treatment. This challenge has spurred the development of control-based imputation methods, which aim to incorporate more realistic scenarios in handling missing data after discontinuation of treatment.

3.2 *Control-Based Imputation Methods*

In placebo-controlled trials, it is reasonable to assume that a patient who drops out of the control group would have a similar response after dropout to that of patients who stay in the trial because there is little biologic difference between taking and not taking a placebo. Therefore, a MAR assumption might be justifiable for the missing data because of dropouts in the control group. For the test drug group, when a patient drops out and stops taking the assigned treatment, it is expected that the unobserved responses after dropout are somewhat similar to those of patients in the control group. In other words, the control group can provide a reference level for the response trajectory of dropouts in the test drug group. As with survival analysis to handle censoring, we can use J2R here to replace the means of responses after dropout in the test drug group with the means of responses of the control group. Specifically, the conditional means of Eq. (12) become

$$\begin{aligned} E(\boldsymbol{Y}_{i0}^{\mathrm{m}(k)}|\boldsymbol{Y}_{i0}^{\mathrm{o}(k)}) &= \boldsymbol{\mu}_0^{\mathrm{m}} + \boldsymbol{\Sigma}^{\mathrm{mo}}(\boldsymbol{\Sigma}^{\mathrm{oo}})^{-1}(\boldsymbol{Y}_{i0}^{\mathrm{o}} - \boldsymbol{\mu}_0^{\mathrm{o}}) \\ E(\boldsymbol{Y}_{i1}^{\mathrm{m}(k)}|\boldsymbol{Y}_{i1}^{\mathrm{o}(k)}) &= \boldsymbol{\mu}_0^{\mathrm{m}} + \boldsymbol{\Sigma}^{\mathrm{mo}}(\boldsymbol{\Sigma}^{\mathrm{oo}})^{-1}(\boldsymbol{Y}_{i1}^{\mathrm{o}} - \boldsymbol{\mu}_1^{\mathrm{o}}) \end{aligned} \tag{15}$$

where the means of missing responses in test drug group $\boldsymbol{\mu}_1^m$ are replaced with $\boldsymbol{\mu}_0^m$ in Eq. (12). Under J2R, the mean of the test drug group at the last time point is as follows:

$$\begin{aligned}\mu_{1T}^{\text{J2R}} &= \sum_{k=1}^{T-1} \pi_{1k} E\left[E(\boldsymbol{Y}_{i1}^{\text{m}(k)} | \boldsymbol{Y}_{i1}^{\text{o}(k)})\right]_T + \pi_{1T}\mu_{1T}^{(\text{T})} \\ &= \sum_{k=1}^{T-I} \pi_{1k}\left[\boldsymbol{\mu}_0^{\text{m}} + \boldsymbol{\Sigma}^{\text{mo}}(\boldsymbol{\Sigma}^{\text{oo}})^{-1}(\boldsymbol{\mu}_1^{\text{o}(k)} - \boldsymbol{\mu}_1^{\text{o}})\right]_T + \pi_{1T}\mu_{1T}^{(\text{T})} \\ &= \sum_{k=1}^{T-1} \pi_{1k}(\mu_{0T} - \mu_{1T}) \\ &\quad + \sum_{k=1}^{T-1} \pi_{1k}\left[\boldsymbol{\mu}_1^{\text{m}} + \boldsymbol{\Sigma}^{\text{mo}}(\boldsymbol{\Sigma}^{\text{oo}})^{-1}(\boldsymbol{\mu}_1^{\text{o}(k)} - \boldsymbol{\mu}_1^{\text{o}})\right]_T + \pi_{1T}\mu_{1T}^{(T)}\end{aligned} \tag{16}$$

where $[\boldsymbol{X}]_T$ is the Tth element of vector $\boldsymbol{X}$. From Eq. (14), the last two terms in Eq. (17) become μ_{1T}. Therefore, we have

$$\theta_T^{\text{J2R}} = \sum_{k=1}^{T-1} \pi_{1k}(\mu_{0T} - \mu_{1T}) + \mu_{1T} - \mu_{0T} = \pi_{1T}(\mu_{1T} - \mu_{0T})$$

where π_{1T} is the proportion of patients in the test drug group who completed the trial. When $\pi_{1T} < 1$, the J2R estimate shrinks the treatment effect more toward 0 than the MAR estimate does. The point and variance estimates can be obtained using the delta-adjusted method [15]:

$$\hat{\theta}_T^{\text{J2R}} = \hat{\pi}_{1T}(\hat{\mu}_{1T} - \hat{\mu}_{0T})$$

$$var(\hat{\theta}_T^{\text{J2R}}) = var(\hat{\theta}_T^{\text{MAR}})\hat{\pi}_{1k}^2 + \left[var(\hat{\theta}_T^{\text{MAR}}) + (\hat{\theta}_T^{\text{MAR}})^2\right]\hat{\pi}_{1T}(1 - \hat{\pi}_{1T})/n_1$$

where $\hat{\theta}_T^{\text{MAR}}$ and $var(\hat{\theta}_T^{\text{MAR}})$ are the point estimate and its variance under from MMRM under MAR; $\hat{\pi}_{1T}$ is the proportion of completers and n_1 is the sample size in the test drug group.

J2R is a relatively easy control-based imputation method to implement; its popularity is also boosted by its conservative nature, which shrinks the estimated treatment effect toward 0. There are other types of control-based imputation methods, including copy reference (CR) and copy incremental in reference (CIR). In contrast to the J2R method, in which the means of responses for dropouts in the test drug jump to the means of responses in the control group, the CR method assumes that the means of responses for dropouts in the test drug group equal the means of the control group both before and after dropout. In CIR, mean changes from the time of dropout in the test drug group are assumed to be similar to the changes in the control group. Formulas and statistical inference for the estimands of CR and CIR can be found in Liu and Pang [15].

3.3 Bayesian Sensitivity Analysis

From the conditional means for the imputation in Eqs. (12) and (16), the assumed mean parameters after dropout are μ_1^m (a subvector of μ_1) under MAR or μ_0^m (a subvector of μ_0) under J2R for the test drug group. This implies that the mean profile of dropouts is the same as the mean profile of those who stay in the study under MAR or that it jumps to the mean profile of the control group under J2R. Both approaches use "deterministic" mean profiles in the sense that we do not expect any variations in the trajectory means after dropout. That assumption can, and should, be checked via a sensitivity analysis, by including uncertainty quantification on the mean parameters after dropout. Here we consider a Bayesian approach to incorporate uncertainty about the assumed means.

Because the primary focus of the analysis is the treatment difference at the last time point, we assume that $\mu_{1T}^m = \mu_{1T} + \delta$ (under the MAR assumption) and $\mu_{1T}^m = \mu_{0T} + \delta$ (under the J2R assumption). We further assume that δ, a sensitivity parameter, follows an $N(\xi, \tau^2)$ prior with known hyperparameters of ξ and τ. As we vary the values of these hyperparameter, we can obtain a quantified measure of how sensitive the final analysis is to the changes in these values. The treatment difference can be derived as follows:

- Under MAR, $\theta_T^{\text{MAR}}(\delta) = \mu_{1T} - \mu_{0T} + (1 - \pi_{1T})\xi$, where π_{1T} is the proportion of completers in the test drug group. It can be estimated by

$$\hat{\theta}_T^{\text{MAR}}(\delta) = \hat{\theta}_T^{\text{MAR}} + (1 - \pi_{1T})\xi$$

  and its variance $\text{var}(\hat{\theta}_T^{\text{MAR}}(\delta)) = \text{var}(\hat{\theta}_T^{\text{MAR}}) + (1 - \hat{\pi}_{1T})^2\tau^2$.
- Under J2R, $\theta_T^{\text{J2R}}(\delta) = \pi_{1T}(\mu_{1T} - \mu_{0T}) + (1 - \pi_{1T})\xi$, it can be estimated by

$$\hat{\theta}_T^{\text{J2R}}(\delta) = \hat{\pi}_{1T}\hat{\theta}_T^{\text{MAR}} + (1 - \hat{\pi}_{1T})\xi$$

  with variance $\text{var}(\hat{\theta}_T^{\text{J2R}}(\delta)) = \text{var}(\hat{\theta}_T^{\text{J2R}}) + (1 - \hat{\pi}_{1T})^2\tau^2$.

In the preceding formulas, $\hat{\theta}_T^{\text{MAR}}$ and $\text{var}(\hat{\theta}_T^{\text{MAR}})$ are the point estimate and variance of the treatment difference from MMRM analysis, respectively; $\text{var}(\hat{\theta}_T^{\text{J2R}})$ can also be obtained using the estimates from the MMRM analysis as described in Sect. 3.2. Therefore, for a given prior $N(\xi, \tau^2)$, the sensitivity analysis of θ_T^{MAR} and θ_T^{J2R} can be performed using the results from the MMRM analysis without using the MI approach. We illustrate the analysis in the next section using examples.

4 Examples

4.1 A Time-to-Event Trial Example

We conduct Bayesian sensitivity analysis on time-to-event data from a randomized clinical trial conducted by AIDS Clinical Trials Group Study 175 (ACTG175) [26]. The study evaluated treatment with either a single nucleoside or two nucleosides in adults infected with human immunodeficiency virus type 1 (HIV-1). These subjects had CD4 cell counts that ranged from 200 to 500 per cubic millimeter. The study randomized 2467 patients to one of four daily regimens: 600 mg of zidovudine; 600 mg of zidovudine plus 400 mg of didanosine; 600 mg of zidovudine plus 2.25 mg of zalcitabine; or 400 mg of didanosine. The primary endpoint was time to a 50% or greater decline in the CD4 cell count, development of AIDS, or death. *J. R. Stat. Society* [27] made the data publicly available. For illustration purposes, we use a subset of the data in this example. The subset contains antiretroviral-naive patients who were assigned to either the monotherapy of zidovudine (ZDV) or the monotherapy of didanosine (ddI) regimen. The analysis compares the hazard ratio of the two treatment groups with a model including the treatment group only.

Data from 461 patients (223 in ZDV and 238 in ddI) are used in the analysis. There are 59 and 44 events observed in the ZDV and ddI groups, respectively. The log-HR estimate from a Cox PH regression is −0.456 (HR: 0.634) with a p-value of 0.022, indicating that patients in the ddI group have a significantly lower hazard than those in the ZDV group.

To evaluate the sensitivity of the analysis to the random censoring assumption that underlies the Cox PH regression model, we conduct MI analysis using the delta-adjusted and J2R methods. We assumed that censored values after month 33 are the administrative type in nature (i.e., censoring is due to the completion of the study) and are therefore treated as censoring at random. Censored values prior to month 33 are treated as non-administrative, or potentially informative, censoring. After exploring both two- and three-component mixture Weibull models, we conclude that a two-component Weibull model provides reasonable fit to the data and a three-component model does not add much noticeable difference. Figure 1 shows the estimated survival curves from a two-component mixture model (smooth lines), which match the non-parametric survival estimate curves from the Cox PH model (jagged lines) very well.

For the bootstrap steps outlined in Sect. 2.3, we set B to 1000 and M to 100 in the sensitivity analysis. With these relatively large B and M values, the results are fairly stable, because almost the same results were obtained by running the analysis using different random seeds. The results are presented in Table 1.

When non-administrative censoring values are imputed under MAR (second row) using $M = 200$ MI, both the point estimate of log-HR (−0.431) and its standard error (0.200) are similar to those from the Cox PH model (−0.456 and 0.200, respectively). MI produces a slightly larger p-value than that from the Cox PH model; this is expected because MI carries additional variation from imputations.

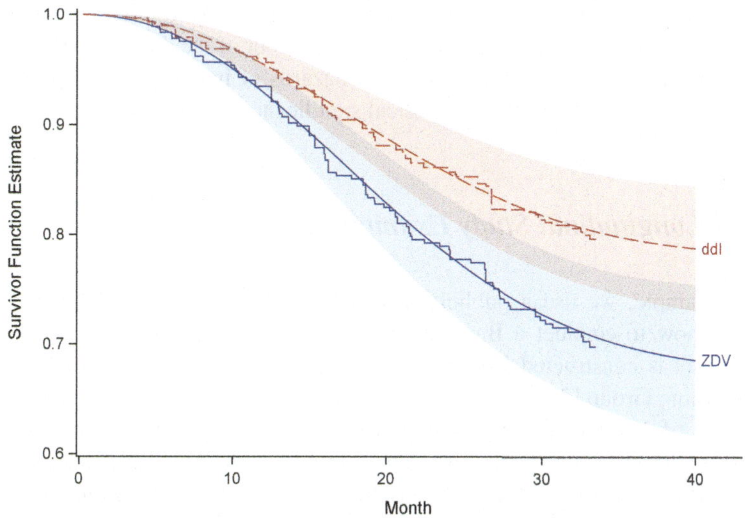

Fig. 1 Estimated survival curves from a two-component mixture model (smoothed line), overlaid with non-parametric curves from a Cox PH model. The top fit is from the ddI group; the bottom fit is from the ZDV group. Shaded regions are pointwise confidence intervals

Table 1 Sensitivity analysis for ACTG175

Method	log-HR	S.E.	p-value
Cox PH	−0.456	0.200	0.022
MAR[a]	−0.431	0.200	0.030
J2R[b]	−0.384	0.180	0.032
δ-adjustment[b]			
$\delta = 1.6$	−0.401	0.200	0.046
$\delta = 1.8$	−0.393	0.200	0.050
$\delta = 2.0$	−0.386	0.201	0.054

[a] Based on MI with $M = 200$
[b] Using $B = 1000$ bootstrap plus $M = 100$ MI approaches

When the non-administrative censoring values are imputed under J2R, both the estimated log-HR and its standard error shrink toward 0. The p-value from the J2R analysis is similar to that from the MI analysis under MAR. This is consistent with what has been reported in the literature regarding J2R analysis for longitudinal trials [15].

We also perform a tipping point analysis using the δ-adjustment method. Increased δ values lead to larger p-values, nudging significant results to insignificant. As shown in Table 1, the tipping point for this study is at $\delta = 1.8$, which produces a p-value of 0.050.

In conclusion, sensitivity analysis based on J2R and δ adjustment (tipping point analysis) implies that finding from the Cox PH model is robust to the random censoring assumption. The result from using control-based imputation (J2R) is significant. The estimated tipping point value of 1.8 supports the significance of the findings: The hazards of patients who dropped out of the ddI group would need to be more than 1.8 times higher than the hazards of patients who remain in the study before we could eliminate statistical significance.

4.2 A Longitudinal Study Example

In this example, we use a publicly available antidepressant drug trial dataset to illustrate how to conduct a Bayesian sensitivity analysis in a longitudinal study. This dataset is constructed from a real clinical trial and is made available by the DIA Working Group [28].

A total of 172 patients were randomized to an active drug and placebo. The primary endpoint is the Hamilton Depression 17-item (HAMD-17) total scores, which were measured at week 0 (baseline) and weeks 1, 2, 4, and 6 of post-randomization. In this analysis, we exclude one patient who has intermittent missing data. Overall, about 24% and 26% of patients in the active drug and placebo groups, respectively, dropped out before week 6 (the primary analysis time point). Figure 2 shows the mean value changes from baseline by treatment group for patients who dropped out in different weeks (missing data pattern). Solid blue lines represent

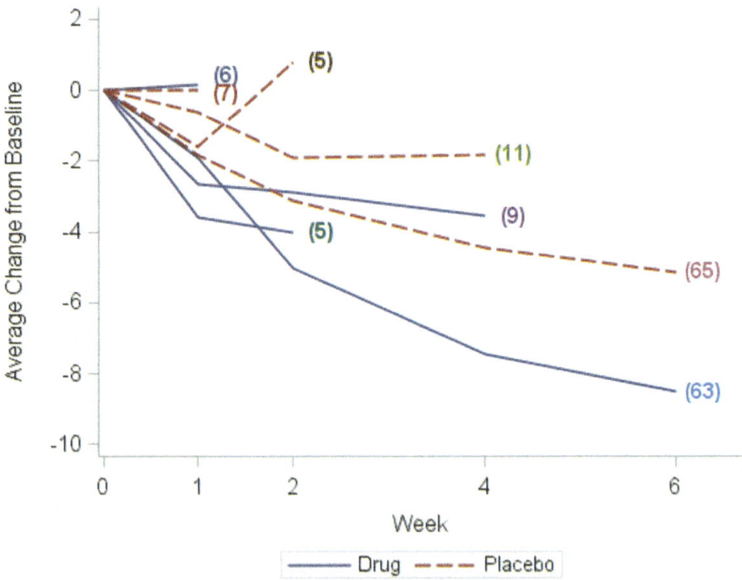

Fig. 2 Mean change from baseline of HAMD-17 by treatment and week of discontinuation (numbers of patients are given in parentheses). Solid blue line indicates drug group, and dashed red line indicates placebo group

Table 2 Primary and Bayesian sensitivity analysis for DIA antidepressant dataset

Method		θ^{MAR}	95% CI[a]	θ^{J2R}	95% CI[a]
Mixed model		−2.90	(−5.12, −0.68)	−2.20	(−3.91, −0.49)
Bayesian approach		−2.90	(−5.12, −0.73)	−2.20	(−3.92, −0.53)
Sensitivity analysis					
τ	ξ				
	0	−2.90	(−5.17, −0.63)	−2.20	(−3.98, −0.42)
1	1	−2.66	(−4.93, −0.39)	−1.96	(−3.74, −0.18)
	2	−2.42	(−4.69, −0.15)	−1.72	(−3.50, 0.06)
	0	−2.90	(−5.32, −0.48)	−2.20	(−4.16, −0.24)
2	1	−2.66	(−5.08, −0.24)	−1.96	(−3.92, −0.00)
	2	−2.42	(−4.84, −0.00)	−1.72	(−3.68, 0.24)
	0	−2.90	(−5.54, −0.26)	−2.20	(−4.43, 0.03)
3	1	−2.66	(−5.30, −0.02)	−1.96	(−4.19, 0.27)
	2	−2.42	(−5.06, 0.22)	−1.72	(−3.95, 0.51)

[a] Confidence interval or credible interval

patients in the drug group, and dashed red lines represent patients in the placebo group. The numbers in parentheses (for weeks 1, 2, and 4) are the numbers of patients from each group who stayed up to that week and then dropped out. The two numbers, 63 and 65, in week 6, are the number of patients in the two groups who completed the study. The trend of the graph indicates that patients who drop out earlier experience a smaller decrease in HAMD-17 scores than those who stay, suggesting that responses for early dropouts could be worse than those of the completers.

The primary analysis is to compare treatment effects as measured by the change from baseline in HAMD-17 total scores at week 6. Table 2 presents analysis results for MAR and J2R using mixed model and Bayesian analysis. The table also includes sensitivity analysis over the range of the hyperparameters (ξ and τ in the normal prior on δ), with $\delta = 0, 1, 2$ and $\tau = 1, 2, 3$.

Table 2 (first two rows) shows that the likelihood-based analysis using the mixed model (with PROC MIXED) and the Bayesian approach with a non-informative prior (with PROC MCMC) lead to almost identical results, for both MAR and J2R. This is expected, because Bayesian and frequentists' inferences on linear mixed models are known to produce similar estimates when non-informative prior distributions are used.

Bayesian sensitivity analysis introduces an additional δ parameter to account for variability of the assumed mean profiles of the dropouts. This uncertainty is reflected in the prior distribution, and changes to the mean and variance of the normal prior of δ can provide sensitivity to assess the treatment difference and its credible interval. In the MAR analysis, the 95% credible intervals shift upwards (toward less significant) as either the ξ or τ values increase. When $\xi = 2$ and $\tau = 3$, the upper credible interval limit becomes positive, implying insignificant results (in the classical statistics sense). Because such CIs occur only when ξ or τ values are large, this implies that the results are fairly robust to the MAR assumption. Here a positive large value of ξ shifts the response after dropout toward worsening, and a large value of τ adds extra variation to the assumed response after dropout. Increasing either ξ or τ to a certain value might tip the analysis to become insignificant. For the J2R analysis, the results turn to insignificant territory more quickly than they do for the MAR analysis. This implies that the J2R analysis is less robust to variations of the assumed profile for the dropouts. Figure 3 shows the treatment difference and corresponding 95% CIs for MAR and J2R for different fixed values of ξ and τ.

5 Summary and Discussions

In clinical trials, censoring or missing data occur at a high frequency for reasons such as patients discontinue the study treatment or decide to leave the trials because of lack of efficacy, tolerability issues, and so on. Many of these causes are related to treatment and observed outcomes, indicating a potentially systematic difference among the patients remaining in the study. Hence censoring and missing data should be handled carefully and with explicitly stated assumptions. Many statistical models make random censoring or MAR assumptions to account for missingness because these assumptions often simplify the modeling difficulties and enable the estimation based on likelihood- or partial-likelihood and testing on the treatment effects. However, these assumptions generally are not verifiable from the observed trial data, casting doubts on the validity of the estimates and the robustness of the analyses. As we apply increasingly complex models and study designs, such reliance on missingness assumptions invites a greater degree of scrutiny. This sentiment is reflected in the recent regulatory guidance documents, which recommend that sensitivity analyses should be conducted to assess the robustness of the analysis results [1, 4].

In this chapter, we reviewed sensitivity analysis methods and strategies for handling missing data for both survival and longitudinal trials. The topics that we covered include control-based imputation and delta-adjusted methods, and we illustrated how to conduct such analysis from a Bayesian perspective that offers flexibility in accounting for variability and in examining sensitivities. It is important to recognize the inappropriateness of applying Rubin's combination rules naively in MI in an uncongenial condition where the imputation model is different from the analysis model. We recommend using a parametric mixture Weibull model to estimate survival function; the simplicity of the model provides computational efficiency without scarifying modeling accuracy. Delta-adjustment can be applied to impute censored time to events, and bootstrap method can be used to estimate variance for treatment comparisons in survival trials. For longitudinal trials that have continuous endpoints, control-based imputation can be implemented using a likelihood-based method. Extension to Bayesian sensitivity analysis focuses on examining uncertainty of the assumed mean profile after dropout, which can provide insight into the robustness of analysis under different missing data assumptions.

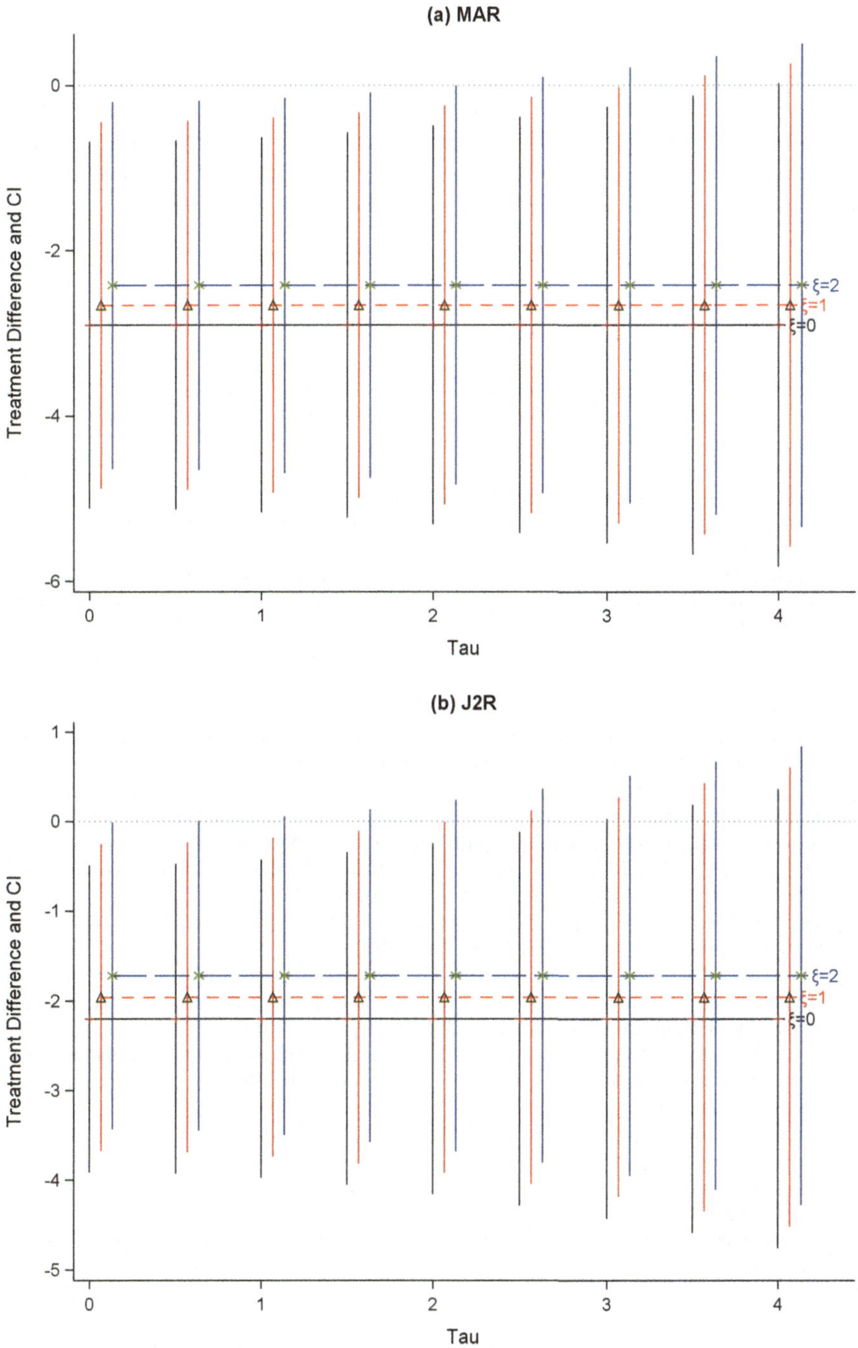

Fig. 3 Bayesian sensitivity analysis of the DIA antidepressant dataset using (**a**) MAR and (**b**) J2R methods. A range of values are selected for the hyperparameters ξ (mean) and τ (standard deviation). The 95% CIs (vertical bars) increase as either the τ (along the X axis) or ξ (superimposed) value increases. The tipping point is to identify large values of the hyperparameters that lead to crossing the zero value of the upper CI. Crossing of the zero threshold occurs faster in J2R than in MAR, indicating the MAR approach is more robust than the J2R approach in modeling variations of assumed profiles for the dropouts

We have illustrated how to use Bayesian methods for sensitivity analysis in survival trials with time to first event and longitudinal trials with continuous outcomes. In the future, it will be worthwhile to investigate the Bayesian approaches for sensitivity analysis in other settings, such as in studies with recurrent times to events and longitudinal trials with categorical and binary outcomes.

References

1. International Council for Harmonization (ICH): Addendum on Estimand and Sensitivity Analysis in Clinical Trials, available via ICH 2019 (2020). https://database.ich.org/sites/default/files/E9-R1_Step4_Guideline_2019_1203.pdf
2. Allison, P.: Survival Analysis Using SAS. SAS Institute, Cary (1995)
3. Little, R., Rubin, D.: Statistical Analysis with Missing Data. Willy, Hoboken (2019)
4. National Research Council (NRC): The Prevention and Treatment of Missing Data in Clinical Trials. The National Academies Press, Washington (2010)
5. Jackson, D., White, I.R., Seaman, S., et al.: Relaxing the independent censoring assumption in the Cox proportional hazards model using multiple imputation. Stat. Med. **33**, 4681–4694 (2014)
6. Zhao, Y., Herring, A.H., Zhou, H., et al.: A multiple imputation method for sensitivity analyses of time-to-event data with possibly informative censoring. J. Biopharm. Stat. **24**, 229–253 (2014)
7. Lu, K., Li, D., Koch, G.G.: Comparison between two controlled multiple imputation methods for sensitivity analyses of time-to-event data with possibly informative censoring. Stat. Biopharm. Res. **7**, 199–213 (2015)
8. Lipkovich, I., Ratitch, B., O'Kelly, M.: Sensitivity to censored-at-random assumption in the analysis of time-to-event endpoints. Pharm. Stat. **15**, 216–229 (2016)
9. Demarqui, F.N., Loschi, R.H., Colosimo, E.A.: Estimating the grid of time-points for the piecewise exponential model. Lifetime Data Anal. **14**, 333–356 (2008)
10. Goodman, M.S., Lib, Y., Tiwari, R.C.: Detecting multiple change points in piecewise constant hazard functions. J. Appl. Stat. **38**, 2523–2532 (2011)
11. Carpenter, J.R., Roger, J.H., Kenward, M.G.: Analysis of longitudinal trials with protocol deviation: a framework for relevant, accessible assumptions, and inference via multiple imputation. J. Biopharm. Stat. **23**, 1352–1371 (2013)
12. Ayele, B.T., Lipkovich, I., Molenberghs, G., Mallinckrodt, C.: A multiple-imputation-based approach to sensitivity analyses and effectiveness assessments in longitudinal clinical trials. J. Biopharm. Stat. **24**, 211–228 (2014)
13. Lu, K.: An analytic method for the placebo-based pattern-mixture model. Stat. Med. **33**, 1134–1145 (2014)
14. Tang, Y.: Short notes on maximum likelihood inference for control-based pattern-mixture models. Pharm. Stat. **14**, 395–399 (2015)
15. Liu, G., Pang, L.: On analysis of longitudinal clinical trials with missing data using reference-based imputation. J. Biopharm. Stat. **26**, 924–936 (2016)
16. Liu, G., Pang, L.: Control-based imputation and delta-adjustment stress test for missing data analysis in longitudinal clinical trials. Stat. Biopharm. Res. *9*, 186–194 (2017)
17. Liao, J., Liu, G.: A flexible parametric survival model for fitting time to event data in clinical trials. Pharm. Stat. **18**, 555–567 (2019)
18. Liu, G., Liao, J.: Analysis of time-to-event data using a flexible mixture model under a constraint of proportional hazards. J. Biopharm. Stat. Res. https://doi.org/10.1080/10543406.2020.1783283

19. Meng, X.L.: Multiple-imputation inferences with uncongenial sources of input. Stat. Sci. **9**, 538–573 (1994)
20. Gao, F., Liu, G., Zeng, D. et al.: Control-based imputation for sensitivity analyses in informative censoring for recurrent event data. Pharm. Stat. **16**, 424–432 (2017)
21. Ibrahim, J., Molenberghs, G.: Missing data methods in longitudinal studies: a review. Test **18**, 1–43 (2009)
22. Mallinckrodt, C., Lane, P., Schnell, D., et al.: Recommendations for the primary analysis of continuous endpoints in longitudinal clinical trials. Drug Inform. J. **42**, 303–319 (2008)
23. SAS: SAS/STAT 15.2 User's Guide. SAS Institute, Cary (2020)
24. O'Kelly, M., Ratitch, B.: Clinical Trials with Missing Data: A Guide for Practitioners. Wiley, New York (2014)
25. Mallinckrodt, C., Bell, J., Liu, G., et al.: Aligning estimators with estimands in clinical trials: putting the ICH E9(R1) guidelines into practice. Ther. Innovation Regul. Sci. **54**, 353–364 (2020)
26. Hammer, S.M., Katzenstein, D.A., Hughes, M.D., et al.: A trial comparing nucleoside monotherapy with combination therapy in HIV-infected adults with CD4 cell counts from 200 to 500 per cubic millimeter. N. Engl. J. Med. **335**, 1081–1090 (1996)
27. Jiang, R., Lu, W., Song, R., Davidian, M.: On estimation of optimal treatment regimes for maximizing t-year survival probability. J. R. Stat. Soc. B **79**, 1165–1185 (2017)
28. Drug Information Association (DIA) Missing Data Working Group: https://www.lshtm.ac.uk/research/centres-projects-groups/missing-data

Bayesian Analysis for Clustered Data under a Semi-Competing Risks Framework

Seong W. Kim, Sehwa Hong, Yewon Han, and Jinheum Kim

Abstract In clinical trials or medical studies, we often encounter diverse survival data such as recurrent event data, clustered data, and competing risks data. In particular, relapse for any disease is quite common, which makes usage of appropriate models indispensable. Conventional models including the logistic regression model are not appropriate in accounting for patients' transitions who die before experiencing a relapse within a time of interest. To circumvent this phenomenon we utilize an illness-death model under a semi-competing risks framework. This model characterizes some non-terminal events like relapse and a terminal event like death. We develop Bayesian methods to analyze clustered data under the semi-competing risks framework. Subsequently, R program codes are provided to analyze publically available breast cancer data. Parameter estimations are performed based on Gibbs sampling within Metropolis–Hastings algorithm.

1 Introduction

In classical time-to-event or survival analysis, subjects are at risk for one fatal event. However, they do not fail from just one certain type of event in some applications, but are under the risk of failing from two or more mutually exclusive types of events. These events are often called competing risks. Thus, one of the events censors the other and vice versa in a competing risks setup [1, 16, 17]. On the other hand, many clinical trials have frequently shown that a terminal event like "death" censors a non-terminal event like "disease diagnosis," but not vice versa under the circumstances that a subject could be simultaneously exposed to both terminal and non-terminal events. We often call these types of data semi-competing risks data [2, 6, 11, 18].

S. W. Kim (✉) · Y. Han
Department of Applied Mathematics, Hanyang University, Ansan, South Korea

S. Hong · J. Kim
Department of Applied Statistics, University of Suwon, Suwon, South Korea

Y. Lio et al. (eds.), *Bayesian Inference and Computation in Reliability and Survival Analysis*, Emerging Topics in Statistics and Biostatistics,
https://doi.org/10.1007/978-3-030-88658-5_12

Further, the terminal event can be regarded as a competing event, and a dependency is formulated between non-terminal and terminal events for model specifications in the semi-competing risks framework. Fig. 1(a) shows a graphical display for the structure regarding semi-competing risks data where primary interest lies in some non-terminal events, the occurrence of which is subject to a terminal event.

We frequently encounter situations that survival data is comprised of several clusters. For instance, failure times of subjects are observed in multi-center clinical trials or group-randomized trials [15], forcing us to incorporate dependencies for survival/failure times within each cluster. There has been a decent amount of literature for analyzing semi-competing risks data under a clustered structure framework [5, 12, 15, 18]. In this chapter we use a Bayesian approach to obtain relevant parameter estimates under the semi-competing risks framework. The rest of the chapter is organized as follows. In Sect. 2 we present several models that are used in our analysis. Modeling strategies are briefly described under the semi-competing risks framework. Section 3 contains data analysis using real breast cancer data collected from multi-institutional clinical trials under the Bayesian framework. Brief concluding remarks are provided in Sect. 4. Some R codes are provided in the Appendix.

2 Models and Methodologies

We conduct univariate analysis in comparison of semi-competing risks analysis. The *univariate logistic analysis* is proceeded with a binary response. That is,

$$\text{logit}P(Y_{ij} = 1|\boldsymbol{X}_{ij}) = \boldsymbol{X}_{ij}^T\beta + V_j,$$

where $Y_{ij} = 0$ or 1 implies whether the ith patient at the jth location is relapsed or not, $\boldsymbol{X}_{ij}$ is a vector of covariates for the ith subject in the jth cluster ($i = 1, 2, \ldots, n_j$; $j = 1, 2, \ldots, J$), and β is the vector of the regression coefficients corresponding to $\boldsymbol{X}_{ij}$. Here we assume that a random effect V_j, specific to cluster j, follows a normal distribution with a mean of zero and variance σ^2. Several possibilities for the working correlation structure of $\boldsymbol{Y}_j = (Y_{1j}, Y_{2j}, \ldots, Y_{n_j j})'$ have been suggested in the clustered logistic models [13].

When a patient is at risk of experiencing non-terminal event during a predetermined (given) time interval, it is quite common to utilize a *standard survival analysis*. Let T_1 denote the time to a non-terminal event, e.g. relapse, and let T_2 denote the time to a terminal event, e.g. death. Then the hazard of relapse can be expressed as

$$h^*(t) = \lim_{\Delta \to 0} \frac{P(t \le T_1 < t + \Delta | T_1 \ge t)}{\Delta}, \; t > 0. \tag{1}$$

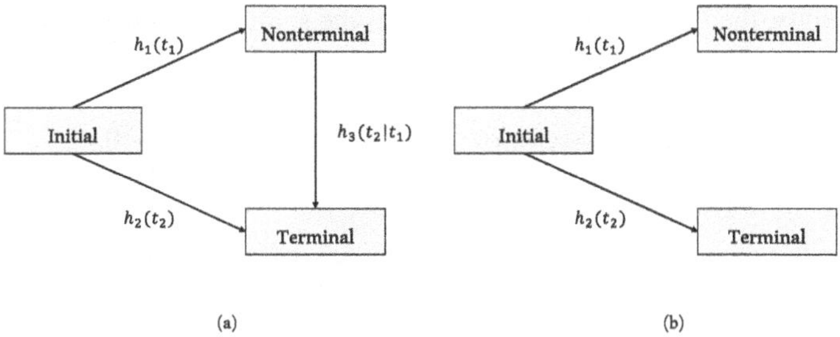

Fig. 1 Graphical representation of (**a**) semi-competing risks and (**b**) competing risks

We often utilize the hazard function for the relapse with a univariate Cox proportional hazars (PH) model, expressed as

$$h^*(t|\boldsymbol{X}_{ij}) = h_0^*(t)\exp\{\boldsymbol{X}_{ij}^T\beta^* + V_j\}. \tag{2}$$

We may perform an analysis by incorporating death not as a censoring mechanism but as a component of the outcome, often called a *composite endpoint*. See Gomez and Lagakos [7] for detailed descriptions. More precisely, let $T_c = \min(T_1, T_2)$ denote the time from discharges to the first relapse or death. This process can be proceeded with a conventional survival analysis for T_c by the following model:

$$h(t_c|\boldsymbol{X}_{ij}) = h_{0c}(t_c)\exp\{\boldsymbol{X}_{ij}^T\beta_c + V_j\}, \tag{3}$$

where h_{0c} is the baseline hazard function corresponding to T_c. Usual estimation procedures for β_c can be applied under the assumption that the remaining forms of censoring are independent. As raised by Haneuse and Lee [10], there is a shortcoming on this approach. That is, the interpretation of β_c should be based on a mixture of the effects of $\boldsymbol{X}_{ij}$ on both relapse and death. Therefore, the primary interest could be drifted away from relapse.

We use the illness-death model to analyze semi-competing risks data. To formalize the model under a semi-competing risks setup, we utilize the illness-death model represented as three transition-specific hazard functions (as depicted in Fig. 1),

$$\begin{aligned}
h_1(t_1) &= \lim_{\Delta\to 0}\frac{P(t_1 \le T_1 < t_1+\Delta|T_1 \ge t_1, T_2 \ge t_1)}{\Delta},\ t_1 > 0,\\
h_2(t_2) &= \lim_{\Delta\to 0}\frac{P(t_2 \le T_2 < t_2+\Delta|T_1 \ge t_2, T_2 \ge t_2)}{\Delta},\ t_2 > 0,\\
h_3(t_2|t_1) &= \lim_{\Delta\to 0}\frac{P(t_2 \le T_2 < t_2+\Delta|T_1 = t_1, T_2 \ge t_2)}{\Delta},\ 0 < t_1 < t_2.
\end{aligned} \tag{4}$$

Subsequently, the Cox PH model [3, 4] under the semi-competing risks framework can be expressed as

$$\begin{aligned} h_1(t_1|\gamma_{ij}, \boldsymbol{X}_{ij}) &= \gamma_{ij} h_{01}(t_1) \exp\{\boldsymbol{X}_{ij}^T \beta_1 + V_{j1}\},\ t_1 > 0, \\ h_2(t_2|\gamma_{ij}, \boldsymbol{X}_{ij}) &= \gamma_{ij} h_{02}(t_2) \exp\{\boldsymbol{X}_{ij}^T \beta_2 + V_{j2}\},\ t_2 > 0, \\ h_3(t_2|t_1, \gamma_{ij}, \boldsymbol{X}_{ij}) &= \gamma_{ij} h_{03}(t_2|t_1) \exp\{\boldsymbol{X}_{ij}^T \beta_3 + V_{j3}\},\ 0 < t_1 < t_2, \end{aligned} \tag{5}$$

where $\gamma_{ij}(> 0)$ is a subject-specific shared frailty which follows Gamma(θ^1, θ^1). Further, note that $h_{01}(t_1)$, $h_{02}(t_2)$, and $h_{03}(t_2|t_1)$ denote the baseline hazard functions. More specifically, $h_{01}(t_1)$ denotes the baseline hazard function for relapse from discharge and β_1 is the vector of log hazard ratios (HRs) that take into account the effect of covariates on the hazard for relapse from discharge. On the other hand, $h_{02}(t_2)$ denotes the baseline hazard for death from discharge. Finally, $h_{03}(t_2)$ corresponds to the conditional baseline hazard function for death, given that a relapse event occurred at time t_1. However, we often face difficulties on choosing or handling the baseline hazard $h_{03}(t_2|t_1)$ in (5) due to complex structure inherited in the model itself. Thus, from a practical standpoint we assume that $h_{03}(t_2|t_1)$ is independent of t_1. Therefore, the third hazard function in (5) can be expressed as

$$h_3(t_2|t_1, \gamma_{ij}, \boldsymbol{X}_{ij}) = \gamma_{ij} h_{03}(t_2) \exp\{\boldsymbol{X}_{ij}^T \beta_3 + V_j\},\ 0 < t_1 < t_2. \tag{6}$$

3 Data and Bayesian Analysis

3.1 Breast Cancer Data

In our analysis we use a dataset from the multi-institutional clinical trials of breast cancer, where a total of 5715 patients with breast cancer was collected by 36 cancer centers in the USA and Europe. This dataset has been initially analyzed by Haibe-Kains et al. [9], and Peng et al. [15] also analyzed this dataset using a semiparametric regression model under the semi-competing risks framework. The dataset is readily available from the supplementary materials of Haibe-Kains et al. [9]. Data from 6 different patient cohorts, containing observations (either censored or completed) of the non-terminal and terminal event times, are gathered from databases collected by six different institutions.

The survival outcomes of interest are the times for relapse-free survival (RFS) defined as the duration from the operation time to the time until relapse is detected, and the time for overall survival (OS) is defined as the duration from the operation time to death. RFS and OS are considered under semi-competing risks, where RFS is the non-terminal event and OS is the terminal event. We are interested in how the clinical information of breast cancer patients affects both two events and the correlation between these two event times. A total of 987 patients was used in our

Table 1 Summary of breast cancer data

	Distribution		Outcome,%			
	N	%	Censored (alive without relapse)	Dead without relapse	Alive with relapse	Dead with relapse
Total	987	100.00	56.84	9.93	12.06	21.18
Acronym of the dataset						
CAL[a]	103	10.44	0.61	6.69	2.43	0.71
NKI[b]	292	29.58	19.15	0.20	2.74	7.50
STNO2[c]	88	8.92	4.66	0.51	1.11	2.63
TRANSBIG[d]	196	19.86	10.84	0.00	3.34	5.67
UCSF[e]	120	12.16	7.29	2.23	0.91	1.72
UNC4[f]	188	19.05	14.29	0.30	1.52	2.94
Estrogen receptor status						
0	296	29.99	14.49	3.75	2.43	9.32
1	691	70.01	42.35	6.18	9.63	11.85
Histological grade						
1	156	15.81	11.85	1.22	1.22	1.52
2	379	38.40	20.97	4.26	6.18	6.99
3	452	45.80	24.01	4.46	4.66	12.66
Nodal status						
0	569	57.65	34.65	3.95	6.89	12.16
1	418	42.35	22.19	5.98	5.17	9.02
Treatment						
0	403	40.83	23.20	1.32	5.98	10.33
1	584	59.17	33.64	8.61	6.08	10.84

[a] *CAL* dataset of breast cancer patients from the University of California, San Francisco, and the California Pacific Medical Center (United States)
[b] *NKI* dataset from National Cancer Institute (the Netherlands)
[c] *STNO* dataset from Stanford/Norway (United States and Norway)
[d] *TRANSBIG* dataset collected by the TransBIG consortium (Europe)
[e] *UCSF* dataset from University of California, San Francisco (United States)
[f] *UNC* dataset from University of North Carolina (United States)

analysis after deleting some missing observations. We have also changed the unit of time from days to years.

Table 1 shows brief summary statistics for breast cancer data. As mentioned above, there are six institutions including CAL (University of California, San Francisco, and the California Pacific Medical Center). Three covariates are used in the analysis. They are *estrogen receptor status*, 0 for negative and 1 for positive; *historical grade*, 1 for low, 2 for intermediate, and 3 for high and *nodal status*. We can see that 33% of patients having had operations showed relapse within about 25 years, and 21% of all patients died. The overall death rate turned out to be 31.1%, and 56.8% of patients have never experienced any events (relapse/death) and censored.

3.2 Bayesian Inference

As described in Sect. 2 we apply three approaches for modeling. They are the logistic regression and survival analysis for univariate analysis, and semi-competing risks analysis. We only present a Bayesian setup for survival analysis in detail. A setup for semi-competing risks analysis is fairly similar, and thus it is omitted. We utilize R package BayesSurv_HReg for the analysis. This would be applied to cluster-correlated, univariate time-to-event data fitting to a Cox PH model with the Weibull baseline hazard.

Let t_{ij} denote the time-to-event of interest for individuals $i = 1, \ldots, n_j$ in location $j = 1, \ldots, J$, subject to right censoring at time c_{ij}. Let $(y_{ij}, \delta_{ij}, \boldsymbol{x}_{ij})$ denote independent observations, where $y_{ij} = \min(t_{ij}, c_{ij})$, $\delta_{ij} = I(t_{ij} \le c_{ij})$, and $\boldsymbol{x}_{ij}$ is a vector of covariates for individual i in location j. Similar to what is presented in (5), the following Cox PH model is assumed:

$$h(t_{ij}|x_{ij}) = h_0(t_{ij}) \exp(\boldsymbol{x}_{ij}^T \beta + V_j), \ t_{ij} > 0,$$

where the V_j's are location-specific random effects and the baseline hazard h_0 is defined parametrically by a Weibull hazard, $h_0(t) = \alpha\kappa t^{\alpha-1}$. For prior specifications we assume the following prior distributions below:

$$\begin{cases} \pi(\beta) & \propto & 1, \\ \pi(\alpha) & \sim & \text{Gamma}(a, b), \\ \pi(\kappa) & \sim & \text{Gamma}(c, d), \\ V_j & \sim & \text{Normal}(0, \sigma^2), \\ \xi = 1/\sigma^2 & \sim & \text{Gamma}(a_N, b_N). \end{cases}$$

We note that a gamma random variable X has the form of $f(x|a, b) \propto x^{a-1} e^{-bx}$. So, the mean and variance of X are given respectively by $\mu_X = a/b$ and $\sigma_X^2 = a/b^2$. Thus, we have $a = (\mu_X/\sigma_X)^2$ and $b = \mu_X/\sigma_X^2$. In order to impose diffuse information on the gamma prior distributions, we set the variance to be 1000. Further, we set the mean value as the MLE of the corresponding parameters. Thus, the resulting hyperparameter values are

$$a = 0.00085, \ b = 0.00092, \ c = 2.749 \times 10^{-6}, \ d = 5.243 \times 10^{-5}.$$

On the other hand, the cluster-specific random effects are assumed to be i.i.d. $N(0, \sigma^2)$. We set $a_N = 0.1$ and $b_N = 0.01$ accordingly. Finally, the number of replication is 500,000 with a thin value of 1000, and we use 10% as the proportion of burn-in samples.

Recall that we have three hazards functions given in (5) for the semi-competing regression models. Since we have patient-specific frailty γ_{ij}, it is assumed that $\gamma_{ij}|\theta \sim \text{Gamma}(\theta^{-1}, \theta^{-1})$. Under a hierarchical structure we assume that θ^{-1}

follows a gamma distribution. Moreover, let $\boldsymbol{V}_j = (V_{j1}, V_{j2}, V_{j3})'$ denote a vector of cluster-specific random effects associated with the hazards functions in (5). Since $\boldsymbol{V}_j$ is assumed to follow a multivariate normal distribution with a mean vector of zeros and variance–covariance matrix Σ_V, we impose an Inverse-Wishart distribution as a prior for Σ_V, which is commonly used in Bayesian framework. Specific choices for the hyperparameters in entire computations are provided in Appendix.

3.3 Results

Table 2 provides the results for three different analysis as mentioned in Sect. 2. We use age, estrogen receptor status, historical grade, nodal status, tumor size (unit: cm), and treatment as independent variables for all three analyses. In Table 2 we provide the odds ratios (OR) and HR along with corresponding 95% HPD intervals. First, the univariate logistic regression utilizes "geeglm" function to conduct the analysis. There are several arguments to reflect covariance structures such as independence, exchangeable, AR(1), and unstructured. We simply select one structure in which the quasi-likelihood correlation information (QIC) is minimized [14]. It turned out that the *exchangeable* case has the smallest QIC value of 1203.2 so that this case has been used. We can see that the OR's for all variables yield reasonable values. For instance, they increase as the historical grade and nodal status increase, while estrogen status decreases. The estimates for the common variance and correlation turned out to be 0.99 and 0.01, respectively.

We have three cases for survival analysis, and their corresponding response variables are relapse, death, and composite endpoint. More specifically, the variables of interest are the event for relapse-free survival (RFS) corresponding to relapse, and an event for overall survival (OS) corresponding to death. Recall that description for the composite endpoint has been explained in Sect. 2. Regarding the results for survival analysis, we have similar outcomes as appeared in the logistic regression. Both the relapse and death rates increase as the level of the historical grade increases. See HR values of 2.19 and 2.30 for the "Relapse column," and 1.66 and 2.04 for the "Death column" in Table 2. Similarly, we have an HR value of 1.24%, which implies that both rates increase as the tumor size increases. There seems to be little association between the age of patients and the relapse rate since the HPD intervals contain a value of 1 for all three cases. However, the relapse rate is higher for younger patients, while the death rate is higher for elderly patients. In view of composite endpoint analysis, the HR value for the third historical grade is a little smaller than those for both relapse and overall survival categories. We provide the values of three different variances for survival analysis. Figure 2 shows the estimated Weibull hazard functions for the three cases.

We used the function called BayesID_HReg to analyze the data under the semi-competing risks framework, where the results are provided in the last three columns of Table 2. Compared to the logistic regression and survival analysis, we have

Table 2 Estimates of odds ratio (OR) and hazards ratio (HR) parameters along with corresponding HPD intervals

	Univariate analysis								Semi-competing risks analysis					
	Logistic regression		Survival analysis											
	Relapse		Relapse		Death		Composite endpoint		Relapse		Death without relapse		Death after relapse	
	OR	95% HPD	HR	95% HPD	HR	95% HPD	HR	95% HPD	HR	95% HPD	HR	95% HPD	HR	95% HPD
Age	0.98	(0.97, 0.99)	0.99	(0.97, 1.00)	1.01	(1.00, 1.02)	1.00	(0.99, 1.01)	0.99	(0.98, 1.01)	1.06	(1.04, 1.08)	1.02	(1.00, 1.04)
Estrogen receptor status	0.85	(0.69, 1.05)	0.77	(0.60, 0.98)	0.53	(0.42, 0.68)	0.73	(0.60, 0.92)	0.61	(0.41, 0.88)	0.29	(0.15, 0.52)	0.32	(0.17, 0.51)
Histological grade2	2.55	(1.87, 3.48)	2.19	(1.47, 3.42)	1.66	(1.09, 2.57)	1.87	(1.34, 2.67)	3.13	(1.82, 5.79)	2.66	(1.17, 6.86)	1.46	(0.64, 3.35)
Histological grade3	2.58	(1.59, 4.18)	2.30	(1.59, 3.64)	2.04	(1.39, 3.20)	1.94	(1.39, 2.80)	4.75	(2.57, 9.55)	3.63	(1.35, 11.11)	2.40	(0.95, 7.44)
Nodal status	1.32	(0.70, 2.47)	1.46	(1.07, 1.99)	1.34	(0.98, 1.80)	1.44	(1.13, 1.86)	1.74	(1.11, 2.74)	2.51	(1.35, 5.08)	1.26	(0.73, 2.40)
Tumor size (cm)	1.31	(1.21, 1.42)	1.24	(1.13, 1.35)	1.25	(1.13, 1.37)	1.20	(1.10, 1.29)	1.50	(1.27, 1.82)	1.46	(1.13, 1.93)	1.59	(1.28, 2.10)
Treatment	0.61	(0.32, 1.16)	0.68	(0.47, 1.01)	0.85	(0.59, 1.26)	0.68	(0.49, 0.94)	0.71	(0.43, 1.06)	3.54	(1.55, 8.00)	1.51	(0.85, 2.82)

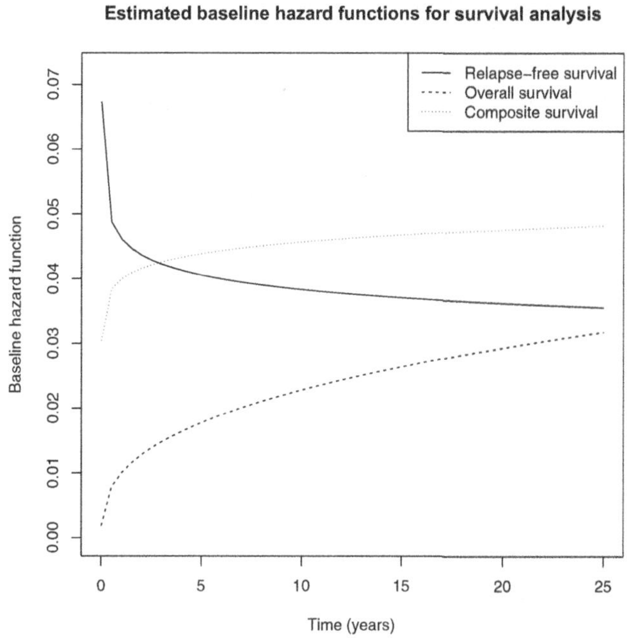

Fig. 2 The hazard functions of survival analysis

several different results under semi-competing risks setup. There is a significant result for age effect with an HR value of 1.06. Also, we have a very significant result for treatment effect. The HR value turned out to be 3.54 with an HPD interval (1.55, 8.00). The three estimated hazards functions defined in (5) are plotted in Fig. 3. The estimates for the three variances of Σ_V are 0.011, 0.012, and 0.011, respectively. Further, the estimates for the three covariances σ_{12}, σ_{13}, and σ_{23} of Σ_V are -4.96×10^{-4}, 9.54×10^{-5}, and -5.95×10^{-4}, respectively.

The assessment of convergence of the Gibbs sampling is carried out based on the methodology of Gelman and Rubin [8]. A total of 3 chains were run from different starting values for the parameters to check convergence. Figure 4 shows trace plots of the estimates of the regression coefficients for the "death without relapse" model in (5). They correspond to three different chains (represented by light gray, gray, and black lines) that were started from initial parameter values reflecting an over-dispersed state. These trace plots show convergence reasonably well. The other trace plots of "relapse" and "death after relapse" categories yielded similar patterns for convergence.

Overall, with regard to relapse through the three approaches, there are significant results in both survival and semi-competing risks analyses for estrogen receptor and nodal status, while the logistic regression yields an insignificant result. This implies that the logistic regression is somewhat inadequate for explaining these risk factors. When we compare the death rate for survival and semi-competing risks

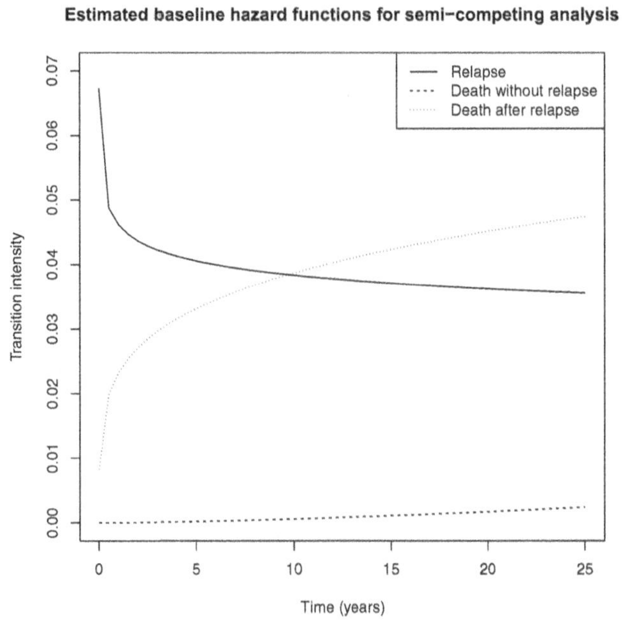

Fig. 3 The hazard functions of semi-competing analysis

analyses, both age and nodal status reveal significant results for semi-competing risks analysis, while they do not seem significant under the survival analysis. Moreover, in contrast to survival analysis, the treatment has a considerable amount of effect on death with semi-competing risks analysis. This is mainly due to the situation that survival analysis contains both "death without relapse" and "death after relapse" in one category, resulting in a lack of appropriate explanation on potential high risks.

4 Concluding Remarks

In this chapter, we analyzed the breast cancer data collected by 36 cancer centers in the USA and Europe with three models: logistics regression, survival analysis, and semi-competing risks analysis. The maximum likelihood approach was applied for the first one while the Bayesian approach was employed for the rest of approaches. For implementing the logistic regression, we used the "geeglm" function reserved in the R package. Furthermore, we used the "BayesSurv_HReg" and "BayesID_HReg" functions reserved in the R package for the survival analysis and the semi-competing risks analysis, respectively. The risk factors affecting the relapse show similar trends for the first two models, while the effect sizes of the historical grade were higher in the semi-competing risks model than other models. For death, the effects

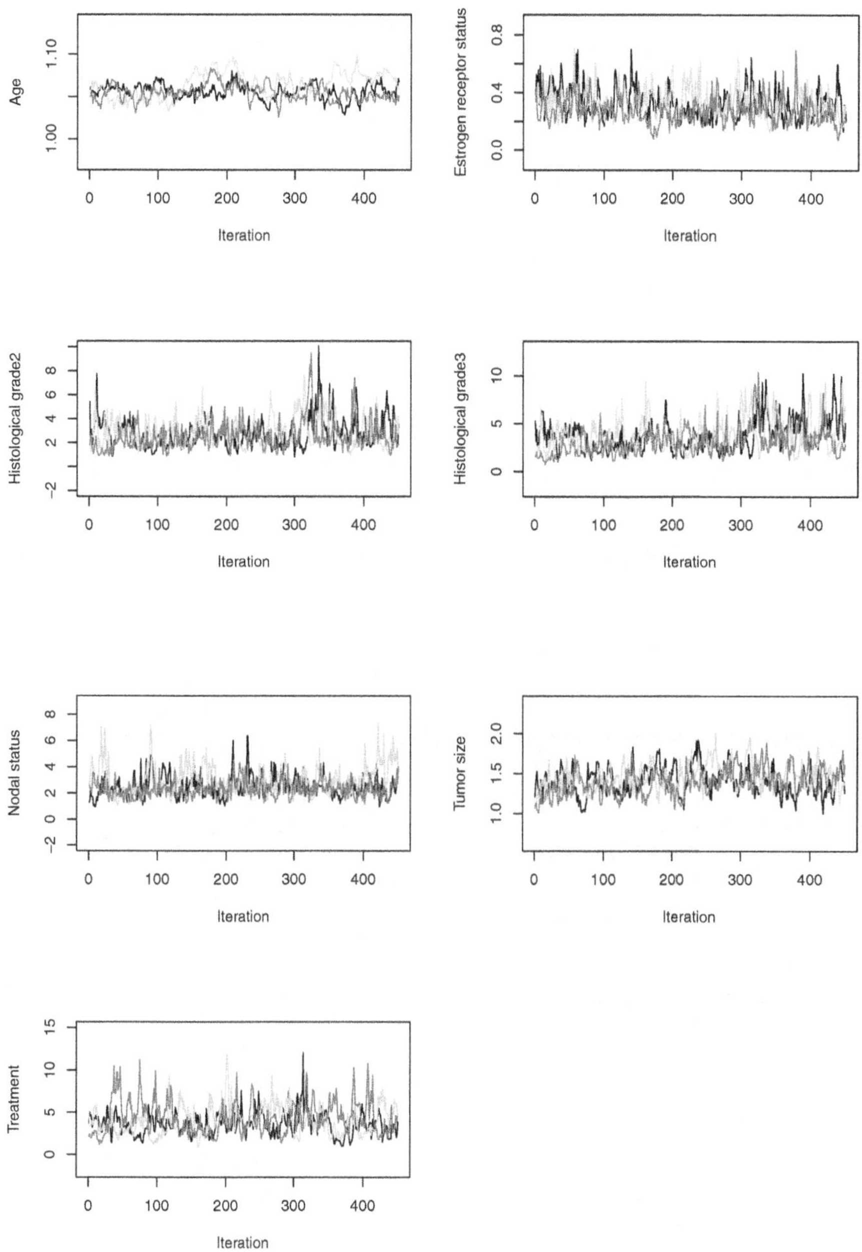

Fig. 4 Trace plots of the estimates of the regression coefficients for the "death without relapse" model

of covariates such as estrogen receptor status, historical status, nodal status, and treatment were considerably different depending on whether the relapse is treated as a censoring or not. Finally, we found that the effects of historical status, nodal status, and treatment on the death were reduced after experiencing the relapse.

Acknowledgments This research was partially supported by Basic Science Research Program through the National Research Foundation of Korea (NRF) funded by the Ministry of Education (NRF-2018R1D1A1B07045804) (Seong W. Kim), and by Basic Science Research Program through the National Research Foundation of Korea (NRF) funded by the Ministry of Education (NRF-2020R1F1A1A01048397) (Jinheum Kim).

Appendix

```
 ## 1. Logistic regression

# Get data from https://www.ncbi.nlm.nih.gov/pmc
/articles/PMC3283537/bin/supp_djr545_jnci-JNCI-11-0924-s02.
csv
breast <- read.csv("breast.csv")
breast <- breast[!is.na(breast$e.rfs) &
                 !is.na(breast$e.os),
                c(1:3, 5:6, 9:13, 16:18)]
obs = which(breast$e.rfs == 0 &
                breast$e.os == 1 &
                breast$t.rfs < breast$t.os)
breast=breast[-obs,]
# Change the units of the date
breast$t.rfs <- breast$t.rfs / 365.25
breast$t.os <- breast$t.os / 365.25

# Age at diagnosis (years)
age <- breast$age
# Estrogen receptor status
er <- breast$er
# Histological grade
grade2 <- breast$grade2
grade3 <- breast$grade3
# Nodal status
node <- breast$node
# Tumor size (cm)
size <- breast$size
# Time for relapse-free survival
t.rfs <- breast$t.rfs
# Event for relapse-free survival
e.rfs <- breast$e.rfs
# Time for overall survival
```

```
t.os <- breast$t.os
# Event for overall survival
e.os <- breast$e.os
# Treatment
treatment <- breast$treatment

# geepack packages are needed to execute geeglm
install.packages("geepack")
library(geepack)

# Change the data type
breast$dataset <- as.factor(breast$dataset)
id = breast$dataset
LR <-
  formula(e.rfs ~  age + er + grade2 +
            grade3 + node + size + treatment)
EX <-
  geeglm(
    LR, id = dataset, data = breast, family = "binomial",
    corstr = "exchangeable"
  )

install.packages("ztable", repos = "http://cran.us.r-
project.org")
library(ztable)
ztable(EX, size=4, digit=2, caption = "table. Exchangeable")
QIC(EX)


 ## 2. Survival Analysis

 # 2-1. Relapse survival

install.packages("SemiCompRisks")
library(SemiCompRisks)

id = breast$dataset
survival_rfs <-
  Formula(t.rfs + e.rfs ~ age + er + grade2
          + grade3 + node + size + treatment)

shape.rfs = rfs[[2]]  # shape parameter
scale.rfs = rfs[[3]]  # scale parameter

sigma = 1000
a.r <- shape.rfs ^ 2 / sigma
b.r <- shape.rfs / sigma
c.r <- scale.rfs ^ 2 / sigma
d.r <- scale.rfs / sigma
```

```
WB.ab_rfs <- c(a.r, b.r)
WB.cd_rfs <- c(c.r, d.r)
Normal.ab_rfs <- c(0.1, 0.01)

hyperParams <-
  list(
    WB = list(WB.ab = WB.ab_rfs, WB.cd = WB.cd_rfs),
    Normal = list(Normal.ab = Normal.ab_rfs)
  )
numReps <- 500000
thin <- 1000
burninPerc <- 0.1

storeV <- TRUE
mhProp_V_var <- 100
mhProp_alpha_var <- 100

mcmc.WB  <-
  list(
    run = list(
      numReps = numReps,
      thin = thin,
      burninPerc = burninPerc
    ),
    storage = list(storeV = storeV),
    tuning = list(mhProp_alpha_var = mhProp_alpha_var,
                  mhProp_V_var =
                    mhProp_V_var)
  ) #MCMC Settings

myModel <- c("Weibull", "Normal")
startValues <-
  initiate.startValues_HReg(survival_rfs, breast,
                             id, model = myModel, nChain = 5)
fit_rfs <-
  BayesSurv_HReg(survival_rfs, breast, id, model = myModel,
                hyperParams, startValues, mcmc.WB)
print(fit_rfs, digits = 2)
summary(fit_rfs)


 # 2-2. Overall survival

survival_os <-
  Formula(t.os + e.os ~ age + er + grade2 + grade3
          + node + size + treatment)

shape.os = os[[2]]
```

```
scale.os = os[[3]]

a.o <- shape.os ^ 2 / sigma
b.o <- shape.os / sigma
c.o <- scale.os ^ 2 / sigma
d.o <- scale.os / sigma

WB.ab_os <- c(a, b)
WB.cd_os <- c(c, d)
Normal.ab_os  <- c(0.1, 0.01)

hyperParams <- list(
  WB = list(WB.ab = WB.ab_os, WB.cd = WB.cd_os),
  Normal = list(Normal.ab = Normal.ab_os)
)

startValues  <-
  initiate.startValues_HReg(survival_os, breast,
                            model = myModel, id, nChain = 5)
fit_os <-
  BayesSurv_HReg(survival_os, breast, id, model = myModel,
             hyperParams, startValues, mcmc.WB)
print(fit_os, digits = 2)
summary(fit_os)

# 2-3. Composite survival

form_cep <-
  Formula(t.c + e.c ~ age + er + grade2 + grade3
          + node + size + treatment)

shape.cps <- cps[[2]]
scale.cps <- cps[[3]]

a.c <- shape.cps ^ 2 / sigma
b.c <- shape.cps / sigma
c.c <- scale.cps ^ 2 / sigma
d.c <- scale.cps / sigma

WB.ab_cps <- c(a.c, b.c)
WB.cd_cps <- c(c.c, d.c)
Normal.ab_cps  <- c(0.1, 0.01)

hyperParams <- list(
  WB = list(WB.ab = WB.ab_cps, WB.cd = WB.cd_cps),
  Normal = list(Normal.ab = Normal.ab_cps)
)

startValues  <-
```

```
  initiate.startValues_HReg(form_cep, breast,
                            model = myModel, id, nChain = 5)
fit_cps <-
  BayesSurv_HReg(form_cep, breast, id,
    model = myModel, hyperParams,
    startValues, mcmc.WB)
print(fit_cps, digits = 2)
summary(fit_cps)



 ## 3. Semi-Competing Risks Analysis

semi_comp <-
  Formula(
    t.rfs + e.rfs |
      t.os + e.os ~ age + er + grade2 + grade3 + node
      + size + treatment |age + er + grade2 + grade3
      + node + size + treatment |age + er + grade2 +
      grade3 + node + size + treatment
  )

a <- shape.rfs ^ 2 / sigma
b <- shape.rfs / sigma
c <- scale.rfs ^ 2 / sigma
d <- scale.rfs / sigma

theta.ab <- c(0.1, 0.01)
WB.ab1 <- c(a, b)
WB.ab2 <- c(a, b)
WB.ab3 <- c(a, b)

WB.cd1 <- c(c, d)
WB.cd2 <- c(c, d)
WB.cd3 <- c(c, d)

Psi_v <- diag(1, 3)
rho_v <- 100

hyperParams <-
  list(
    theta = theta.ab,
    WB = list(
      WB.ab1 = WB.ab1, WB.ab2 = WB.ab2,
      WB.ab3 = WB.ab3, WB.cd1 = WB.cd1,
      WB.cd2 = WB.cd2, WB.cd3 = WB.cd3
    ),
    MVN = list(Psi_v = Psi_v, rho_v = rho_v)
  )
```

```
numReps     <- 500000
thin        <- 1000
burninPerc <- 0.1
nGam_save <- 0
storeV     <- rep(TRUE, 3)

mhProp_theta_var  <- 0.1
mhProp_Vg_var     <- c(100, 100, 100)
mhProp_alphag_var <- c(100, 100, 100)


mcmc.WB  <-
  list(
    run = list(
      numReps = numReps, thin = thin,
      burninPerc = burninPerc
    ),
    storage = list(nGam_save = nGam_save, storeV = storeV),
    tuning = list(
      mhProp_theta_var = mhProp_theta_var,
      mhProp_Vg_var = mhProp_Vg_var,
      mhProp_alphag_var = mhProp_alphag_var
    )
  )

myModel_semi <- c("Markov", "Weibull", "MVN")

startValues_semi  <-
  initiate.startValues_HReg(semi_comp, breast,
                            myModel_semi, id, nChain =
                              5)
fit_semicomp <-
  BayesID_HReg(semi_comp, breast, id,
               model = myModel_semi, hyperParams,
               startValues_semi, mcmc.WB)
print(fit_semicomp, digits = 2)
summary(fit_semicomp)
```

References

1. Andersen, P.K., Geskus, R.B., de Witte, T., Putter, H.: Competing risks in epidemiology: possibilities and pitfalls. Int. J. Epidemiol. **41**, 861–870 (2012)
2. Barrett, J.K., Siannis, F., Farewell, V.T.: A semi-competing risks model for data with interval-censoring and informative observation: an application to the MRC cognitive function and aging study. Stat. Med. **30**, 1–10 (2011)
3. Cox, D.R.: Models and life-tables regression. J. R. Stat. Soc. Ser. B **34**, 187–220 (1972)
4. Cox, D.R.: Partial likelihood. Biometrika **62**, 269–276 (1975)

5. Emura, T., Murotani, K.: An algorithm for estimating survival under a copula-based dependent truncation model. Test **24**, 734–751 (2015)
6. Fine, J.P., Jiang, H., Chappell, R.: On semi-competing risks data. Biometrika **88**, 907–919 (2001)
7. Gómez, G., Lagakos, S.W.: Statistical considerations when using a composite endpoint for comparing treatment groups. Stat. Med. **32**, 719–738 (2013)
8. Gelman, A., Rubin, D.B.: Inference from iterative simulation using multiple sequences. Stat. Sci. **7**, 457–472 (1992)
9. Haibe-Kains, B., Desmedt, C., Loi S., Culhane, A.C., Bontempi, G., Quackenbush, J., Sotiriou, C.: A three-gene model to robustly identify breast cancer molecular subtypes. J. Nat. Cancer Inst. **104**, 311–325 (2012)
10. Haneuse, S., Lee, K.H.: Semi-competing risks data analysis: accounting for death as a competing risk when the outcome of interest is nonterminal. Cardiovasc. Qual. Outcomes **9**, 322–331 (2016)
11. Jazić, I., Schrag, D., Sargent, Daniel J., Haneuse, S.: Beyond composite endpoints analysis: semicompeting risks as an underutilized framework for cancer research. J. Nat. Cancer Inst. **108**, 48–55 (2016)
12. Lee, K.H., Dominici, F., Schrag, D., Haneuse, S.: Hierarchical models for semi-competing risks data with application to quality of end-of-life care for pancreatic cancer. J. Am. Stat. Assoc. **111**, 1075–1095 (2016)
13. Liang K.-Y., Zeger, S.L.: Longitudinal data analysis for discrete and continuous outcomes. Biometrics **42**, 121–130 (1986)
14. Pan, W.: Akaikes information criterion in generalized estimating equations. Biometrics **57**, 120–125 (2001)
15. Peng, M., Xiang, L., Wang, S.: Semiparametric regression analysis of clustered survival data with semi-competing risks. Comput. Stat. Data Anal. **124**, 53–70 (2018)
16. Putter, H., Fiocco, M., Geskus, R.B.: Tutorial in Biostatistics: competing risks and multi-state models. Stat. Med. **26**, 2389–2430 (2007)
17. Tsiatis, A.A.: Competing risks. Encycl. Biostat. **2**, 1025–1035 (2005)
18. Xu, J., Kalbfleisch, J.D., Tai, B.: Statistical analysis of illness-death processes and semi-competing risks data. Biometrics **66**, 716–725 (2010)

Survival Analysis for the Inverse Gaussian Distribution: Natural Conjugate and Jeffrey's Priors

Erin P. Eifert, Kalanka P. Jayalath, and Raj S. Chhikara

Abstract This study focuses on the use of a Bayesian method to analyze survival data that follow an inverse Gaussian (IG) distribution. Both IG parameters are assumed to be unknown, and the natural conjugate and Jeffrey's priors are used in the Bayesian procedure. As the closed-form posteriors of these parameters are intractable due to censored data, a flexible Gibbs sampler is used to derive them computationally. The Gibbs sampler is also used to estimate the average remaining time of the censored units. A comprehensive simulation study is conducted to assess the effects of natural conjugate hyperparameter settings at differing levels of skewness, as measured by the shape parameter ($\phi = \frac{\lambda}{\mu}$), as well as compare behavior of the two priors. Results are compared for point and interval estimates, coverage probabilities, and kernel density estimates. A practical example is included to illustrate the procedure.

1 Introduction

The Inverse Gaussian distribution (IG) originated as a model for the first passage time in Brownian motion, which models the random movement of particles in a fluid and for which the position of a particle at any time is governed by the Gaussian distribution. Schrödinger [16] first derived the distribution of the first passage time of the particle to a defined point. The name inverse Gaussian was coined by Tweedie [19] as a result of the inverse relationship between the cumulant generating functions associated with modeling the distance of the particle and the time until the particle has been in motion to the defined point.

The Gaussian process underlying Brownian motion is inherent to varied physical, biological, and other progressive change in developmental environments. As such the application of IG as a statistical model has been far and wide in fields

E. P. Eifert · K. P. Jayalath (✉) · R. S. Chhikara
University of Houston, Houston, TX, USA
e-mail: erin.p.eifert@outlook.com; jayalath@uhcl.edu; chhikara@uhcl.edu

Y. Lio et al. (eds.), *Bayesian Inference and Computation in Reliability and Survival Analysis*, Emerging Topics in Statistics and Biostatistics,
https://doi.org/10.1007/978-3-030-88658-5_13

ranging from business to science and engineering. Its use in modeling lifetime and performing survival analysis, in particular, is found suitable and beneficial. For references see Chhikara and Folks [6], Seshadri [17], among other related works in literature.

1.1 Parameterizations

Tweedie [18] proposed different parameterizations for the IG distribution. The most common parameterization, noted as IG(μ, λ), has probability density function,

$$f(x;\mu,\lambda) = \sqrt{\frac{\lambda}{2\pi}} x^{-\frac{3}{2}} \exp\left(-\frac{\lambda(x-\mu)^2}{2\mu^2 x}\right), \tag{1}$$

where μ is the mean of the distribution and λ is a shape parameter. This form has two primary advantages. First, a substantial body of work exists on the statistical properties of its parameters μ and λ. As detailed in Chhikara and Folks [6], there are many analogies of sampling distributions and statistical inferential methods for these parameters and those of the normal distribution. Parameter μ represents the mean of the population and thus has a more intuitive meaning and appeal for making population inference.

An alternate parameterization that utilizes the reciprocal of the mean, $\theta = \frac{1}{\mu}$, is denoted here as IG(θ, λ) and has probability density function,

$$f(x;\theta,\lambda) = \sqrt{\frac{\lambda}{2\pi}} x^{-\frac{3}{2}} \exp\left(-\frac{\lambda x}{2}\left(\theta - \frac{1}{x}\right)^2\right). \tag{2}$$

While this parameterization offers somewhat less meaningful interpretation of parameters for IG, the parameter θ has a physical meaning as it represents the mean displacement in unit time for Brownian motion. Moreover, the use of the reciprocal mean facilitates easier development of some Bayesian forms, such as the natural conjugate prior.

A third parameterization, proposed by Tweedie [18], makes use of a third parameter, ϕ, where $\phi = \frac{\lambda}{\mu}$. While this form of the density function is not directly used here, this shape parameter plays an important role in this study. It is a measure of the skewness of the distribution, with a lower value of ϕ indicating a more skewed distribution and a more symmetric distribution associated with a higher value. The parameter ϕ is a unitless quantity and is invariant under a scale transformation of random variable X. Though μ is the mean for IG, it acts as a scale parameter where X/μ is distributed as IG($1, \phi$), a form of standard IG involving one parameter only. In fact, this feature of IG implies that ϕ is intrinsically the shape parameter for a family of two-parameter IG(μ, λ).

1.2 Development of Bayesian Models

Many of the earliest Bayesian developments attributed to Palmer [15] are described in Chhikara and Folks [6]. Because of many useful statistical properties available for the IG(μ, λ) parameterization given in Eq. (1), Palmer focused to work with that form. The natural conjugate prior for this form does not always exist when both parameters were unknown. Rather than transforming the density to another parameterization, Palmer [15] suggested, whenever possible, to limit the parameter space of μ such that the prior existed. Along with a development of the conjugate prior, Palmer also developed the joint posterior for Jeffrey's prior. While the prior was improper, it was shown that the posterior could be normalized to form a proper density. While a closed form for the marginal distribution of μ was given, a tractable form of the marginal posterior for λ could not be derived.

Padgett [14] later developed Bayesian estimators for the reliability function, using both Jeffrey's and the natural conjugate priors, assuming μ to be known. An approximation for the marginal posterior density of λ was developed by Achcar et al. [1] and the method for which was outlined by Kadane and Tierney [11].

Banerjee and Bhattacharyya [3] considered both a locally uniform prior and the natural conjugate prior for the IG(θ, λ) parameterization and developed the posterior joint distributions associated with both priors, as well as the marginal posterior distributions of both parameters. Ahmad and Jaheen [2] later developed estimators for both parameters and the reliability function, based on approximations by Lindley [13] and Kadane and Tierney [11]. This instance is one of the few available in the literature where the hyperparameters specified by Banerjee and Bhattacharyya [3] are given values and utilized. As the goal of the work was to evaluate the performance of the estimators, the hyperparameters were set to values that would minimize their effect on the estimate.

Betrò and Rotondi [4] developed Bayesian forms using a third parameterization. Palmer [4, 15] argued against the use of the IG(θ, λ) parameterization and preferred the one specified by Tweedie [18] that uses parameters μ and $\phi = \frac{\lambda}{\mu}$. Their work developed a prior that, while not technically a conjugate prior, possessed the mathematical tractability for the prior and posterior closed forms as well as posterior moments for both parameters.

1.2.1 Bayesian Survival Analysis

Using the IG(μ, λ) parameterization and assuming a known μ, Ismail and Auda [9] developed kernel density estimates for λ and the total remaining time of a Type-II right censored process using a Gibbs sampler. Two estimation procedures were used, the first being a Bayesian estimation using Jeffrey's prior, and the second considering a fiducial approach. Jayalath and Chhikara [10] extended the work of Ismail and Auda [9] by assuming both parameters unknown and considering any form of right censoring, including progressively right censored data. The Bayesian analysis was performed with a locally uniform prior and was again compared with that obtained using the fiducial approach.

The present study also makes use of Gibbs sampler to estimate the two unknown parameters, as well as the average remaining time under right censoring. The priors currently used are the natural conjugate prior for the IG(θ, λ) parametrization developed by Banerjee and Bhattacharyya [3], and the Jeffrey's prior as given in Palmer [15] and Ahmad and Jaheen [2]. The effectiveness of both priors is examined for different levels of skewness and at different levels of censoring. Further, the impact of hyperparameters on the posterior distributions for the natural conjugate prior is also examined.

1.2.2 Natural Conjugate Prior

For the IG(θ, λ) parameterization, the natural conjugate prior is [3]

$$f_c(\theta, \lambda) = K_1 \lambda^{\frac{n'}{2}-1} \exp\left(-\frac{\lambda n'\alpha'}{2}\left[1 + \frac{\beta'}{\alpha'}\left(\theta - \frac{1}{\beta'}\right)^2\right]\right), \quad \theta > 0, \lambda > 0, \tag{3}$$

where $n' > 1, \alpha' > 0$, and $\beta' > 0$ are hyperparameters. The normalization constant K_1 is given by

$$K_1 = \frac{\left(\frac{\beta'}{\alpha'}\right)^{\frac{1}{2}} \left(\frac{n'\alpha'}{2}\right)^{\frac{n'}{2}}}{S_{n'-1}(\xi')\mathrm{B}\left(\frac{n'-1}{2}, \frac{1}{2}\right)\Gamma\left(\frac{n'}{2}\right)}, \text{ where} \xi' = \left(\frac{n'-1}{\alpha'\beta'}\right)^{\frac{1}{2}}. \tag{4}$$

Here, $S_{n'-1}(\cdot)$ is the Student's t-distribution with $n' - 1$ degrees of freedom, while $\mathrm{B}(\cdot, \cdot)$ and $\Gamma(\cdot)$ represent the Beta and Gamma distributions, respectively. The joint posterior distribution is then given by

$$f_c(\theta, \lambda|\mathbf{x}) = K_2 \lambda^{\frac{n''}{2}-1} \exp\left(-\frac{\lambda n''\alpha'}{2}\left[1 + \frac{\beta''}{\alpha''}\left(\theta - \frac{1}{\beta''}\right)^2\right]\right), \quad \theta > 0, \lambda > 0, \tag{5}$$

where

$$K_2 = \frac{\left(\frac{\beta''}{\alpha''}\right)^{\frac{1}{2}} \left(\frac{n''\alpha''}{2}\right)^{\frac{n''}{2}})}{S_{n''-1}(\xi'')\mathrm{B}\left(\frac{n''-1}{2}, \frac{1}{2}\right)\Gamma\left(\frac{n''}{2}\right)} \text{ and } \xi'' = \left(\frac{n''-1}{\alpha''\beta''}\right)^{\frac{1}{2}}. \tag{6}$$

The quantity u is defined as the reciprocal of the MLE for λ,

$$u = \frac{1}{n}\sum_{i}^{n}\frac{1}{x_i} - \frac{1}{\bar{x}} \tag{7}$$

and $\overline{x} = \sum_{i=1}^{n} x_i/n$ is the MLE of μ. The quantities n'', α'', and β'' are defined as

$$n'' = n + n' \tag{8}$$

$$\alpha'' = \frac{1}{n''}\left[nu + n'\alpha' + \frac{nn'\beta'}{\overline{x}n''\beta''}\left(1 - \frac{\overline{x}}{\beta'}\right)^2\right] \tag{9}$$

$$\beta'' = (n\overline{x} + n'\beta')/n''. \tag{10}$$

The marginal distributions of θ and λ are, respectively,

$$f_c(\theta|\mathbf{x}) = K_2\Gamma\left(\frac{n''}{2}\right)\left(\frac{n''\alpha''}{2}\right)^{-\frac{n''}{2}}\left[1 + \frac{\beta''}{\alpha''}\left(\theta - \frac{1}{\beta''}\right)^2\right]^{-\frac{n''}{2}}, \quad \theta > 0 \tag{11}$$

and

$$f_c(\lambda|\mathbf{x}) = \frac{\left(\frac{\lambda n''\alpha''}{2}\right)^{\frac{n''-1}{2}} \Phi\left[\left(\frac{n''\lambda}{\beta''}\right)^{\frac{1}{2}}\right]}{\lambda\Gamma\left(\frac{n''-1}{2}\right) S_{n'-1}(\xi'')} \exp\left(-\frac{\lambda n''\alpha''}{2}\right), \quad \lambda > 0. \tag{12}$$

Some discussion on setting the values of the hyperparameters of n', α', and β' is warranted here. Note that n' acts as a weighting parameter in relation to the sample size. If its value is set to a minimal value, as it was in the work of Ahmad and Jaheen [2], the effect of the hyperparameters will also be minimal. As n' increases, however, the effect of the hyperparameters becomes more prominent. The expression for β'' in Eq. (10) provides an example of the weighting effected by n'. That is, the hyperparameter β' is weighted against the sample mean, $\overline{x}$, in the posterior distribution. Thus, a difference in setting for β' can shift the resulting posterior curve, resulting in an inverse shift in the estimate for θ, which then translates to a direct shift for μ. The hyperparameter α' has a similar effect on the marginal posterior density of λ, in that it is weighted against the reciprocal of the MLE for λ. This effect, however, is not as straightforward as that of β' to its distribution parameter θ, because the sample mean and analogous hyperparameter β' also affect the resulting marginal distribution for λ.

In practice, the advantage of an informative prior such as the natural conjugate prior is to enable, when possible, the incorporation of information about the data and the system that produces it in the modeling process. It is in this way that the natural conjugate prior associated with the IG(θ, λ) parameterization has a particular advantage. Previous researchers, such as Palmer [15] and Betrò and Rotondi [4], have argued against the use of the IG(θ, λ) parameterization and its associated natural conjugate prior, for reasons pertaining to both physical meaning and the breadth of knowledge of the original IG(μ, λ) form. Palmer [15], for example, preferred a form of the natural conjugate prior where the parameter space for μ was limited and the prior existed. Both Palmer [15] and Betrò and Rotondi [4] used four hyperparameters, but in neither case did these directly relate to some obvious characteristic of the distribution. The hyperparameters used in this work have more intuitive meanings, which, in the presence of true prior information, make setting much easier and their effects more discernible.

1.2.3 Jeffrey's Prior

The log likelihood of the IG(μ, λ) parameterization, given in Eq. (1), is expressed as

$$l(\mu, \lambda) = \frac{n}{2}\ln(\lambda) - \frac{n}{2}\ln(2\pi) - \frac{3}{2}\sum_{i=1}^{n}\ln(x_i) - \frac{\lambda}{2\mu^2}\sum_{i=1}^{n}x_i + \frac{n\lambda}{\mu} - \frac{\lambda}{2}\sum_{i=1}^{n}\frac{1}{x_i}. \quad (13)$$

The Jeffrey's prior, $g_j(\mu, \lambda)$, defined as being proportional to $[\det I(\mu, \lambda)]^{\frac{1}{2}}$, is expressed as

$$g_j(\mu, \lambda) \propto (\mu^3\lambda)^{-\frac{1}{2}}, \quad \mu > 0, \lambda > 0. \quad (14)$$

The joint posterior is given by

$$g_j(\mu, \lambda|\mathbf{x}) \propto \frac{\lambda^{\frac{(n-1)}{2}}}{\mu^{\frac{3}{2}}} \exp\left(-\frac{\lambda}{2\mu^2}\sum_{i=1}^{n}x_i + \frac{n\lambda}{\mu} - \frac{\lambda}{2}\sum_{i=1}^{n}\frac{1}{x_i}\right), \quad \mu > 0, \lambda > 0. \quad (15)$$

While the prior is improper, this posterior can be normalized to form a proper density. The marginal posterior distribution of μ is given by

$$g_j(\mu|\mathbf{x}) \propto \mu^{-\frac{3}{2}}\left(\frac{1}{2\mu^2}\sum_{i=1}^{n}x_i - \frac{n}{\mu} + \frac{1}{2}\sum_{i=1}^{n}\frac{1}{x_i}\right)^{-\frac{n+1}{2}}, \quad \mu > 0. \quad (16)$$

When both parameters are unknown, a closed form for the marginal posterior distribution of λ is not derivable. Achcar et al. [1] derived an approximation using methods outlined by [11]. The marginal density may then be approximated by

$$g_j(\lambda|\mathbf{x}) \propto \frac{(\Psi^*)^{\frac{1}{2}}\lambda^{\frac{(n-1)}{2}}\exp\left(-\frac{\lambda}{2}\sum_{i=1}^{n}\frac{1}{x_i}\right)}{(\hat{\mu}^*)^{\frac{3}{2}}\exp\left(\frac{\lambda}{2\hat{\mu}^{*2}}\sum_{i=1}^{n}x_i - \frac{n\lambda}{\hat{\mu}^*}\right)}, \quad \lambda > 0, \quad (17)$$

where $\hat{\mu}^* = \frac{-2n\lambda + \sqrt{4n^2\lambda^2 + 24\lambda\sum_{i=1}^{n}x_i}}{6}$, $\Psi^* = -\frac{1}{\frac{\partial^2 L_\lambda(\mu)}{\partial\mu^2}}\Big|_{\mu=\hat{\mu}^*}$, and $\frac{\partial^2 L_\lambda(\mu)}{\partial\mu^2} = \frac{1}{n}\left(\frac{3}{2\mu^2} - \frac{3\lambda}{\mu^4}\sum_{i=1}^{n}x_i + \frac{2n\lambda}{\mu^3}\right)$.

2 Gibbs Sampling Algorithm

Consider a random sample of size n such that r units are observed, leaving $n - r$ units to be right censored. Let $\mathbf{y}' = (x_{r+1}^+, x_{r+2}^+, \ldots, x_n^+)$ designate the censored values and let $\tilde{\mathbf{y}}' = (x_{r+1}, x_{r+2}, \ldots, x_n)$ designate the true values of the censored units. Then, the average remaining time is given by

$$\overline{T} = \frac{1}{\mathbf{1}'\mathbf{1}}(\tilde{\mathbf{y}}'1 - \mathbf{y}'\mathbf{1}), \tag{18}$$

where $\mathbf{1}$ is a $(n - r) \times 1$ column vector of ones. The Gibbs sampling algorithm previously employed by Jayalath and Chhikara [10] is adopted here and summarized as follows:

1. Determine initial estimates for μ and λ, respectively. As noted in Jayalath and Chhikara [10], given the absence of a closed-form solution for the maximum likelihood estimator that includes both the observed and censored observations, these estimates are generated iteratively [7]. Set $\hat{\mu}_{MLE} = \mu_1^{(0)}$ and $\hat{\lambda}_{MLE} = \lambda_1^{(0)}$.
2. Set the hyperparameters for the natural conjugate prior.
3. Generate $n - r$ random variates from a uniform distribution bounded by the IG CDF value of the given censored value and 1, that is, $u_{i+1} \sim U[F_{IG}(x_{i+1}^+; \mu_1^{(0)}, \lambda_1^{(0)}), 1]$. Replace the censored values with the inverse CDF values associated with the generated random variates, that is, $x_{i+1}^{(0)} = F_{IG}^{-1}(u_{i+1}; \mu_1^{(0)}, \lambda_1^{(0)})$.
4. Given the new samples for censored observations, obtain the marginal posteriors for both the prior distributions. Update the estimates of μ and λ (say, $\mu_1^{(1)}$ and $\lambda_1^{(1)}$) by sampling from these posterior distributions. For the natural conjugate prior, a sample from the posterior distribution of θ will be obtained and its reciprocal used.
5. Generate the chain by repeating steps 3 and 4 k times, each time by generating random variates using the newly sampled parameters in step 4.
6. Calculate the average remaining time, $\overline{T}_1^{(k)}$, using the last set of simulated observations: $x_{r+1}^{(k)}, x_{r+2}^{(k)}, \ldots, x_n^{(k)}$ obtained using updated parameters $\mu_1^{(k)}$ and $\lambda_1^{(k)}$.
7. Repeat steps 3–6 above for a total of m repetitions, resulting m posteriors estimates for μ and λ, as well as m average remaining time $\overline{T}$ estimates.

Three measures were employed to ensure sufficient convergence of the Gibbs algorithm. Trace plots were first periodically checked to ensure that the sample space was evenly and thoroughly explored. To ensure a sufficient chain length and number of chains, the variance between and within each chain was compared using the scale reduction factor developed by Brooks and Gelman [5] and Gelman et al. [8]. For each set of data, the mean and two-tailed 90% confidence bounds were calculated, with the mean representing the point estimate of the simulation sample. The confidence bounds provide both a measure of the frequency with which the true value was captured in the interval as well as the relative precision of the estimate, as measured by the coverage probability and the average size of the interval, respectively.

Further, kernel density estimates were obtained from the parameter estimates using 1000 random samples in each simulation. These plots provide a visual description of the marginal posterior distributions and may also be compared with the sampling distribution of the MLE values for each estimated parameter. If the hyperparameters shift the posterior distribution of the natural conjugate prior, the effect will be particularly evident in these plots.

3 Monte-Carlo Simulation

This section presents the results of Monte-Carlo simulation studies conducted to investigate the use of two priors for the Bayesian survival analysis for IG in its different parameter settings. Also, the effects of the conjugate hyperparameters are examined and the relative performance of the two priors is evaluated. Following the simulation strategy outlined in Sect. 3.1, the Gibbs sampler was applied on 1000 randomly generated right censored IG samples from each of the six parametric cases considered. Inspection of trace plots, autocorrelation plots, and calculation of the scale reduction factor indicate that convergence was reasonably achieved with $k = 750$ iterations and $m = 1000$ repetitions.

3.1 Selection of Hyperparameters

First, to study the effect of the conjugate hyperparameters, the six cases were divided by two different levels of skewness as measured by $\phi = \frac{\lambda}{\mu}$. For each level of skewness, the variability was increased by a multiple of 2 for standard deviation $\sigma = \sqrt{\mu^3/\lambda}$. Each case was evaluated using 1000 randomly generated samples of size $n = 25$ from the given IG(μ, λ) distribution. From each sample, 20% of the observations were right censored. The weighting hyperparameter for the conjugate prior, $n' = 5$, which is 20% of the sample size for all simulations. This setting was chosen so that the effects of α' and β' could be assessed without completely overshadowing the influence of the data.

The six cases are summarized as follows:

Case 1: $\phi = 0.2, \alpha' = 1, \beta' = 5$

(1a) $\mu = 2.5, \lambda = 0.5$
(1b) $\mu = 5, \lambda = 1$ (Control)
(1c) $\mu = 10, \lambda = 2$

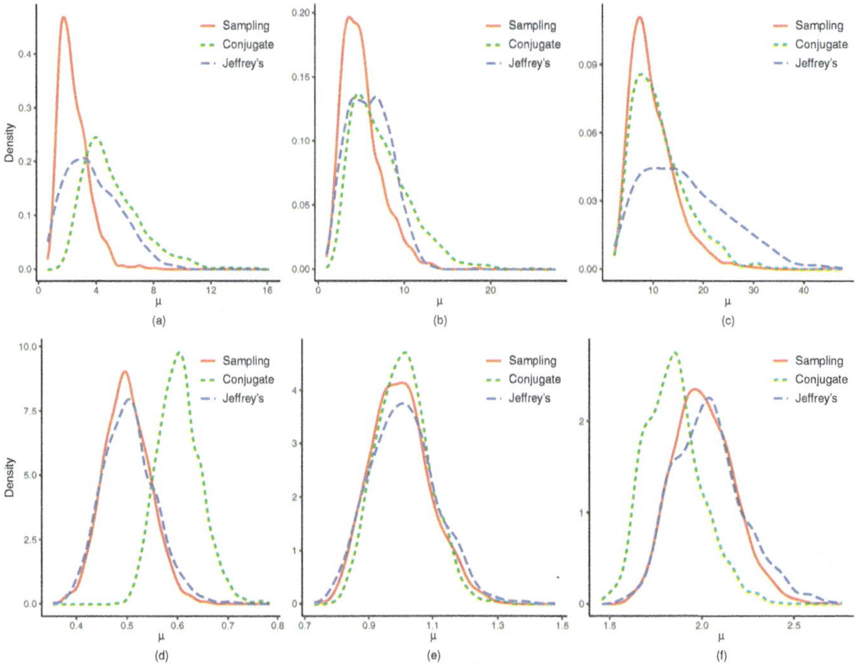

Fig. 1 Kernel Density Plots for μ, showing hyperparameter effects: Cases 1a, 1b, and 1c (top panel) and 2a, 2b, and 2c (bottom panel)

Case 2: $\phi = 5, \alpha' = 0.2, \beta' = 1$

(2a) $\mu = 0.5, \lambda = 2.5$
(2b) $\mu = 1, \lambda = 5$ (Control)
(2c) $\mu = 2, \lambda = 10$

These cases are arranged such that cases 1b and 2b with $\beta' = \mu$ and $\alpha' = \lambda^{-1}$ serve as control cases, where the hyperparameters are set to match with the parameters of the generated IG data. The other cases would then demonstrate how the change in the hyperparameters would affect the posterior density compared to that when a non-informative prior is the basis for the posterior density.

3.1.1 Simulation Results

The simulation results are shown in Table 1. The table provides the point estimates, their standard errors, the coverage probabilities, and the average width of the 90% confidence interval for each of the parameters μ, λ, and T. The true value for $\overline{T}$ was calculated as the mean of the actual average remaining time over the 1000 samples simulated.

Kernel density plots for the posteriors of μ are shown in Fig. 1. For the two control cases depicted in Fig. 1b and e, the two Kernel densities are fairly similar,

Table 1 Simulation results for estimation of μ, λ, and $\overline{T}$

	Conjugate prior				Jeffrey's prior			
True	Mean	Std. err.	Coverage	Interval length	Mean	Std. err.	Coverage	Interval length
Case 1a ($\phi = 0.2$)								
$\mu = 2.5$	5.16	0.0681	0.968	13.29	3.80	0.0594	0.904	9.09
$\lambda = 0.5$	0.567	0.00495	0.907	0.493	0.609	0.00661	0.867	0.582
$\overline{T} = 6.13$	15.57	0.379	0.992	42.61	11.19	0.288	0.889	34.64
Case 1b ($\phi = 0.2$)								
$\mu = 5$	7.32	0.111	0.967	17.49	5.96	0.078	0.906	10.61
$\lambda = 1$	1.068	0.00860	0.935	0.937	1.210	0.0128	0.880	1.150
$\overline{T} = 12.81$	21.64	0.569	0.934	61.23	16.67	0.367	0.868	46.97
Case 1c ($\phi = 0.2$)								
$\mu = 10$	11.30	0.171	0.907	24.89	16.43	0.271	0.905	42.54
$\lambda = 2$	1.825	0.0123	0.902	1.601	2.419	0.0262	0.866	2.307
$\overline{T} = 25.39$	32.13	0.828	0.876	91.80	49.30	1.30	0.895	155.79
Case 2a ($\phi = 5$)								
$\mu = 0.5$	0.604	0.00134	0.448	0.227	0.504	0.00165	0.871	0.167
$\lambda = 2.5$	2.026	0.0147	0.761	1.815	3.014	0.0366	0.857	3.030
$\overline{T} = 0.197$	0.267	0.00218	0.999	0.458	0.193	0.00194	0.948	0.296
Case 2b ($\phi = 5$)								
$\mu = 1$	1.008	0.00265	0.926	0.307	1.009	0.00332	0.865	0.330
$\lambda = 5$	5.422	0.0476	0.912	5.038	6.040	0.0687	0.859	6.010
$\overline{T} = 0.395$	0.398	0.00355	0.984	0.657	0.383	0.00379	0.946	0.586
Case 2c ($\phi = 5$)								
$\mu = 2$	1.845	0.00483	0.815	0.646	2.304	0.00602	0.912	0.666
$\lambda = 10$	6.924	0.0409	0.545	6.208	12.36	0.153	0.861	12.409
$\overline{T} = 0.771$	0.669	0.00632	0.951	1.14	0.769	0.00743	0.963	1.18

indicating no effect on the posterior distributions due to skewness. However, the posteriors in each case differ from one another with respect to the control primarily due to a shift resulting from the use of conjugate priors. Though, no obvious effect on posterior density is seen due to an increase in standard deviation, the estimate of μ is much higher than the true value when the standard deviation is small, as seen in cases 1(a) and 2(a) of Table 1. As expected, the interval sizes are increased with increase in the standard deviations of underlying IG sampling distributions. Overall, the posterior density of λ is notably taller for the conjugate prior than Jeffrey's prior, as seen in Fig. 2. For $\overline{T}$, its posteriors depicted in Fig. 3 for the two priors are pretty much similar in their shape.

It is seen from Table 1 that the natural conjugate prior performs better in higher skewness ($\phi = 0.2$) scenarios than it does with more symmetric ($\phi = 5$) scenarios. The effect of β' on the marginal posterior of μ is most prominently seen in the more symmetric cases where $\phi = 5$; there is a noticeable shift in the kernel density

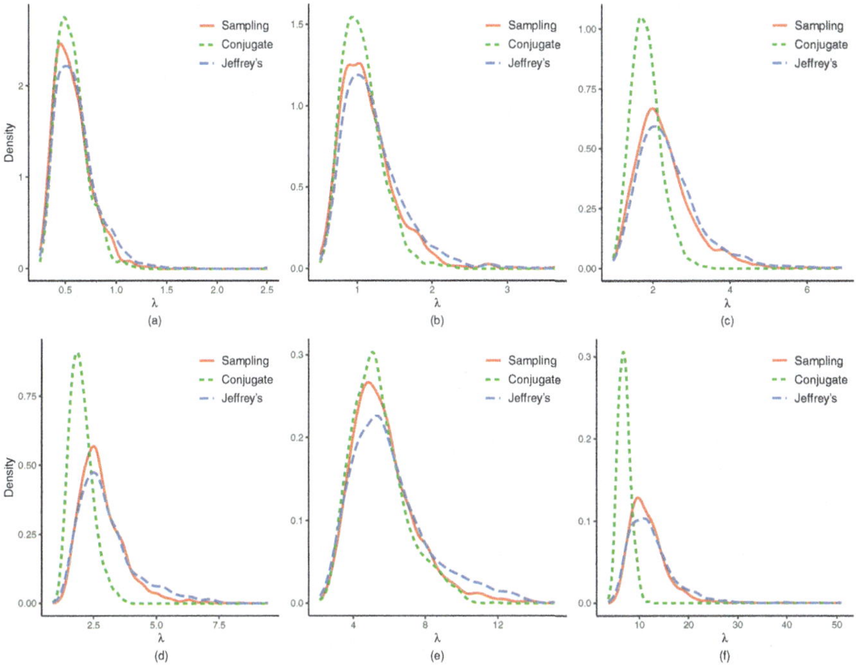

Fig. 2 Kernel Density Plots for λ, observing hyperparameter effects: Cases 1a, 1b, and 1c (top panel) and 2a, 2b, and 2c (bottom panel)

curves of the conjugate prior cases (Fig. 1d and f). This effect is also evident in the coverage probabilities for the two non-control cases 2a and 2c since these are noticeably below the 90% for which the intervals were obtained. For the more skewed ($\phi = 0.2$) cases, while a slight shift kernel density is visible in cases 1a and 1c, this shift does not lead to less coverage of the true parameter within the intervals.

The effect of the hyperparameters on the posterior distributions of λ is more complex. As with the effect observed in the posterior of μ, the effect of the hyperparameters on the posterior distribution of λ is more pronounced in the more symmetric cases of 2a and 2c depicted in Fig. 2d and f. This may be due to the way both α' and β' affect the posterior marginal distribution of λ, as seen from the complex expressions in Eqs. (9) and (12). If α' is the only hyperparameter affecting the marginal posterior, then the effect would be similar to that of how β' affects for μ. However, as Eq. (9) shows, both α' and β' affect the posterior for λ. When the chosen value of β' is close to the sample mean, last term in Eq. (9) approaches zero. Any deviation of β', whether positive or negative, from the true mean will increase the value of α'', resulting in a leftward shift of the density for λ given in Eq. (12). Thus, when smaller α' values should lead to a rightward shift, as in cases 1a and

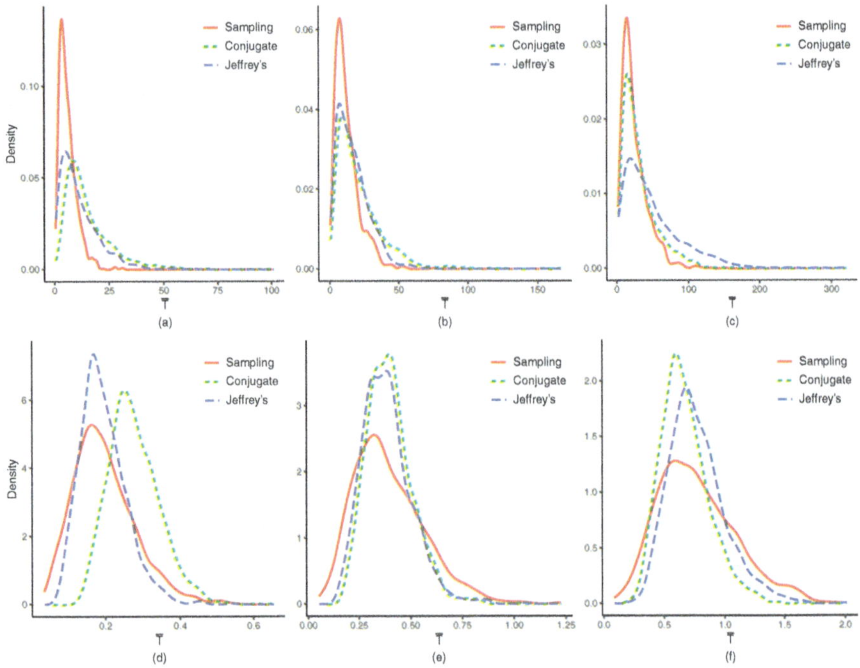

Fig. 3 Kernel Density Plots for $\overline{T}$, observing hyperparameter effects: Cases 1a, 1b, and 1c (top panel) and 2a, 2b, and 2c (bottom panel)

2a, the deviation of β' from the true mean has a competing effect on the posterior density. This is seen in the density plots for cases 1a and 2a. In case 1a, no shift is readily obvious. In case 2a, the shift is in the negative direction, indicating that the effect of β' was much greater than that of α'. Conversely, when the value of α' leads to a leftward shift in the posterior density for λ, as in cases 1c and 2c, this leftward shift is combined with the leftward shift that results from setting β' at values that differ from the true value of μ. While this effect is evident in both cases 1c and 2c, the combined shift is more pronounced in the more symmetric case.

The kernel density estimates for $\overline{T}$ given in Fig. 3 show that the posterior distributions have a tendency to shift in the same direction as that of μ. However, this shift is less pronounced for $\overline{T}$ than for μ. The coverage probabilities indicate that the true average time is captured in the interval at a much higher percentage than the true value of μ did in the symmetric cases. This is particularly evident in Case 2a, where the true value of μ is within the bounds of the interval only 44.8% of the time, while for the same case, the true average time is captured in all but one sample. In general, the difference in coverage probabilities for the two priors appears to follow the difference in the length of the interval where the wider interval generally resulted in higher coverage.

3.2 Comparison at Different Censoring Levels

To further evaluate the performance of the two priors, two additional levels of censoring were considered, having censored observations approximately 10% ($n - r = 3$) and 40% censoring ($n - r = 10$). This is done only for the control cases 1b and 2b discussed earlier in the simulation study. Again, 1000 randomly generated IG samples from each case are considered. The results for the simulations at different censoring levels are presented in Table 2. The Kernel density plots are depicted in Figs. 4, 5, and 6.

In general, it is seen in Table 2 and also the 20% censored results shown in Table 1 (see cases 1b and 2b), neither prior performed consistently better across all censoring levels. The estimates of the two parameters μ and λ from each prior do not vary appreciably across censoring levels. This indicates some robustness of the suggested procedures when the level of censoring varied for the cases considered. The natural conjugate prior did produce higher coverage probabilities in every scenario, but this can be attributed in some cases to wider intervals, which are seen as heavier tails in the kernel density plots shown in Figs. 4 and 5. In the cases with a higher level of skewness ($\phi = 0.2$), Jeffrey's prior produces estimates for μ that are closer to the true value, smaller intervals, and coverage probabilities that are slightly lower than the nominal 90% level. In the cases of more symmetric distributions ($\phi = 5$), the estimates for both priors across all censoring levels provide better estimates for the true value. For the parameter λ, the natural conjugate prior produces estimates closer to the true value, as well as higher coverage probabilities

Table 2 Simulation results for estimation of μ, λ, and $\overline{T}$ for different censoring levels

	Conjugate prior				Jeffrey's prior			
True	Mean	Std. err.	Coverage	Interval size	Mean	Std. err.	Coverage	Interval size
$\phi = 0.2$, 10% censoring								
$\mu = 5$	7.05	0.105	0.949	15.63	5.997	0.0748	0.899	10.32
$\lambda = 1$	1.07	0.0082	0.933	0.929	1.20	0.0120	0.882	1.119
$\overline{T} = 15.47$	25.77	0.694	0.938	74.70	20.54	0.455	0.895	61.83
$\phi = 0.2$, 40% censoring								
$\mu = 5$	7.12	0.097	0.981	18.46	5.455	0.0765	0.883	10.76
$\lambda = 1$	1.09	0.0087	0.929	0.965	1.30	0.0151	0.845	1.289
$\overline{T} = 8.99$	13.51	0.288	0.940	37.00	10.12	0.212	0.841	27.64
$\phi = 5$, 10% censoring								
$\mu = 1$	1.0086	0.00252	0.924	0.294	1.0100	0.00311	0.878	0.318
$\lambda = 5$	5.43	0.0457	0.938	4.876	5.98	0.0646	0.874	5.740
$\overline{T} = 0.382$	0.388	0.00332	0.995	0.774	0.373	0.00351	0.983	0.704
$\phi = 5$, 40% censoring								
$\mu = 1$	1.0083	0.00294	0.924	0.347	1.0061	0.00387	0.854	0.374
$\lambda = 5$	5.55	0.0539	0.906	5.510	6.35	0.0834	0.843	6.651
$\overline{T} = 0.413$	0.420	0.00410	0.946	0.558	0.406	0.00464	0.861	0.491

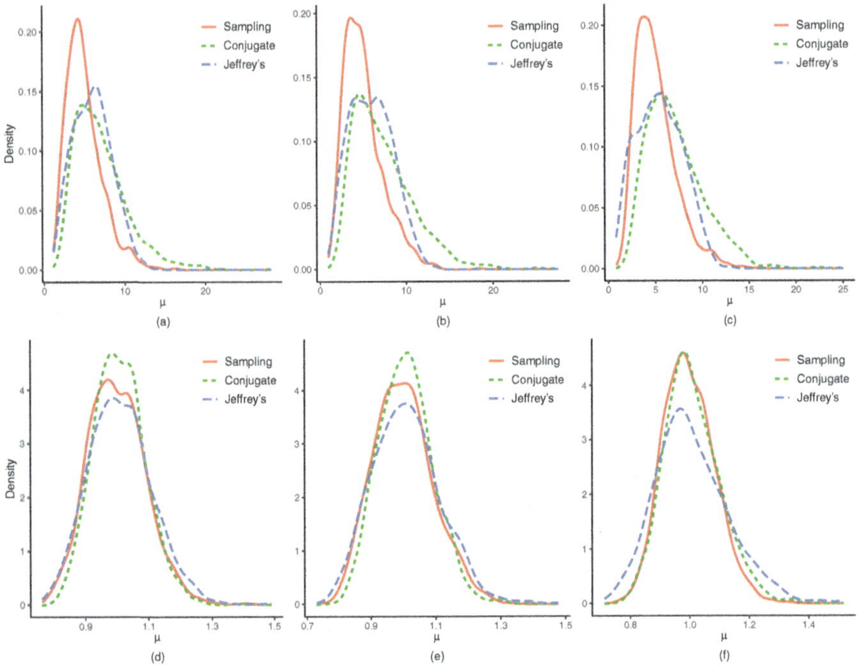

Fig. 4 Kernel Density Plots for μ at different censoring levels. Top panel: $\phi = 0.2$, at 10% censoring (**a**), 20% censoring (**b**), and 40% censoring (**c**). Bottom panel: $\phi = 5$, at 10% censoring (**d**), 20% censoring (**e**), and 40% censoring (**f**)

and smaller intervals than Jeffrey's prior. The performance of estimated $\overline{T}$ is very comparable for both the priors and different censoring levels, certainly when $\phi = 5$.

Figure 4a–c show density curves of μ for the highly skewed ($\phi = 0.2$) cases. Here, both posteriors provide similar curves but are shifted to the right from the sampling distribution. For the density curves of the symmetric cases (Fig. 4d–f), the posterior curves more closely match the shape of the sampling distribution. In general, the density curves show that the level of censoring hardly affects the posterior distributions. Figure 5 shows the density curves of the shape parameter λ. While the natural conjugate prior results in lighter tails for all cases, the two priors differ in how well each approximates the true sampling distributions. Jeffrey's prior appears to better approximate the true sampling distributions in skewed cases while the conjugate prior appears to perform better in the more symmetric cases. However, the higher level of censoring seems to affect the performance of the Jeffrey's prior negatively for λ estimates, as seen in the progressively shorter peaks for each level of censoring in Fig. 5d–f.

Of the three estimates, $\overline{T}$ has the least consistent results in terms of coverage probabilities, particularly in the more symmetric cases. In these cases, the kernel density estimates in Fig. 6 show that both priors behave similarly but in lower censoring cases (Fig. 6d and e) the curves have highly peaked densities than the true

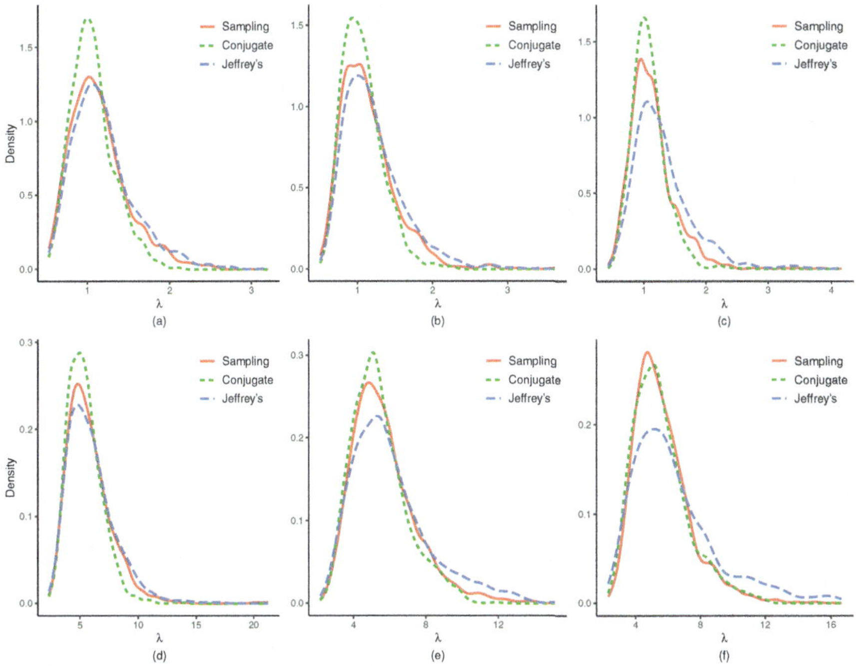

Fig. 5 Kernel Density Plots for λ at different censoring levels. Top panel: $\phi = 0.2$, at 10% censoring (**a**), 20% censoring (**b**), and 40% censoring (**c**). Bottom panel: $\phi = 5$, at 10% censoring (**d**), 20% censoring (**e**), and 40% censoring (**f**)

sampling distributions. However, the sampling distribution is comparatively much more peaked than the two Bayesian posterior in the skewed ($\phi = 0.2$) cases. In the higher skewness cases, Jeffrey's prior provides estimates that are closer to the true value and contain shorter intervals. While the kernel density curves for these cases are nearly identical for the high dense regions, the heavier tails can be noticed for the conjugate prior, which would translate to a larger average interval width.

4 Illustrative Example

For illustration, the Gibbs sampler was employed with the deep-groove ball bearing data originally reported by Lieblein and Zelen [12] and used by Ismail and Auda [9] and Jayalath and Chhikara [10]. The data given below provides the number of revolutions in millions prior to failure.

17.88	28.92	33.00	41.52	42.12	45.60	48.48	51.84	51.96	54.12	55.56	67.80
68.64	68.64	68.88	84.12	93.12	98.64	105.12	105.84	127.92	128.04	173.40	

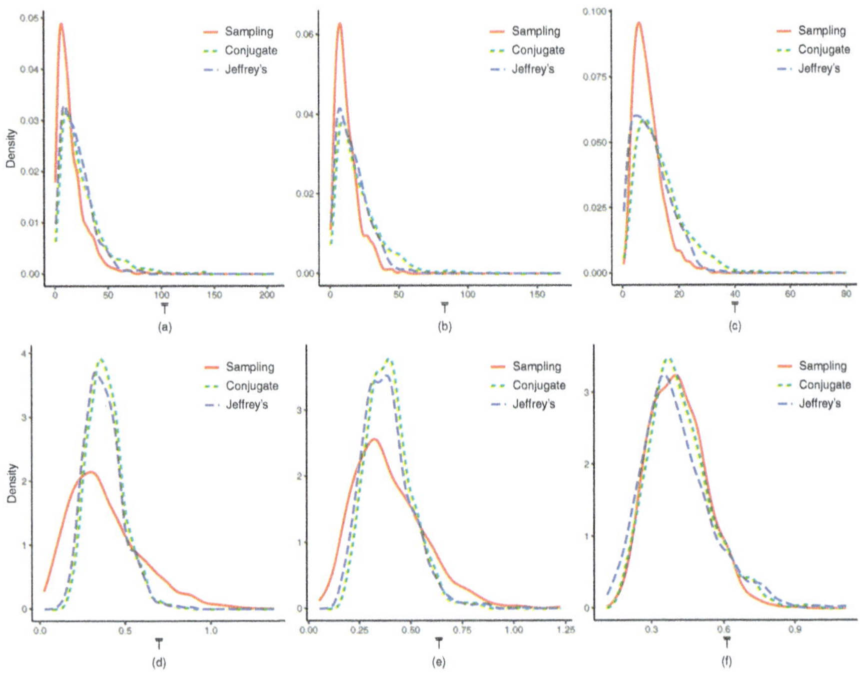

Fig. 6 Kernel Density Plots for $\overline{T}$ at different censoring levels. Top panel: $\phi = 0.2$, at 10% censoring (**a**), 20% censoring (**b**), and 40% censoring (**c**). Bottom panel: $\phi = 5$, at 10% censoring (**d**), 20% censoring (**e**), and 40% censoring (**f**)

The MLE values of μ and λ are 72.21 and 231.68, respectively, and thus $\hat{\phi} = 3.208$ and therefore the distribution is not heavily skewed. Due to a lack of information about the process parameters, a bootstrap approach was used to set the natural conjugate hyperparameters. Specifically, the natural conjugate hyperparameters β' and α' were obtained using the MLE's of μ and λ, respectively, from 10,000 bootstrap samples of the complete data. In order to verify the robustness of the selection of hyperparameters, the sample mean and all three quartiles of both the bootstrap distributions were used to set the hyperparameters. The resulting values of α' and β' are shown in Table 3. In all the cases, the weighting parameter n' was kept at 5.

The algorithm was applied at three different censoring levels, corresponding roughly to 10%, 20%, and 35% censoring. The highest censoring level, which censors $n - r = 8$ observations, corresponds to that used by Ismail and Auda [9] and Jayalath and Chhikara [10] in previous applications of the Gibbs sampler to these data. Comparisons could then be made regarding the estimate, the size of the confidence interval, and consistency between different censoring levels.

The results for this data set are shown in Table 3. At all censoring levels, the estimates for μ and $\overline{T}$ are remarkably consistent, regardless of the prior or choice of hyperparameters used in estimation. And the same holds true for the intervals

Table 3 Estimates for ball bearing lifetime data

	Conjugate prior (First quartile)		Conjugate prior (Median)		Conjugate prior (Third quartile)		Conjugate prior (Mean)		Jeffrey's prior	
	$\alpha' = 1/200, \beta' = 67$		$\alpha' = 1/251, \beta' = 72$		$\alpha' = 1/321, \beta' = 77$		$\alpha' = 1/272, \beta' = 72$			
Parameter	Estimate	90% CI	Estimate	90% CI	Estimate	90% CI	Estimate	90% CI	Estimate	90% CI
Censored observations: $n - r = 3$										
μ	72.67	(59.84, 88.57)	74.15	(60.01, 95.17)	74.89	(63.05, 91.84)	73.70	(60.98, 88.97)	74.74	(60.85, 92.29)
λ	215.06	(122.07, 316.69)	228.25	(133.24, 345.23)	229.99	(131.02, 348.59)	229.65	(137.40, 351.14)	229.97	(131.36, 359.48)
$\overline{T} = 37.28$	40.91	(9.40, 97.33)	40.12	(9.69, 91.02)	43.37	(10.34, 100.99)	40.02	(10.45, 86.87)	40.40	(9.88, 91.70)
Censored observations: $n - r = 5$										
μ	75.05	(61.68, 92.60)	76.09	(62.31, 95.42)	77.68	(63.73, 97.47)	76.78	(63.45, 95.97)	77.71	(61.58, 100.86)
λ	205.29	(117.59, 312.96)	210.02	(121.70, 328.39)	213.49	(120.10, 322.20)	214.07	(119.85, 332.30)	213.24	(117.91, 335.41)
$\overline{T} = 29.42$	42.97	(14.10, 92.81)	45.63	(14.90, 97.65)	46.43	(14.65, 97.39)	46.51	(14.60, 99.13)	45.60	(16.00, 89.56)
Censored observations: $n - r = 8$										
μ	69.09	(56.54, 85.95)	70.18	(58.44, 85.55)	71.90	(58.82, 90.35)	70.22	(57.90, 87.11)	70.21	(56.82, 89.83)
λ	235.21	(132.06, 359.71)	239.84	(131.70, 374.15)	245.28	(138.11, 387.24)	249.58	(139.21, 389.34)	256.07	(138.08, 406.20)
$\overline{T} = 45.65$	35.23	(15.15, 66.81)	35.46	(15.83, 66.26)	38.44	(15.21, 72.53)	35.31	(15.11, 68.19)	34.39	(15.94, 59.94)

for these parameters. When the first quartile MLE values of the bootstrap sample are used for the hyperparameters, the shift in λ is most noticeable. As noted in Sect. 3.1 for cases 1c and 2c, when α' and β' set to be smaller than the MLE or true parameter value of the data, the effect on the estimate of λ is compounded, resulting in the observed shift. When the third quartile values are used, the estimate is much more in line with that obtained when Jeffrey's prior or the conjugate prior with hyperparameters set to the median and mean of the bootstrap sample for lower censoring levels. As illustrated with cases 1a and 2a in Sect. 3.1, this is an expected result, as overestimated hyperparameters help improve the precision of the posterior estimates, leading to a more robust result.

The results at the higher censoring levels may be compared with the vague prior results reported in [10]. For λ, the first quartile and median-based hyperparameters give results similar to those reported in their work. While the μ estimates are very similar, the $\overline{T}$ is slightly underestimated for all prior selections, including the Jeffrey's prior. This underestimation may be a result of Type-II rightly censored data with a high level of censoring.

It is also interesting to note that while a shift is observed in some parameter estimates due to the use of various prior settings, in comparison to the large shifts evident in the earlier simulations, the estimates are still reasonable, and the confidence intervals cover the MLE of the data in all cases. The relative scale of the deep-groove data provides a possible explanation for the increased robustness of this example, as the most extreme hyperparameter value represents a no more than 40% increase over the MLE of the associated parameter, compared to the halving or doubling of the true value that occurred in the cases of Sect. 3.1.

5 Concluding Remarks

When the hyperparameters were set within the neighborhood of the true values, both priors investigated provided similar estimates for the IG distribution parameters and the average remaining lifetime. Neither prior appeared to outperform the other consistently in terms of accuracy of the estimate and width of the associated confidence interval, although Jeffrey's prior tended to have slightly lower coverage probabilities when compared to a natural conjugate prior with appropriate hyperparameters, but this difference is often associated with shorter confidence intervals.

The setting of the hyperparameters for the natural conjugate prior deserves particular attention. When the hyperparameters are set outside the neighborhood of the true values, the resulting marginal posterior distributions for the parameters will shift, and the estimation of those parameters will get affected. Thus, in the absence of appropriate information, a non-informative prior such as Jeffrey's would be preferred in estimation of the inverse Gaussian parameters. That said, the estimate of average remaining lifetime estimate did appear to be relatively robust to the effects of inappropriately set hyperparameters, even when the estimates for the distribution parameters were noticeably affected. Further, if the use of an informative prior is desired, but some uncertainty remains in the setting of hyperparameters, the estimates produced by the natural conjugate prior are somewhat more stable when the hyperparameters are slightly overestimated relative to the values of μ and λ. That may be due to the fact that those overestimated hyperparameters tend to offset the right censoring effect of right skewed IG data. In this work, the role of n', the weighting hyperparameter, was not investigated in depth, but the mathematical derivation would indicate that as uncertainty around the values of α' and β' increases, the value of n' should be decreased, thereby limiting the influence of poorly set hyperparameters on the posterior estimates.

Acknowledgments The authors thank the anonymous referees and the editor for their constructive and very useful comments and suggestions on an earlier manuscript which led to a substantial improvement.

References

1. Achcar, J.A., Bolfarine, H., Rodrigues, J.: Inverse Gaussian distribution: a Bayesian approach. Braz. J. Probab. Stat. **5**(1), 81–93 (1991)
2. Ahmad, K.E., Jaheen, Z.F. Approximate Bayes estimators applied to the inverse Gaussian lifetime model. Comput. Math. Appl. **29**(12), 39–47 (1995)
3. Banerjee, A.K., Bhattacharyya, G.K.: Bayesian results for the inverse Gaussian distribution with an application. Technometrics **21**(2), 247–251 (1979)
4. Betrò, B., Rotondi, R.: On Bayesian inference for the inverse Gaussian distribution. Stat. Probab. Lett. **11**(3), 219–224 (1991)
5. Brooks, S.P., Gelman, A.: General methods for monitoring convergence of iterative simulations. J. Comput. Graph. Stat. **7**(4), 434–455 (1998)
6. Chhikara, R.S., Folks, J.L.: The Inverse Gaussian Distribution: Theory, Methodology, and Applications. Taylor & Francis (1989)
7. Delignette-Muller, M.L., Dutang, C., et al.: fitdistrplus: an R package for fitting distributions. J. Stat. Softw. **64**(4), 1–34 (2015)
8. Gelman, A., Stern, H.S., Carlin, J.B., Dunson, D.B., Vehtari, A., Rubin, D.B.: Bayesian Data Analysis. Chapman and Hall/CRC (2013)
9. Ismail, S.A., Auda, H.A.: Bayesian and fiducial inference for the inverse Gaussian distribution via Gibbs sampler. J. Appl. Stat. **33**(8), 787–805 (2006)
10. Jayalath, K.P., Chhikara, R.S.: Survival analysis for the inverse Gaussian distribution with the Gibbs sampler. J. Appl. Stat. 1–20 (2020)
11. Kadane, J.B., Tierney, L.: Accurate approximations for posterior moments and marginal densities. J. Am. Stat. Assoc. **81**(393), 82–86 (1986)
12. Lieblein, J., Zelen, M.: Statistical investigation of the fatigue life of deep-groove ball bearings. J. Res. Nat. Bur. Stand. **57**(5), 273–316 (1956)
13. Lindley, D.V.: Approximate Bayesian methods. Trabajos de Estadistica Y de Investigacion Operativa **31**, 223–245 (1980)
14. Padgett, W.J.: Bayes estimation of reliability for the inverse Gaussian model. IEEE Trans. Reliab. **R-30**(4), 384–385 (1981)
15. Palmer, J.M.: Certain Non-Classical Inference Procedures Applied at the Inverse Gaussian Distribution. Ph.D. Thesis, Oklahoma State University (1973)
16. Schrödinger, E.: Zur theorie der fall-und steigversuche an teilchen mit brownscher bewegung. Phys. Z. **16**, 289–295 (1915)

17. Seshadri, V.: The Inverse Gaussian Distribution: Statistical Theory and Applications, vol. 137. Springer, Berlin (2012)
18. Tweedie, M.: Statistical properties of inverse Gaussian distributions. I. Ann. Math. Stat. **28**(2), 362–377 (1957)
19. Tweedie, M.C.: Inverse statistical variates. Nature **155**(3937), 453–453 (1945)

Bayesian Inferences for Panel Count Data and Interval-Censored Data with Nonparametric Modeling of the Baseline Functions

Lu Wang, Lianming Wang, and Xiaoyan Lin

Abstract Both panel count data and interval-censored data arise commonly in real-life studies when subjects are examined at periodic follow-ups. Interval-censored data are studied when the exact times of the events are of interest and these exact times are not directly observed but are only known to fall within some intervals formed by the observation times. Panel count data are under investigation when the exact times of the recurrent events are not of interest but the counts of the recurrent events occurring within the time intervals are available and of interest. A novel unified Bayesian approach is developed for analyzing panel count data under the Gamma frailty Poisson process model and interval-censored data under Cox's proportional hazards model and the proportional odds model. The baseline functions in these models share the same property of being nondecreasing positive functions and are modeled nonparametrically by assigning a Gamma process prior. Efficient Gibbs samplers are developed for the posterior computation under these three models for the two types of data. The proposed methods are evaluated in a simulation study and illustrated by three real-life data applications.

1 Introduction

Panel count data frequently occur in epidemiological and social-behavioral studies. In such studies, subjects experience multiple recurrences of an event of interest such as smoking or infections, but they are monitored or observed only at finite discrete time points instead of continuously. A consequence of such designs is that the exact occurrence times of the events are not observed and only the numbers of the

---

L. Wang
Department of Mathematics, Western New England University, Springfield, MA, USA
e-mail: lu.wang@wne.edu

L. Wang (✉) · X. Lin
Department of Statistics, University of South Carolina, Columbia, SC, USA
e-mail: wangl@stat.sc.edu; lin@stat.sc.edu

Y. Lio et al. (eds.), *Bayesian Inference and Computation in Reliability and Survival Analysis*, Emerging Topics in Statistics and Biostatistics,
https://doi.org/10.1007/978-3-030-88658-5_14

occurrences of the events within the time windows are available, which leads to the panel count data structure. The primary interests for panel count data are to estimate the mean function of the counting process and/or the covariate effects on the counts. Sun and Kalbfleisch [28] first studied nonparametric estimation of the mean function of panel count data and adopted the isotonic regression technique to estimate the mean function. Wellner and Zhang [34] investigated two likelihood methods based on a non-homogeneous Poisson process without considering covariates and showed that their methods are robust to the misspecification of the Poisson process [34, 35]. To account for overdispersion and the within-subject correlation, Zhang and Jamshidian [41] and Yao et al. [38] introduced gamma frailty Poisson process model and developed EM algorithms for their estimation. It is observed that the estimation methods based on the gamma frailty Poisson models are also quite robust to misspecification of the gamma frailty distribution [14, 37].

In many situations, the event of interest is not recurrent for a subject, such as death or HIV infection. In such cases, the resulting counting process becomes a 0-1 process and the panel count data reduce to interval-censored survival data [34]. Among all of the survival models, Cox's proportional hazards (PH) model [4] is unquestionably the most popular and widely used semiparametric regression model in the literature. It specifies that covariates have a multiplicative effect on the hazard function of the failure time of interest. Many approaches have been developed for the regression analysis of interval-censored data under the PH model. For example, Finkelstein [7] proposed a Newton–Raphson algorithm to fit the model, Satten [23] proposed a marginal likelihood approach, Goggins et al. [9] developed a Monte Carlo EM algorithm, Satten et al. [23] proposed estimating equations, Pan [22] proposed a generalized gradient projection method, Pan [21] developed a multiple imputation method, Cai and Betensky [3] developed a penalized likelihood approach, Zhang et al. [40] proposed a sieve maximum likelihood method, Sinha et al. [27] proposed a Bayesian method by modeling the baseline hazard function with a piecewise constant function, and Wang et al. [29] developed a computational efficient EM algorithm. Yi et al. [39] considered time-dependent covariates in the model and proposed a MCEM algorithm for the estimation. Zhong [42] proposed a maximum approximate Bernstein likelihood estimation of the baseline density function and the regression coefficients.

Besides Cox's model, the semiparametric proportional odds (PO) model is another popular survival model, which specifies that covariates have a multiplicative effect on the unspecified baseline odds function. Unlike the PH model, the ratio of the hazard functions converges to unity as time increases under the PO model. This model is closely related to logistic regression model for binary data with time varying intercept. Each regression parameter in the PO model can be interpreted as the log odds ratio of the failure event due to 1 unit increase in the corresponding covariate when keeping all other covariates at fixed values. In contrast to the flourishing work on the PH model, the research on the PO model is quite limited, especially for interval-censored data. For general interval-censored data using the PO model, Huang and Rossini [15] proposed a sieve maximum likelihood estimator, Shen [24] used monotone splines with variable orders and knots for approximating the baseline odds function and proposed a sieve maximum likelihood estimator, Wang and Lin [31] proposed a Bayesian approach based on the work of Lin and Wang [18] utilizing the relationship between the PO model and the probit model, and Wang et al. [32] further proposed two new simpler Bayesian computational algorithms based on the relationships between the standard logistic distribution and the normal distributions.

In all these three semiparametric models, the baseline functions, more specifically the baseline mean function in the Gamma frailty Poisson model for panel count data and the baseline cumulative hazards function in the PH model and the baseline odds function in the PO model for interval-censored data, are all unspecified nondecreasing functions taking zero at the initial time point 0. In many existing approaches, they are approximated by linear combinations of spline functions [12, 13, 38] or by a step-function with fixed jump sizes at every observation time points [43]. Different from previous researches, we treat these baseline functions as random from a Bayesian perspective and assign them a Gamma process prior. The Gamma process can be thought of as arising from a compound Poisson process of gamma-distributed increments in which the Poisson rate tends to infinity while the sizes of the increments tend to zero in proportion [17]. Based on the Gamma process prior for the baseline functions, we develop new Bayesian estimation methods for analyzing both panel count data and interval-censored survival data.

Using a Gamma process to model nondecreasing functions is not uncommon in the literature. For example, Kalbfleisch [16] used the Gamma process to model the cumulative hazard function under the PH model for right-censored data. Ferguson and Phadia [6] used the processes neutral to the right as prior distributions for the unknown cumulative distribution function (CDF) F and provided theoretic justification of their estimation of F for right-censored data. However, as mentioned in Wellner and Zhang [36], most of those methods are limited to special cases where all subjects have the same number of observation times. For example, Groeneboom and Wellner [10] and Huang [14] developed methods for cases when each subject is only observed once or twice. The proposed method solves this problem by creating a fine partition of the time space and defining a Gamma process on these intervals. The proposed approach allows individuals to have different numbers of observation times and even different observation schemes. It can also accommodate missing observation points, which are common in real-life studies.

The organization of the rest of this chapter is as follows. Section 2 provides detailed description of the data, models, and the observed likelihoods. Section 3 proposes to model the baseline functions under the considered models nonparametrically through a Gamma process. Section 4 introduces a novel data augmentation that is essential for the posterior computation under the three considered models. Section 5 presents the proposed Gibbs samplers for both panel count data and interval-censored data, respectively. Section 6 evaluates the performance of proposed Bayesian approach for analyzing the two types of data through a simulation study. Section 7 provides illustrations of the proposed methods via three real-life data applications. Section 8 gives some concluding remarks and discussions.

2 Models and the Observed Likelihoods

2.1 Gamma Frailty Poisson Process for Panel Count Data

Suppose that there are n independent subjects in a study. For subject i, the counting process of the recurrent event of interest $N_i(t)$ is only observed at discrete examination time points $\{t_{ij}, j = 1, ..., J_i\}$, where J_i is the total number of examination time points for subject i. Conditioning on an unobserved frailty ϕ_i, we assume a non-homogeneous Poisson process for $N_i(t)$ with the following conditional mean function:

$$E(N_i(t)|\phi_i) = \mu_0(t)\exp(\mathbf{x}_i'\boldsymbol{\beta})\phi_i,$$

where $\mu_0(t)$ is an unspecified nondecreasing baseline mean function with $\mu_0(0) = 0$, $\mathbf{x}_i$ is a $p \times 1$ vector of time-independent covariates, and $\phi_i \sim \mathcal{G}a(v, v)$ is a frailty with mean 1 and variance v^{-1}. The purpose of introducing the unobserved frailty ϕ_i is to account for the within-subject correlation between the counts for subject i. Even though the above proposed model is conditional on the frailty, μ_0 here can be still interpreted as the marginal baseline mean function since $E\{N_i(t)\} = E[E\{N_i(t)|\phi_i\}] = E\{\mu_0(t)\phi_i\} = \mu_0(t)$ when $\mathbf{x} = 0$. For the same reason, $\exp(\beta_j)$ also has a marginal interpretation and can be interpreted as the multiplicative effect on the mean function due to 1 unit increase in the jth covariate while keeping all other covariates at fixed values.

Define $Z_{ij} = N_i(t_{ij}) - N_i(t_{ij-1})$, the count of recurrent events within time interval $(t_{ij-1}, t_{ij}]$, the properties of the non-homogeneous Poisson process guarantee that Z_{ij}'s are conditionally independent Poisson random variables given ϕ_i and

$$Z_{ij}|\phi_i \sim \text{Poisson}\Big[\{\mu_0(t_{ij}) - \mu_0(t_{ij-1})\}\exp(\mathbf{x}_i'\boldsymbol{\beta})\phi_i\Big]$$

for $j = 1, \cdots, J_i$ and $i = 1, \cdots, n$. Under the assumption that the observational process and the recurrent event process are conditionally independent given the time-independent covariates, the observed data likelihood takes the form

$$L_{obs} = \prod_{i=1}^{n} \int g(\phi_i|v) \prod_{j=1}^{J_i} \mathcal{P}(Z_{ij}|\mu_{ij}) d\phi_i,$$

where $g(.|v)$ is the probability density function (PDF) of $\mathcal{G}a(v, v)$ and $\mathcal{P}(.|\mu_{ij})$ is the probability mass function of the Poisson distribution with mean equal to $\mu_{ij} = \{\mu_0(t_{ij}) - \mu_0(t_{ij-1})\}\exp(\mathbf{x}_i'\boldsymbol{\beta})\phi_i$. A similar stochastic model was proposed by Sinha [26], which assumes that all the subjects are examined at the same set of time points.

2.2 The PH and PO Models for General Interval-Censored Data

We consider the PH and PO models for general interval-censored data in this subsection. Let T_i denote the survival time of interest and $\mathbf{x}_i$ a $p \times 1$ vector of potential covariates for subject i, for $i = 1, \cdots, n$. Due to the study design of examining subjects periodically, T_i is not exactly observed but is known to fall within some observed interval $(L_i, R_i]$, with $0 \leq L_i < R_i \leq \infty$ for $i = 1, \cdots, n$. This general interval $(L_i, R_i]$ yields a left-censored observation when $0 = L_i < R_i < \infty$, a strictly interval-censored observation when $0 < L_i < R_i < \infty$, and a right-censored observation when $0 < L_i < R_i = \infty$. Under the assumption that the failure time and the observation process are independent conditional on the covariates, the observed data likelihood takes the form

$$L_{obs} = \prod_{i=1}^{n} \{1 - S(R_i|\mathbf{x}_i)\}^{\delta_{i1}} \{S(L_i|\mathbf{x}_i) - S(R_i|\mathbf{x}_i)\}^{\delta_{i2}} S(L_i|\mathbf{x}_i)^{\delta_{i3}}, \tag{1}$$

where $S(.|\mathbf{x})$ is the survival function of the failure time given covariate $\mathbf{x}$, and δ_{i1}, δ_{i2}, and δ_{i3} are binary censoring indicators for left-censored, interval-censored, and right-censored observations, respectively, with the constraint $\delta_{i1} + \delta_{i2} + \delta_{i3} = 1$ for each i.

The survival function $S(t|\mathbf{x})$ takes the form $S(t|\mathbf{x}) = \exp\{-\mu_0(t)\exp(\mathbf{x}'\boldsymbol{\beta})\}$ under the PH model and $S(t|\mathbf{x}) = \{1 + \mu_0(t)\exp(\mathbf{x}'\boldsymbol{\beta})\}^{-1}$ under the PO model, where $\mu_0(\cdot)$ can be interpreted as the baseline cumulative hazard function and the baseline odds function under the PH and PO models, respectively.

It is known that the survival function in the PO model can be rewritten as the marginal survival function of the frailty PH model with the frailty following a $\mathcal{G}a(1, 1)$ distribution, i.e.,

$$S(t|\mathbf{x}) = \{1 + \mu_0(t)\exp(\mathbf{x}'\boldsymbol{\beta})\}^{-1} = \int_0^{\infty} \exp\{-\mu_0(t)\exp(\mathbf{x}'\boldsymbol{\beta})\phi\}\exp(-\phi)d\phi.$$

This fact suggests that we can rewrite the observed likelihood (1) under the PH and PO models as the following unified form:

$$L_{obs} = \prod_{i=1}^{n} \int_0^{\infty} [1 - S(R_i|\mathbf{x}_i, \phi_i)]^{\delta_{i1}} [S(L_i|\mathbf{x}_i, \phi_i) \\ - S(R_i|\mathbf{x}_i, \phi_i)]^{\delta_{i2}} S(L_i|\mathbf{x}_i, \phi_i)^{\delta_{i3}} g(\phi_i) d\phi_i,$$

where $S(t|\mathbf{x}, \phi) = \exp\{-\mu_0(t)\exp(\mathbf{x}'\boldsymbol{\beta})\phi\}$ is the conditional survival function of the failure time given covariate $\mathbf{x}$ and frailty ϕ, ϕ_i's are i.i.d. frailties with a density function g, and g takes degenerated Point mass distribution at 1 for the PH model and $\mathcal{G}a(1, 1)$ for the PO model.

3 Modeling the Baseline Functions Nonparametrically

The baseline mean function in the Poisson process model, the baseline cumulative hazard function in the PH model, and the baseline odds function in the PO model are all unspecified nondecreasing functions taking 0 at time 0. We model these unknown functions μ_0 nonparametrically here by assigning them a Gamma process prior.

Gamma process is a Lévy process with gamma-distributed increments. It has been extensively studied and applied in various studies since its introduction by Doksum [5] as one of the processes neutral to the right. For example, Nozer [20] used a Gamma process to model the hazard rate process in a dynamic environment; Lawless and Crowder [17] extended the Gamma process model by incorporating random effect to explore its use as a degradation model; Wang [33] introduced a nonparametric estimation of the shape function in the Gamma process for degradation data; Sinha et al. [25] assumes the wear process is a Gamma process and developed a Bayesian analysis of a stochastic wear process model to fit survival data that might have a large number of ties, etc.

Specifically, we assign a Gamma process prior $\mathcal{GP}(H_0, \eta)$ for μ_0, where H_0 is the expected function of μ_0 and η quantifies the uncertainty level of this guess. The larger value of η, the closer μ_0 is to H_0. This prior implies the following two facts. First, for any $t > 0$, $\mu_0(t)$ is a random variable and has a Gamma distribution $\mathcal{G}a(\eta H_0(t), \eta)$. Second, the increments in non-overlapping time intervals are independent of each other. That is, $\mu_0(t+s)-\mu_0(t)$ is independent of $\mu_0(t)$ and

$$\mu_0(t+s) - \mu_0(t) \sim \mathcal{G}a(\eta\{H_0(t+s) - H_0(t)\}, \eta)$$

for any $t > 0$ and $s > 0$.

Now consider a fine partition of the time space based on the observed times, i.e., all t_{ij}'s for panel count data and all L_i's and R_i's for interval-censored data. Basically, they are intervals over the time line upon which any observed interval can be written as a union of some of these partitioned intervals. For panel count data, let k_{ij} denote the position of t_{ij} in the set of $\{s_0, \cdots, s_M\}$ for each i and j. It is easy to see that $t_{ij} = s_{k_{ij}}$ and the interval $(t_{ij-1}, t_{ij}]$ can be written as a finite union of some partition intervals $(t_{ij-1}, t_{ij}] = \bigcup_{l=0}^{k_{ij}-k_{ij-1}-1} (s_{k_{ij-1}+l}, s_{k_{ij-1}+l+1}]$. For interval-censored data, define k_{i1} and k_{i2} to be the positions of L_i and R_i in the set of $\{s_0, \cdots, s_M\}$ for each i. Then the observed interval $(L_i, R_i]$ can be rewritten as $\bigcup_{l=0}^{k_{i2}-k_{i1}-1} (s_{k_{i1}+l}, s_{k_{i2}+l+1}]$ for each i.

Define $\lambda_m = \mu_0(s_m) - \mu_0(s_{m-1})$ as the increment of the baseline mean function for panel count data and the baseline cumulative hazard or odds function for interval-censored data on interval $(s_{m-1}, s_m]$, for $m = 1, \cdots, M$. It is known that λ_m follows a Gamma distribution $\mathcal{G}a(\{H_0(s_m) - H_0(s_{m-1}\}\eta, \eta)$. Since the Gamma process is robust to the choice of H_0, we can simply choose $H_0(t) = at$. Note that the linear function of H_0 does not imply that μ_0 is necessarily a linear function. For panel count data, the increment of baseline mean function for subject i in the jth time interval is $\mu_0(t_{ij}) - \mu_0(t_{ij-1}) = \sum_{l=1}^{k_{ij}-k_{ij-1}} \lambda_{k_{ij-1}+l}$. So the conditional likelihood after incorporating the Gamma process for μ_0 for panel count data can be written as

$$
\begin{aligned}
L_{PC1} \propto \Big(\prod_{i=1}^{n}\Big[\prod_{j=1}^{J_i}\Big(\sum_{l=1}^{k_{ij}-k_{ij-1}} \lambda_{k_{ij-1}+l}\Big)^{Z_{ij}} e^{\mathbf{x}_i'\boldsymbol{\beta} Z_{ij}} \phi_i^{Z_{ij}} \\
\times \exp\Big\{-\Big(\sum_{l=1}^{k_{ij}-k_{ij-1}} \lambda_{k_{ij-1}+l}\Big)e^{\mathbf{x}_i'\boldsymbol{\beta}}\phi_i\Big\}\Big] \qquad (2) \\
\times g(\phi_i|v)\Big)\prod_{m=1}^{M} g\{\lambda_m|a(s_m - s_{m-1})\eta, \eta\}.
\end{aligned}
$$

For interval-censored data, subject i only has one observed interval $(L_i, R_i]$, and the increment of the cumulative baseline hazard or the baseline odds function on this observed interval is $\mu_0(R_i) - \mu_0(L_i) = \sum_{m=k_{i1}+1}^{k_{i2}} \lambda_m$. Thus, the conditional likelihood functions given the frailties ϕ_i's under PH and PO models after incorporating the Gamma process prior for μ_0 take the form

$$
\begin{aligned}
L_{IC1} \propto \Big(\prod_{i=1}^{n}\Big[1 - \exp\Big\{-\Big(\sum_{m=1}^{k_{i2}} \lambda_m\Big)\exp(\mathbf{x}_i'\boldsymbol{\beta})\phi_i\Big\}\Big]^{\delta_{i1}} \\
\times \Big[\exp\Big\{-\Big(\sum_{m=1}^{k_{i1}} \lambda_m\Big)\exp(\mathbf{x}_i'\boldsymbol{\beta})\phi_i\Big\}\Big]^{\delta_{i3}} \\
\times \Big[\exp\Big\{-\Big(\sum_{m=1}^{k_{i1}} \lambda_m\Big)\exp(\mathbf{x}_i'\boldsymbol{\beta})\phi_i\Big\} \qquad (3) \\
- \exp\Big\{-\Big(\sum_{m=1}^{k_{i2}} \lambda_m\Big)\exp(\mathbf{x}_i'\boldsymbol{\beta})\phi_i\Big\}\Big]^{\delta_{i2}} \exp(-\phi_i)\Big) \\
\times \prod_{m=1}^{M} g\{\lambda_m|a(s_m - s_{m-1})\eta, \eta\}.
\end{aligned}
$$

4 Data Augmentation

4.1 For Panel Count Data

The summation of λ_m's inside the product of the L_{pc1} in (2) brings much trouble in Bayesian posterior computation. To solve this problem, we transform the summation into a multiplication by introducing multinomial latent variables. This idea is based on the fact that for $(u_1, \ldots, u_K) \sim \text{Multinomial}\{1, (\frac{1}{K}, \ldots, \frac{1}{K})\}$, integrating the product term $\prod_{l=1}^{K}[\lambda_l]^{u_l}$ with respect to $(u_1, \ldots, u_K)$ leads to $\sum_{l=1}^{K} \lambda_l$. Specifically, for $i = 1, \ldots, n$ and $j = 1, \ldots, J_i$, we introduce $\mathbf{u}_{ij} = (u_{ij1}, \cdots, u_{ijn_{ij}}) \sim \text{Multinomial}\{1, (\frac{1}{n_{ij}}, \ldots, \frac{1}{n_{ij}})\}$, where $n_{ij} = k_{ij} - k_{ij-1}$. The augmented likelihood function has the following simple multiplication form:

$$L_{PCC} \propto \Big(\prod_{i=1}^{n}\Big[\prod_{j=1}^{J_i}\Big(\prod_{l=1}^{k_{ij}-k_{ij-1}} \lambda_{k_{ij-1}+l}^{u_{ijl}}\Big)^{Z_{ij}} e^{\mathbf{x}_i'\boldsymbol{\beta} z_{ij}} \phi_i^{Z_{ij}} \times \exp\Big\{-\Big(\sum_{l=1}^{k_{ij}-k_{ij-1}} \lambda_{k_{ij-1}+l}\Big) e^{\mathbf{x}_i'\boldsymbol{\beta}} \phi_i\Big\}\Big] \times g(\phi_i|\upsilon)\Big) \prod_{m=1}^{M} g\{\lambda_m | a(s_m - s_{m-1})\eta, \eta\}. \tag{4}$$

This augmented data likelihood is the product of Poisson probability mass functions multiplied by the gamma densities of the frailties and the increments of the baseline mean function μ_0. We will treat this augmented likelihood as the complete data likelihood, based on which a Gibbs sampler is to be developed. Note that integrating out the latent variables u_{ijk}'s in the augmented likelihood in (4) leads to the conditional likelihood in (2).

4.2 For Interval-Censored Data

The data augmentation below is based on the connection between the PH and a latent non-homogeneous Poisson process as in Lin et al. [19] and Wang et al. [29]. Let $N_i(t)$ denote a latent non-homogeneous Poisson process with the following conditional cumulative intensity function: $\mu_0(t)\exp(\mathbf{x}_i'\boldsymbol{\beta})\phi_i$ for subject i given frailty ϕ_i, and let T_i denote the time of the first jump of the counting process, i.e., $T_i = \inf\{t : N_i(t) > 0\}$ for each i. Then it is clear that the conditional probability that the first jump has not happened yet at time t is

$$P(T_i > t\,|\phi_i) = P(N_i(t) = 0\,|\phi_i) = \exp\{-\mu_0(t)\exp(\mathbf{x}_i'\boldsymbol{\beta})\phi_i\},$$

which suggests that T_i has a frailty PH model with frailty ϕ_i for each i.

Define $o_{i1} = R_i I(\delta_{i1} = 1) + L_i I(\delta_{i2} = 1)$ and $o_{i2} = R_i I(\delta_{i2} = 1) + L_i I(\delta_{i3} = 1)$ for each i. Let $Z_i = N(o_{i1})$ and $W_i = N(o_{i2}) - N(o_{i1})$ depending on the availability of o_{i1} and o_{i2} from the observed interval $(L_i, R_i]$ for each i. Based on the properties of Poisson process, one has

$$Z_i \sim \text{Poisson}(\mu_0(o_{i1})\exp(\mathbf{x}_i'\boldsymbol{\beta})\phi_i)$$

and

$$W_i \sim \text{Poisson}(\{\mu_0(o_{i2}) - \mu_0(o_{i1})\} \exp(\mathbf{x}_i' \boldsymbol{\beta})\phi_i).$$

Conditional on the latent variables Z_i's, W_i's, and ϕ_i's, the augmented data likelihood is

$$\begin{aligned}
L_{IC2} = &\Bigg(\prod_{i=1}^{n} \mathcal{P}(Z_i | \mu_0(o_{i1}) \exp(\mathbf{x}_i' \boldsymbol{\beta})\phi_i) [\mathcal{P}(W_i | \{\mu_0(o_{i2}) \\
&- \mu_0(o_{i1})\} \exp(\mathbf{x}_i' \boldsymbol{\beta})\phi_i)]^{\delta_{i2}+\delta_{i3}} \\
&\times \exp(-\phi_i) \Bigg) \prod_{m=1}^{M} g\{\lambda_m | a(s_m - s_{m-1})\eta, \eta\} \\
\propto &\Bigg(\prod_{i=1}^{n} \Big\{ \Big(\sum_{m=1}^{k_{i1}} \lambda_m \Big) e^{\mathbf{x}_i' \boldsymbol{\beta}} \phi_i \Big\}^{Z_i} \exp\Big\{ - \Big(\sum_{l=1}^{k_{i1}} \lambda_m \Big) e^{\mathbf{x}_i' \boldsymbol{\beta}} \phi_i \Big\} \\
&\times \Big\{ \Big(\sum_{m=k_{i1}+1}^{k_{i2}} \lambda_m \Big) e^{\mathbf{x}_i' \boldsymbol{\beta}} \phi_i \Big\}^{W_i(\delta_{i2}+\delta_{i3})} \\
&\times \exp\Big\{ - \Big(\sum_{m=k_{i1}+1}^{k_{i2}} \lambda_m \Big) e^{\mathbf{x}_i' \boldsymbol{\beta}} \phi_i (\delta_{i2} + \delta_{i3}) \Big\} \exp(-\phi_i) \Bigg) \\
&\times \prod_{m=1}^{M} g\{\lambda_m | a(s_m - s_{m-1})\eta, \eta\}
\end{aligned}$$

subject to the following constraints $Z_i > 0$ when $\delta_{i1} = 1$, $Z_i = 0$ and $W_i > 0$ when $\delta_{i2} = 1$, and $Z_i = W_i = 0$ when $\delta_{i3} = 1$. Here $\mathcal{P}(\cdot|\gamma)$ denote the Poisson probability mass function with the mean parameter γ. Integrating out the Z_i's and W_i's in L_{IC2} leads to the conditional likelihood L_{IC1} in (3).

Taking advantage of the fact that the sum of independent Poisson random variables is still a Poisson random variable, we decompose both Z_i and W_i as a sum of k_{i1} and $k_{i2} - k_{i1}$ conditionally independent Poisson random variables given ϕ_i as follows:

$$Z_{im} \sim \text{Poisson}(\lambda_m \exp(\mathbf{x}_i' \boldsymbol{\beta})\phi_i), \ \text{for } m = 1, \ldots, k_{i1},$$

and

$$W_{im} \sim \text{Poisson}(\lambda_m \exp(\mathbf{x}_i' \boldsymbol{\beta})\phi_i) \text{ for } m = k_{i1} + 1, \ldots, k_{i2},$$

where $\sum_{m=1}^{k_{i1}} Z_{im} = Z_i$ and $\sum_{m=k_{i1}+1}^{k_{i2}} W_{im} = W_i$ for each i. Conditional on the latent variables Z_{im}'s, W_{im}'s, and ϕ_i's, the augmented data likelihood takes the following form:

$$
\begin{aligned}
L_{ICC} \propto & \Bigg(\prod_{i=1}^{n} \Big[\prod_{m=1}^{k_{i1}} \{\lambda_m \exp(\mathbf{x}_i'\beta)\phi_i\}^{Z_{im}} \exp\{-\lambda_m \exp(\mathbf{x}_i'\boldsymbol{\beta})\phi_i\} \Big] \exp(-\phi_i) \\
& \times \Big[\prod_{m=k_{i1}+1}^{k_{i2}} \{\lambda_m \exp(\mathbf{x}_i'\boldsymbol{\beta})\phi_i\}^{W_{im}\delta_{i2}} \exp\{-\lambda_m \exp(\mathbf{x}_i'\boldsymbol{\beta})\phi_i(\delta_{i2}+\delta_{i3})\} \Big] \Bigg) \\
& \times \prod_{m=1}^{M} g\{\lambda_m | a(s_m - s_{m-1})\eta, \eta\}
\end{aligned} \tag{5}
$$

Integrating out the Z_{im}'s and W_{im}'s out of L_{ICC} leads to the augmented likelihood L_{IC2}. The augmented likelihood L_{ICC} has a simple form of the product of Poisson probability mass functions and Gamma densities and will be used as the complete data likelihood for our Bayesian computation for dealing with interval-censored data.

5 Bayesian Computation

5.1 Prior Specification

For the purpose of providing flexible modeling while also allowing for efficient posterior computation, we assign conventional vague priors for all of the parameters in the Bayesian approach. Specifically, we assign a multivariate normal $\mathcal{N}(\mu_0, \Sigma_0)$ prior for the regression coefficients $\boldsymbol{\beta}$, with mean vector zero and large independent variances. Practically, the very noninformative prior can balance both the skeptical and the enthusiastic views about the effects of covariates [26]. We adopt independent $\mathcal{G}a(1, 1)$ priors for v, a, and η, respectively.

5.2 Gibbs Sampler for Panel Count Data

Based on the complete data likelihood L_{PCC} in (4) and the prior specifications, we develop the following Gibbs sampler for analyzing panel count data.

1. Sample λ_m, for $m = 1, \ldots, M$, from

$$\lambda_m \sim \mathcal{G}a\left(a(s_m - s_{m-1})\eta + \sum_{A_m} u_{ijl} Z_{ij},\ \eta + \sum_{i=1}^{n} \exp(\mathbf{x}_i'\boldsymbol{\beta})\phi_i\right),$$

where $A_m = \{(i, j, l) : k_{ij-1} + l = m,\ j = 1, \cdots, J_i,\ i = 1, \ldots, n\}$.

2. For $i = 1, \ldots, n$, sample ϕ_i from

$$\mathcal{G}a\left(\sum_{j=1}^{J_i} Z_{ij} + v, \{\sum_{j=1}^{J_i} \sum_{l=1}^{k_{ij}-k_{ij-1}} \lambda_{k_{ij-1+l}} \exp(\mathbf{x}_i'\boldsymbol{\beta})\} + v\right).$$

3. Sample $(U_{ij1}, \ldots, U_{ijn_{ij}}) \sim \text{Multinomial}(1, (p_{ij1}, \ldots, p_{ijn_{ij}}))$ for $i = 1, \ldots, n$ and $j = 1, \ldots, J_i$, where

$$p_{ijl} = \frac{\lambda_{k_{ij-1}+l}}{\sum_{l=1}^{k_{ij}-k_{ij-1}} \lambda_{k_{ij-1}+l}} \qquad l = 1, \ldots, n_{ij}.$$

4. Sample $\boldsymbol{\beta}$ by using adaptive rejection metropolis sampling (ARMS) from the following full conditional distribution:

$$L(\boldsymbol{\beta}|.) \propto \exp\left[\sum_{i=1}^{n}\left\{\mathbf{x}_i'\boldsymbol{\beta}\sum_{j=1}^{J_i} Z_{ij} - (\sum_{j=1}^{J_i}\sum_{l=1}^{k_{ij}-k_{ij-1}} \lambda_{k_{ij-1}+l})\phi_i \exp(\mathbf{x}_i'\boldsymbol{\beta})\right\}\right.$$
$$\left. -(\boldsymbol{\beta} - \boldsymbol{\mu}_0)'\Sigma_0^{-1}(\boldsymbol{\beta} - \boldsymbol{\mu}_0)/2\right].$$

5. Sample v by using ARMS from the following full conditional distribution:

$$L(v|.) \propto \exp(-v)\{\frac{v^v}{\Gamma(v)}\}^n(\prod_{i=1}^{n} \phi_i)^{v-1} \exp(-v\sum_{i=1}^{n} \phi_i).$$

6. Sample a by using ARMS from the following full conditional distribution:

$$L(a|.) \propto \frac{\eta^{a\eta s_M} \exp(-a)}{\prod_{m=1}^{M} \Gamma\{a(s_m - s_{m-1})\eta\}} \prod_{m=1}^{M} \lambda_m^{a(s_m - s_{m-1})\eta - 1}.$$

7. Sample η by using ARMS from the following full conditional distribution:

$$L(\eta|.) \propto \frac{\eta^{a\eta s_M} \exp(-\eta \sum_{m=1}^{M} \lambda_m) \exp(-\eta)}{\prod_{m=1}^{M} \Gamma\{a(s_m - s_{m-1})\eta\}} \prod_{m=1}^{M} \lambda_m^{a(s_m - s_{m-1})\eta - 1}.$$

5.3 Gibbs Sampler for Interval-Censored Data

Based on the complete data likelihood L_{ICC} in (5) and the prior specifications, we develop the following Gibbs sampler for analyzing interval-censored data under the PO model. First set all $Z_i's$, $Z_{im}'s$, $W_i's$, and $W_{im}'s$ to be 0 for the initialization and then iterate the following steps.

1. Sample λ_m for $m = 1, \ldots, M$, from $\mathcal{G}a(b_m, c_m)$ with

$$b_m = \sum_i^n \{Z_{im} I(m \le k_{i1}) + W_{im}\delta_{i1} I(k_{i1} < m \le k_{i2})\} + a(s_m - s_{m-1})\eta,$$

and

$$c_m = \sum_i^n \exp(\mathbf{x}_i'\boldsymbol{\beta})\phi_i\{I(m \le k_{i1}) + I(k_{i1} < m \le k_{i2})(\delta_{i2} + \delta_{i3})\} + \eta.$$

2. For $i = 1, \ldots, n$, sample ϕ_i from

$$\mathcal{G}a\Bigg(Z_i + W_i\delta_{i2} + 1, \left\{1 + (\sum_{m=1}^{k_{i1}} \lambda_m)\delta_{i1} + (\sum_{m=1}^{k_{i2}} \lambda_m)(\delta_{i2} + \delta_{i3})\right\} \exp(\mathbf{x}_i'\boldsymbol{\beta})\Bigg).$$

3. Sample $\boldsymbol{\beta}$ by using ARMS

$$L(\boldsymbol{\beta}|.) \propto \exp\Bigg(\sum_{i=1}^{n}\Big[\{Z_i + W_i(\delta_{i2} + \delta_{i3})\}\mathbf{x}_i'\boldsymbol{\beta}$$
$$-\Big\{\Big(\sum_{m=1}^{k_{i1}} \lambda_m\Big) + \Big(\sum_{m=k_{i1}+1}^{k_{i2}} \lambda_m\Big)(\delta_{i2} + \delta_{i3})\Big\}\phi_i \exp(\mathbf{x}_i'\boldsymbol{\beta})\Big]\Bigg).$$

4. Sample $Z_i's$, $Z_{im}'s$, $W_i's$, and $W_{im}'s$ in the following manner.
   (a) If $\delta_{i1} = 1$ (i.e. left-censored) sample Z_i from a truncated Poisson distribution; and conditional on Z_i, sample $(Z_{i1}, \ldots, Z_{ik_{i1}})$ from a multinomial distribution. Specifically,

$$Z_i \sim \text{Poisson}\left\{(\sum_{l=1}^{k_{i1}} \lambda_l) \exp(\mathbf{x}_i'\boldsymbol{\beta})\phi_i\right\} I(Z_i > 0),$$

$$(Z_{i1}, \ldots, Z_{ik_{i1}})|Z_i \sim \text{Multinomial}\Big\{Z_i, (p_{i1}, \ldots, p_{ik_{i1}})\Big\},$$

$$p_{il} = \frac{\lambda_l}{\sum_{h=1}^{k_{i1}} \lambda_h}, \qquad l = 1, \ldots, k_{i1}.$$

(b) If $\delta_{i2} = 1$ (i.e. interval-censored) sample:

$$W_i \sim \text{Poisson}\Big\{\big(\sum_{l=k_{i1}+1}^{k_{i2}} \lambda_l\big) \exp(\mathbf{x}_i'\boldsymbol{\beta})\phi_i\Big\} I(W_i > 0),$$

$$W_{i1}, \ldots, W_{i(k_{i2}-k_{i1})} | W_i \sim \text{Multinomial}\Big\{W_i, (q_{i1}, \ldots, q_{i(k_{i2}-k_{i1})})\Big\},$$

$$q_{il} = \frac{\lambda_l}{\sum_{h=k_{i1}+1}^{k_{i2}} \lambda_h}, \qquad l = k_{i1} + 1, \ldots, k_{i2}.$$

5. Sample a by using ARMS

$$L(a|.) \propto \frac{\eta^{a\eta s_M} \exp(-a)}{\prod_{m=1}^{M} \Gamma\{a(s_m - s_{m-1})\eta\}} \prod_{m=1}^{M} \lambda_m^{a(s_m - s_{m-1})\eta - 1}.$$

6. Sample η by using ARMS

$$L(\eta|.) \propto \frac{\eta^{a\eta s_M} \exp(-\eta) \exp(-\eta \sum_{m=1}^{M} \lambda_m)}{\prod_{m=1}^{M} \Gamma\{a(s_m - s_{m-1})\eta\}} \prod_{m=1}^{M} \lambda_m^{a(s_m - s_{m-1})\eta - 1}.$$

As for the PH model, step 2 is skipped and the rest of this Gibbs sampler is kept the same with all ϕ_is being fixed as 1.

6 Simulation Study

A simulation study is conducted to evaluate the proposed approach. To generate simulated data for each subject, we set 50 evenly allocated examination time points on time interval (0, 10] to imitate the pre-decided research time span and observation scheme. Then we randomly remove 20% of examination time points for each of the subject. This design is very common in real-life studies, where participants often miss or skip some scheduled examinations. At each of these examination times, the count of recurrent events is observed for panel count data and the status of the failure time event is determined. In this way, subjects have different numbers of examination times and various gap times for adjacent examination times.

6.1 Panel Count Data

To generate panel count data, the counting process associated with subject i is generated from the following model:

$$Z_{ij}|\phi_i = N_i(t_{ij})-N_i(t_{ij-1}) \sim \text{Poisson}\left[\{\mu_0(t_{ij})-\mu_0(t_{ij-1})\}\exp(x_{i1}\beta_1+x_{i2}\beta_2)\phi_i\right],$$

where x_{i1} is continuous variable that follows a normal distribution $N(0, 0.5^2)$ and x_{i2} is a binary variable that follows the Bernoulli distribution Bernoulli(0.5). The true regression coefficients are $\beta_1 = \{-1, 1\}$, $\beta_2 = \{-1, 1\}$. The distribution of ϕ_i is $\mathcal{G}a(1, 1)$. Two different baseline mean functions are considered: $\mu_0(t) = \log(1 + t) + t^{1.5}$ and $\mu_0(t) = t + \sin(t)$. For each setting, 100 data sets with sample size $n = 100$ are generated.

We applied the proposed Gibbs sampler in Sect. 5 for each simulated data set. For comparison, we implemented the Bayesian approach developed by Wang and Lin [30] under the same model, which approximates the baseline mean function with the monotone spline. We set the degree to be 3 and used 18 equally spaced interior knots over the time domain in our simulation for the monotone spline specification of this comparison method. Table 1 presents the frequentist operating characteristics of the

Table 1 Estimation of regression parameters for panel count data based on 100 simulated data sets from the proposed method based on the Gamma process (GP) and the comparison Bayesian method using monotone spline (SP) [30]. Empirical bias (BIAS), the average of the estimated standard errors (ESD) and standard deviation (ESD) of β, and the empirical coverage probabilities associated with 95% confidence probability (CP95)

		$\mu_0(t) = log(1 + t) + t^{1.5}$				$\mu_0(t) = t + \sin(t)$			
Method	(β_1,β_2)	BIAS	ESD	SSD	CP95	BIAS	ESD	SSD	CP95
GP	(−1,−1)	0.0217	0.2072	0.1715	0.98	0.0014	0.2228	0.2526	0.94
		0.0066	0.2128	0.2186	0.97	0.0145	0.2343	0.2567	0.94
SP		0.0427	0.2056	0.1697	0.97	−0.0185	0.2246	0.2501	0.95
		0.0030	0.2133	0.2218	0.93	0.0142	0.2341	0.2568	0.94
GP	(−1,1)	0.0250	0.2092	0.2119	0.93	−0.0366	0.2249	0.2403	0.93
		−0.0216	0.2126	0.2283	0.95	−0.0099	0.2323	0.2567	0.96
SP		0.0370	0.2111	0.2167	0.92	−0.0607	0.2277	0.2394	0.93
		−0.0168	0.2135	0.2301	0.92	−0.0089	0.2347	0.2545	0.96
GP	(1,−1)	−0.0038	0.1934	0.2096	0.93	0.0074	0.2101	0.2329	0.91
		0.0017	0.2032	0.2076	0.92	−0.0164	0.2194	0.2196	0.95
SP		0.0039	0.1933	0.2026	0.93	−0.0148	0.2106	0.2250	0.90
		0.0111	0.1994	0.2116	0.94	−0.0158	0.2211	0.2272	0.95
GP	(1,1)	0.0160	0.1997	0.2009	0.95	0.0248	0.2112	0.2284	0.93
		0.0355	0.2091	0.2005	0.94	−0.0016	0.2150	0.1986	0.97
SP		0.0170	0.1947	0.2013	0.91	−0.0034	0.2103	0.2245	0.94
		0.0295	0.2107	0.2075	0.91	−0.0050	0.2175	0.1981	0.97

estimates of the regression parameters. Bias is calculated as the difference between the average of the posterior means and the true parameter value; ESE is the average of the estimated posterior standard errors; SSD is the sample standard deviation of the posterior means; and CP95 is the empirical coverage probability based on the 95% credible intervals. Overall, the proposed method and the comparison method have similar performance. The results indicate that the proposed method performs well in terms of the estimation of the regression parameters because the estimates show very little bias, ESD and SSD are close to each other, and the coverage probabilities are all close to the nominal value 0.95.

6.2 *Interval-Censored Data under the PH and PO Models*

To generate interval-censored data under the PH and PO models, we generate the failure time T from

$$F(t|\mathbf{x}) = 1 - \exp\{-\Lambda_0(t)\exp(x_1\beta_1 + x_2\beta_2)\}$$

under the PH model and from

$$F(t|\mathbf{x}) = \frac{\Lambda_0(t)\exp(x_1\beta_1 + x_2\beta_2)}{1 + \Lambda_0(t)\exp(x_1\beta_1 + x_2\beta_2)},$$

under the PO model, where $\Lambda_0(t) = \log(1+t) + t^{1.5}$, x_1 is a $N(0, 1)$ random variable, and x_2 is a $Bernoulli(0.5)$ random variable. The true values of β_1 and β_2 are taken to be $\{0, 1\}$ and $\Lambda_0(t)$ is the baseline cumulative hazards function and baseline odds function for the PH and PO models, respectively.

The observed interval $(L_i, R_i]$ was then determined by the two adjacent examination times (including 0 and ∞) that bracket the generated failure time t_i. For each parameter configuration, 100 independent data sets were generated each with sample size $n = 200$. On average, the simulated data contain 11.1% to 23.1% of left-censored observations, 31.0% to 38.9% of interval-censored observations, and 19.9% to 36.1% of right-censored observations across all the setups.

We applied the proposed approach in Sect. 5.3 for the simulated data under the right PH and PO models, and the estimation results are summarized in Table 2. As seen in Table 2, the proposed method performs well overall in estimating the regression parameters with small biases, close values of ESD and SSD, and coverage probability close to 95% in general. Noticing that the results for interval-censored data are not as good as the results for panel count data as seen in Table 1. It is not surprising because that the Poisson counts are observed for all the subjects in panel count data but are latent for all the subjects when dealing with interval-censored data. In short, panel count data have much more information than corresponding interval-censored data.

Table 2 Estimation of regression parameters for interval-censored data based on 100 simulated data sets from the proposed Bayesian method. BIAS: the empirical bias; ESD: the average of the estimated standard errors; SSD: standard deviation of β; CP95: the empirical coverage probabilities associated with 95% confidence probability

		$\hat{\beta}_1$				$\hat{\beta}_2$			
Model	(β_1,β_2)	BIAS	ESD	SSD	CP95	BIAS	ESD	SSD	CP95
PH	(1,1)	−0.0539	0.0905	0.0961	0.88	−0.0495	0.1490	0.1416	0.97
PO		−0.0827	0.1301	0.1226	0.92	−0.0517	0.2221	0.2380	0.94
PH	(1,0)	−0.0438	0.0897	0.0731	0.95	−0.0066	0.1398	0.1259	0.97
PO		−0.0547	0.1309	0.1151	0.96	−0.0368	0.2172	0.2297	0.95
PH	(0,1)	0.0041	0.0764	0.0751	0.94	−0.0096	0.1492	0.1685	0.92
PO		0.0053	0.1287	0.1226	0.96	−0.0205	0.2268	0.2287	0.93
PH	(0,0)	0.0017	0.0737	0.0696	0.97	0.0015	0.1359	0.1495	0.93
PO		0.0006	0.1251	0.1267	0.95	−0.0162	0.2182	0.2298	0.93

7 Real-life Data Application

7.1 The Patent Study

The proposed method is first illustrated by an application to an industrial economics data set from the R package "pglm." The data set is extracted from a larger data set that is collected by Hall et al. [11] to study the relationship between patenting and research and development activity at the firm level by the US manufacturing sector during the 1970s. This data set contains 346 firms in the USA, among which 147 are in the scientific sector. From 1970 to 1979, the number of patents that were granted each year is recorded for every firm. The data set also includes the firm's book value of capital in 1972 and its annual research and development (R & D) spending for each firm.

The counts of the granted patents during the study period have formed the structure of panel count data. Our primary objective in this analysis is to assess the relationship between the mean number of patents and the characteristics of the firm. Three covariates are considered, with x_1 being a binary variable indicating if the firm is in the scientific sector, x_2 being the standardized book value of capital of the firm in 1972, and x_3 the standardized average annual research and development (R & D) spending for the firm. We standardized x_2 and x_3 before fitting the model in order to avoid collinearity. For the purpose of comparison, we also analyzed this data set with GFNPM [38] by using R package "PCDSpline." GFNPM is a maximum likelihood approach based on an expectation–maximization (EM) algorithm. This approach adopted a monotone spline to approximate the baseline mean function in gamma frailty non-homogeneous Poisson process model.

As shown in Table 3, the estimates of the regression coefficients from both methods are in accordance with each other. All these three covariates, being in

Table 3 Patent data analysis from the proposed approach (GFGP) and GFNPM. Summarized results are the point estimates (Point), the standard errors (SE), and the 95% credible (confidence) intervals for all the regression parameters and the frailty variance parameter υ

	GFGP			GFNPM		
	Point	SE	CI95	Point	SE	CI95
$\hat{\beta}_1$	0.537	0.146	(0.240,0.834)	0.561	0.127	(0.311, 0.798)
$\hat{\beta}_2$	1.032	0.148	(0.812,1.427)	1.130	0.122	(0.818, 1.303)
$\hat{\beta}_3$	0.617	0.144	(0.335,0.801)	0.795	0.144	(0.483, 1.005)
$\hat{\upsilon}$	0.549	0.037	(0.480,0.624)	0.555	0.037	(0.485, 0.630)

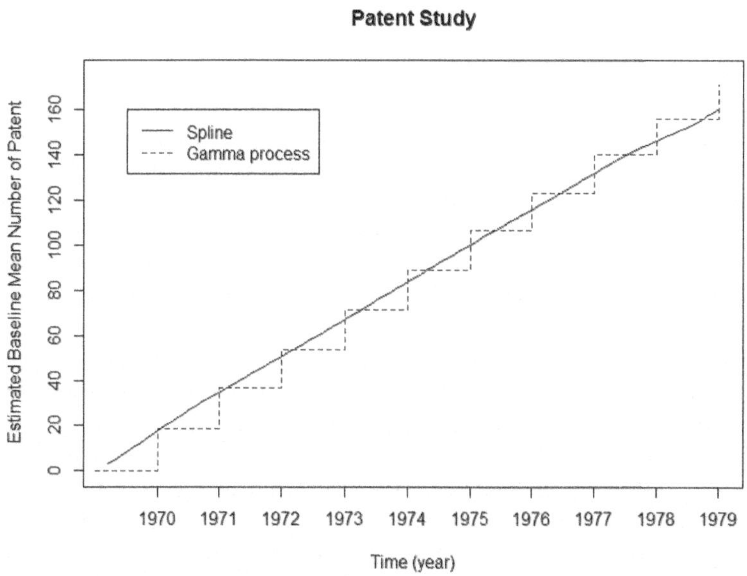

Fig. 1 The estimated baseline mean functions of patent counts obtained from the proposed method that uses the Gamma process to model the baseline mean function (Gamma process) and GFNPM that uses the monotone spline to model the baseline mean function (Spline)

scientific sector, book value of capital, and the R & D spending, have a significant positive effect on the mean number of granted patents. It is especially worthy-noting that the firms in the scientific sector are granted $\exp(0.537) - 1 = 71\%$ more patents than the firms not in the scientific sector. In Fig. 1, we superimpose the estimated baseline mean functions of patent counts between 1970 and 1979 obtained by both methods. The two estimated curves are very close to each other, indicating that the proposed method provides a similar estimation of the baseline mean function as GFNPM.

7.2 The Bladder Tumor Study

We also apply the proposed method to the most widely used panel count data example in the literature, which arose from a bladder cancer study conducted by the Veterans Administration Cooperative Urological Research Group [2]. In this randomized clinical trial study, all the 118 patients had experienced superficial bladder tumors when they entered the trial. They were randomized into one of three treatment groups: placebo, thiotepa, and pyridoxine. During the study at each follow-up visit, new tumors since the last visit were counted, measured, and then removed transurethrally. The number of follow-up clinical visits and follow-up times varied noticeably from patient to patient. The primary objective of the study was to determine if any treatment could significantly reduce the recurrence of bladder tumor.

This data set has been analyzed extensively using many different approaches in the literature. Following Wellner and Zhang [35], we focus on 116 patients in the study, who had at least one follow-up observation after the study enrollment. Following the literature, we consider the following four covariates, x_1 and x_2 being the baseline number of bladder tumors and the size of the largest bladder tumors at the beginning of the trial, respectively, and x_3 and x_4 being the binary variables indicating whether a patient was assigned to the treatment of pyridoxine pills or thiotepa installation, respectively.

Table 4 shows the results from the proposed approach and two other competitive frequentist approaches, i.e. GFNPM [38] and WZ [35]. The results from these two competitors are directly drawn from their papers. As seen in Table 4, the estimates of the parameters from GFGP and GFNPM are close to each other but quite different from the results from the WZ approach. The main reason is that the proposed approach and the GFNPM are based on the same frailty non-homogeneous Poisson model that accounts for the within-subject correlation, while the WZ approach is based on the non-homogeneous Poisson model without accounting for the within-subject correlation. Yao et al. [38] pointed out that the GFNPM approach will produce the same results as those based on the non-homogeneous Poisson model when there is no within-subject correlation. The results in Table 4 suggest that the within-subject correlation is not ignorable for this data set. These explain the consistency of the results from the proposed method and GFNPM as well as the discrepancy of their results from the WZ approach.

As seen in Table 4, the results from all these three methods indicate that the number of initial bladder tumors was positively related to the recurrence of the tumor while the size of the largest tumor at the enrollment did not have a significant effect. It also reveals that the thiotepa instillation treatment significantly reduced the recurrence rate of bladder tumors, while the treatment of pyridoxine pills did not have a significant effect. Figure 2 plots the estimated mean functions of bladder tumor counts for the control and the other two treatment groups controlling the other two covariates at 0. It is clear that the estimated mean functions for the control and the pyridoxine treatment groups are close to each other and they are higher than the one for the thiotepa treatment group.

Table 4 Bladder tumor data analysis from the proposed approach (GFGP), the GFNPM approach [38], and the WZ approach [35]. Summarized results are the point estimates (Point), the standard errors (SE), and the 95% credible (confidence) intervals for the regression parameters and the frailty variance parameter υ

	GFGP			GFNPM			WZ		
	Point	SE	CI95	Point	SE	CI95	Point	SE	CI95
$\hat{\beta}_1$	0.333	0.107	(0.131, 0.550)	0.336	0.106	(0.128, 0.544)	0.207	0.078	(0.054, 0.360)
$\hat{\beta}_2$	0.001	0.122	(−0.224, 0.244)	0.012	0.120	(−0.223, 0.247)	−0.036	0.086	(−0.133, 0.205)
$\hat{\beta}_3$	−0.021	0.427	(−0.851, 0.833)	−0.033	0.409	(−0.835, 0.769)	0.066	0.431	(−0.779, 0.911)
$\hat{\beta}_4$	−1.152	0.427	(−2.051, −0.261)	−1.140	0.435	(−1.993, −0.287)	−0.797	0.360	(−1.503, −0.091)
$\hat{\upsilon}$	0.326	0.058	(0.225, 0.453)	0.351	0.062	(0.229, 0.473)	–	–	–

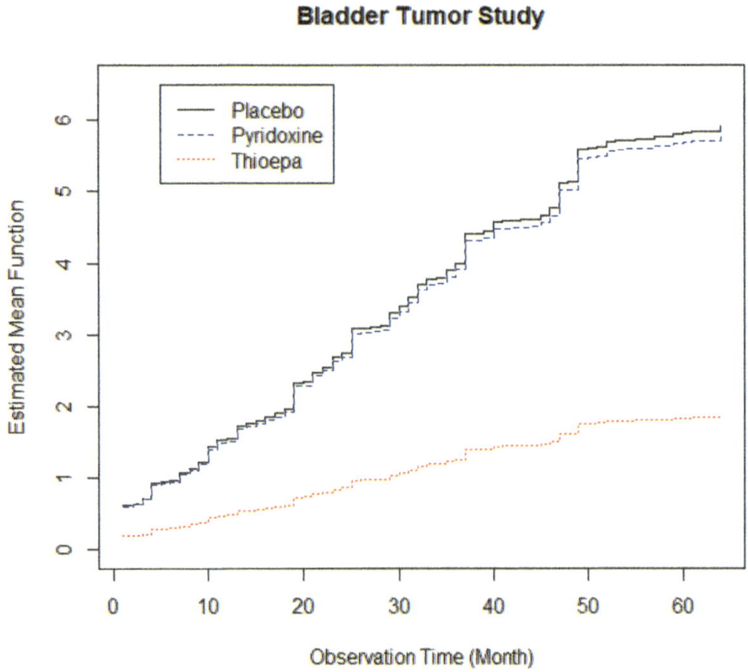

Fig. 2 The estimated mean functions for different treatment groups in the bladder tumor study

7.3 Breast Cosmesis Data

We illustrate the proposed approach on interval-censored data by analyzing the most commonly used interval-censored data set in the literature, the breast cosmesis data [7]. The data came from a study of 94 early breast cancer patients who were treated with adjuvant therapy following tumorectomy. The primary goal of this study was to identify if treating patients with primary radiation therapy and adjuvant chemotherapy could have better long-term cosmetic results than treating with radiotherapy alone. Among all patients, 48 patients were treated with radiation therapy combined with chemotherapy and 46 patients were treated with radiation therapy alone. In this study, patients were examined periodically and actual examination times differed from patient to patient since some of them missed their visits. The response variable of interest was the time (in months) until the appearance of breast retraction. Since the exact onset time of breast retraction was not observed due to the study design, only interval-censored data were available.

We apply the proposed Bayesian approach (GFGP) and compare it with the results obtained by fitting the semiparametric Turnbull (SPT) model with a modified ICM algorithm [1, 22]. The results from the two methods are shown in Table 5. As seen in Table 5, all the credible (confidence) intervals are above 0 under the PH and PO models, indicating that chemotherapy increases the hazards and odds of

Table 5 The results for breast cosmesis data analysis from the proposed approach (GFGP) and the semiparametric Turnbull (SPT) model [1]. Summarized results are the point estimates (Point), the standard errors (SE), and the 95% credible (confidence) interval for the treatment effect

	GFGP			PST		
Model	Estimate	SE	CI95	Estimate	SE	CI95
PH	0.814	0.232	(0.340, 1.257)	0.797	0.345	(0.121, 1.473)
PO	0.798	0.337	(0.142, 1.469)	0.902	0.406	(0.106, 1.698)

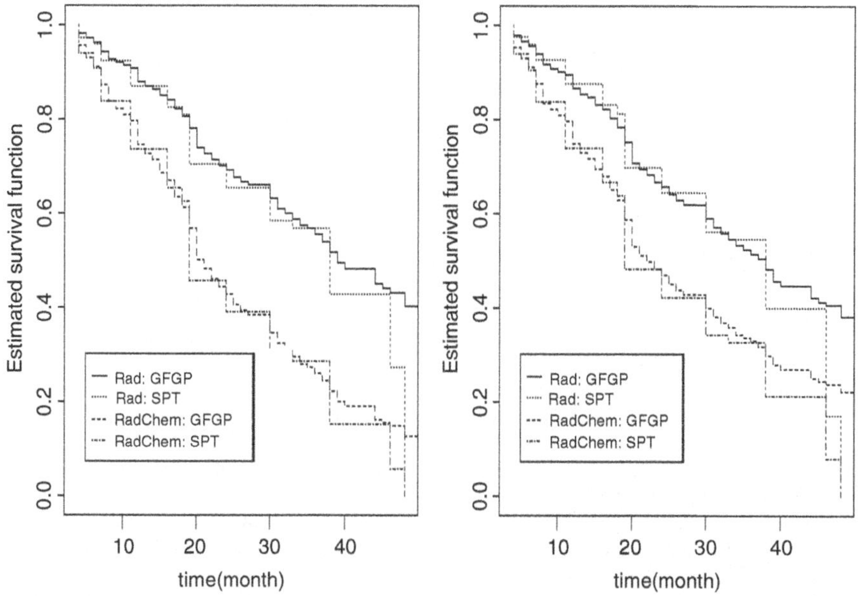

Fig. 3 The estimated survival functions obtained from the proposed approach (GFGP) and the semiparametric Turnbull (SPT) model under PH model (left) and PO model (right)

breast retraction for patients who have been previously treated with radiotherapy. This suggests that the combined therapy is not better than the radiation therapy alone. Figure 3 exhibits the estimated survival functions of appearance of retraction under the PH and PO models. Again, these plots suggest that treating patients with radiotherapy alone has a higher survival rate than the combined therapies. This conclusion agrees with the analysis of Finkelstein and Wolfe [8] and Lin and Wang [18].

8 Discussion

This chapter develops a new Bayesian estimation approach for panel count data and interval-censored data. This unified approach is based on the fact that the two types of data can be connected by a non-homogeneous frailty Poisson process. The Poisson process is observed for penal count data but is latent for interval-censored data. The proposed approach further models the baseline mean, cumulative hazards, and odds functions nonparametrically by assigning them a Gamma process prior, providing additional flexibility. Efficient Gibbs samplers are developed based on innovative data augmentations. This approach has appealing numerical performance in terms of providing efficient, accurate, and reliable estimation of regression coefficients under each model. Since the Gamma process is a discrete process modeling the jumps, it can only provide an estimate of the baseline function as a step function. When the number of jumps is large, the computation is expensive since it tries to estimate the size of each jump. In order for readers to reproduce our results, we provide the computing codes for the real-life data applications on the following website: https://github.com/luwstat/Computing-sources-for-data-application.

References

1. Anderson-Bergman, C.: icenReg: regression models for interval censored data in R. J. Stat. Softw. **81**, 1–23 (2017)
2. Byar, D.P,, Blackard, C.: Comparisons of placebo, pyridoxine, and topical thiotepa in preventing recurrence of stage I bladder cancer. Veterans Administration Cooper. Urol. Res. Group **10**, 556–561 (1977)
3. Cai, T., Betensky, R.A.: Hazard regression for interval-censored data with penalized spline. Biometrics **59**, 570–579 (2003)
4. Cox, D.R.: Regression models and life tables. J. R. Stat. Soc. B **34**, 187–220 (1972)
5. Doksum, K.: Tailfree and neutral random probabilities and their posterior distributions. Ann. Probab. **2**(2), 183–201 (1974)
6. Ferguson, S.T., Phadia, G.E.: Bayesian nonparametric esti-mation based on censored data. Ann. Stat. **1**(1), 163–186 (1979)
7. Finkelstein, D.M. : A proportional hazards model for interval-censored failure time data. Biometrics **42**(4), 845–854 (1986)
8. Finkelstein, D.M., Wolfe, R.A.: A semiparametric model for regression analysis of interval-censored failure time data. Biometrics **41**, 731–740 (1985)
9. Goggins, W., et al.: A Markov chain Monte Marlo EM algorithm for analyzing interval-censored data under the Cox proportional hazards model. Biometrics **54**, 1498–1507 (1998)
10. Groeneboom, P., Wellner, J.A.: Information Bounds and Nonparametric Maximum Likelihood Estimation. Birkhauser, Basel (1992)
11. Hall, B., Zvi, G., Jerry, H.: Patents and R and D: Is there a Lag? Int. Econ. Rev. **27**, 265–283 (1986)
12. Hua, L., Zhang, Y: Spline-based semiparametric projected generalized estimating equation method for panel count data. Biostatistics **13**, 440–454 (2012)
13. Hua, L., Zhang, Y., Zhang, Y., Tu, W.: A spline-based semiparametric sieve likelihood method for over-dispersed panel count data. Can. J. Stat. **42**, 217–245 (2014)
14. Huang, J.: Efficient estimation for the Cox model with interval censoring. Int. Econ. Rev. **24**, 540–568 (1996)
15. Huang, J., Rossini, J.A.: Sieve estimation for the proportional odds model with interval-censoring. J. Am. Stat. Assoc. **92**, 960–967 (1997)
16. Kalbfleisch, D.J.: Non-parametric Bayesian analysis of survival time data. J. R. Stat. Soc. B **40**, 214–221 (1978)

17. Lawless, J., Crowder, M.: Covariates and random effects in a gamma process model with application to degradation and failure. Lifetime Data Anal. **10**, 213–227 (2004)
18. Lin, X., Wang, L.: A semiparametric probit model for case 2 interval- censored failure time data. Stat. Med. **29**, 972–981 (2010)
19. Lin, X., et al.: A Bayesian proportional hazards model for general interval-censored data. Lifetime Data Anal. **21**, 470–490 (2015)
20. Nozer, D.S.: Survival in dynamic envirnoments. Stat. Sci. **10**(1), 86–103 (1995)
21. Pan, W.: A multiple imputation approach to Cox regression with interval- censored data. Biometrics **56**(1), 199–203 (2000)
22. Pan, W.: Extending the iterative convex minorant algorithm to the Cox model for interval-censored data. J. Comput. Graph. Stat. **8**(1), 109–120 (1999)
23. Satten, G.A.: Rank based inference in the proportional hazards model for interval-censored data. Biometrika **83**, 355–370 (1996)
24. Shen, X.T.: Proportional odds regression and sieve maximum likelihood estimation. Biometrika **85**, 165–177 (1998)
25. Sinha, A., Chi, Z., Chen, M.: Bayesian inference of hidden gamma wear process model for survival data with ties. Stat. Sin. **25**, 1613–1635 (2015)
26. Sinha, D.: A Bayesian approach for the analysis of panel-count data with dependent termination. Biometrics **60**, 34–40 (2004)
27. Sinha, D., Chen, M H., Ghosh, S.K.: Bayesian analysis and model selection for interval-censored survival data. Biometrics **55**, 585–590 (1999)
28. Sun, J., Kalbfleisch, J.D.: Estimation of the mean function of point processes based on panel count data. Stat. Sin. **5**, 279–290 (1995)
29. Wang, C.S., McMahan, L., Hudgens, M.G., Qureshi, Z.P.: A flexible, computationally efficient method for fitting the proportional hazards model to interval-censored data. Biometrics **72**, 222–231 (2016)
30. Wang, J., Lin, X.: A Bayesian approach for semiparametric regression analysis of panel count data. Lifetime Data Anal. **26**, 402–420 (2020)
31. Wang, L., Lin, X.: A Bayesian approach for analyzing case 2 interval-censored data under the semiparametric proportional odds model. Stat. Probab. Lett. **81**, 876–883 (2011)
32. Wang, L., Lin, X., Cai, B.: Bayesian semiparametric regression analysis of interval-censored data with monotone splines. In: Chen, D., Sun, J., Peace, K. (eds.) Interval-Censored Time-to-Event Data: Methods and Applications, pp. 149–165 (2012)
33. Wang, X.: Nonparametric estimation of the shape function in a Gamma process for degradation data. Can. J. Stat. **37**(1), 102–118 (2009)
34. Wellner, A.J., Zhang, Y.: Two estimators of the mean of a counting process with panel count data. Ann. Stat. **28**(3), 779–814 (2000)
35. Wellner, A.J., Zhang, Y.: Two likelihood-based semiparametric estimation methods for panel count data with covariates. Ann. Stat. **35**(5), 2105–2142 (2007)
36. Wellner, J.A., Zhang, Y.: Large sample theory for an estimator of the mean of a counting process with panel count data (1998)
37. Xu, D., Zhao, H., Sun, J.: Joint analysis of interval-censored failure time data and panel count data. Lifetime Data Anal. **24**, 94–109 (2018)
38. Yao, B., Wang, L., He, X.: Semiparametric regression analysis of panel count data allowing for within-subject correlation. Comput. Stat. Data Anal. **97**, 47–59 (2016)
39. Yi, F., Tang, N., Sun, J.: Regression analysis of interval-censored failure time data with time-dependent covariates. Comput. Stat. Data Anal. **144**, 106848 (2020)
40. Zhang, Y., Hua, L., Huang, J.: A spline-based semiparametric maximum likelihood estimation method for the Cox model with interval-censored data. Scand. J. Stat. **37**, 338–354 (2010)
41. Zhang, Y., Jamshidian, M.: The gamma-frailty poisson model for the nonparametric estimation of panel count data. Biometrics **59**, 1099–1106 (2003)
42. Zhong, G.: Maximum approximate Bernstein likelihood estimation in proportional hazard model for interval-censored data. Stat. Med. (2020). https://doi.org/10.1002/sim.8801
43. Zhu, L., et al.: A semiparametric likelihood-based method for regression analysis of mixed panel-count data. Biometrics **74**, 488–497 (2018)

Bayesian Approach for Interval-Censored Survival Data with Time-Varying Coefficients

Yue Zhang and Bin Zhang

Abstract Interval-censored data arise when the failure time cannot be observed exactly but can only be determined to lie within an interval. Interval-censored data are very common in medical and epidemiological studies. In this chapter, we discuss a Bayesian approach for correlated interval-censored data under a dynamic Cox regression model. Some methods that incorporate right censoring have been developed for time-to-event data with temporal covariate effects. However, interval-censored data analysis under the same circumstance is much less developed. In this chapter, we introduce a piecewise constant coefficients estimate based on a dynamic Cox regression model under the Bayesian framework. The dimensions of coefficients are automatically determined by the reversible jump Markov chain Monte Carlo algorithm. Meanwhile, we use a shared frailty factor for unobserved heterogeneity or for statistical dependence between observations. Two illustrative examples are given to demonstrate the methods' performance. A summary is provided to discuss the methods introduced in this chapter.

1 Introduction

Interval censoring occurs in studies where the event time cannot be observed but can only be determined to lie within an interval. It is a common censoring scheme in many applications, including medical studies, epidemiological studies, etc. For example, if we are interested in the time to tumor onset for patients with

Y. Zhang (✉)
Department of Bioinformatics and Biostatistics, School of Life Sciences and Biotechnology, Shanghai Jiao Tong University, Shanghai, PR China
e-mail: yue.zhang@sjtu.edu.cn

B. Zhang
Division of Biostatistics and Epidemiology, Cincinnati Children's Hospital Medical Center, Cincinnati, OH, USA
e-mail: Bin.Zhang@cchmc.org

Y. Lio et al. (eds.), *Bayesian Inference and Computation in Reliability and Survival Analysis*, Emerging Topics in Statistics and Biostatistics,
https://doi.org/10.1007/978-3-030-88658-5_15

periodic follow-ups, then the exact time to tumor onset is hard to record. Instead, the time is known to fall between certain visits. There are extensive literature about interval-censored data. In recent years, survival analysis with time-varying covariate effects has drawn much attention from researchers in both statistics and medical fields. Time-varying coefficients are of great interest due to their flexibility in capturing the temporal covariate effects. Different methods have been proposed in order to estimate the temporal effects. One difficulty in analysis for interval-censored data is that the regression parameters and the baseline survival or hazard function need to be estimated simultaneously due to the lack of partial likelihood. Wang et al. [28] applied reversible jump Markov chain Monte Carlo (MCMC) to automatically determine the dimension of coefficients as well as the baseline hazard function. In addition to temporal effects, data structure could be more complicated when the survival events are correlated. This could happen when certain correlation exists between individuals, e.g., clustered data or spatial data. This chapter focuses on Bayesian approach for correlated interval-censored data with time-varying coefficients.

The remainder of this chapter is organized as follows. Section 2 discusses the Bayesian approach for clustered interval-censored data with time-varying covariate effects. The general data structure will be introduced, and a frailty Cox regression model is proposed to account for the correlation within each cluster. Prior specifications and posterior computation will be described in detail. Section 3 considers spatially correlated interval-censored data using Bayesian approach. The priors on the regression coefficients, the frailties, and the other parameters in the models will be specified, and posterior inference details will be provided. Section 4 includes two illustrative examples. They are analyzed using the methods described in Sects. 2 and 3. Concluding remarks can be found in Sect. 5. Bibliographic notes are provided at the end.

2 Bayesian Approach for Clustered Interval-Censored Data

In this section, we focus on the Bayesian approach for clustered interval-censored data with time-varying covariate effects. Clustered data are very natural in medical studies when grouped data are observed where subjects in the same group may share some information that is not observed. For clustered interval-censored data, the correlation between different failure times can be described by a frailty, a commonly used factor for statistical dependence between observations.

2.1 Model and the likelihood

Assume that there are n clusters in a study and m_i subjects in each cluster, $i = 1, 2, \dots, n$. Hence there are a total of $N = \sum_{i=1}^{n} m_i$ subjects in the study. Let $T_{i,j}$

denote the survival time for the jth subject in the ith cluster, $j = 1, \ldots, m_i$. The p-dimensional vector $\boldsymbol{x}_{i,j}$ represents the p covariates, and ω_i denotes the unobserved frailty random variable for the ith cluster. For interval-censored data, the unobserved event time $T_{i,j}$ is located in the censoring interval $(L_{i,j}, R_{i,j}]$. The contribution of the jth subject in the ith cluster to the observed data likelihood is

$$\Pr(T_{i,j} \in (L_{i,j}, R_{i,j}]|\omega_i, \boldsymbol{x}_{i,j}) = \Pr(T_{i,j} > L_{i,j}|\omega_i, \boldsymbol{x}_{i,j}) - \Pr(T_{i,j} > R_{i,j}|\omega_i, \boldsymbol{x}_{i,j}).$$

Under the Cox model with time-varying regression coefficients, the hazard function for the jth subject in the ith cluster can be written as

$$\lambda(t|\omega_i, \boldsymbol{x}_{i,j}) = \lambda_0(t)\omega_i \exp\left\{\boldsymbol{x}_{i,j}^T \boldsymbol{\beta}(t)\right\},$$

where $\lambda_0(t)$ is an unknown baseline hazard function common to all the subjects and $\boldsymbol{\beta}(t)$ is the p-dimensional regression coefficient function of main interest. This is a shared frailty model, which is a common type of the frailty model used for within-cluster dependence. Note that the "shared frailty" implies that individuals in the same cluster share the common frailty. The frailty ω_i is assumed to follow a parametric distribution, which can either take the form of finite mean frailty distributions including but not limited to the gamma or the log-normal distribution or take the form of infinite mean distributions such as the positive stable distribution Ibrahim et al. [14].

In the above model, both $\lambda_0(t)$ and $\boldsymbol{\beta}(t)$ are assumed to be left continuous step functions, where both the number of jumps and the locations of the jumps are random and are estimated. A fine time grid is specified as $\mathcal{T} = \{0 = \tau_0 < \tau_1 < \tau_2 < \ldots \tau_k < \ldots < \tau_K < \infty\}$. It contains all the potential jump points of the functions. The length of each time interval may be taken to be sufficiently small to approximate any hazard and coefficient function. Let $\lambda_k = \lambda_0(\tau_k)$ and $\boldsymbol{\beta}_k = \boldsymbol{\beta}(\tau_k)$ denote the baseline hazard function and the coefficient function evaluated at each grid point k, $k = 1, \ldots, K$; $dN_{i,j,k}$ indicates whether or not the event time $T_{i,j}$ falls within the kth interval of the grid, i.e., $dN_{i,j,k} = \boldsymbol{I}(T_{i,j} \in (\tau_{k-1}, \tau_k])$; $Y_{i,j,k}$ denotes the at-risk variable. If $dN_{i,j,k} = 1$ for some value k, $Y_{i,j,l} = 1$ for $l < k$, and $Y_{i,j,l} = 0$ for $l > k$, while $Y_{i,j,k} = (T_{i,j} - \tau_{k-1})/\Delta_k$ for $l = k$, where $\Delta_k = \tau_k - \tau_{k-1}$ is the width of the kth interval. The augmented likelihood function for the jth subject of the ith cluster is

$$\ell_{i,j}(\Theta|\{dN_{i,j,k}, Y_{i,j,k}\}_{k=1}^K, \omega_i, \boldsymbol{x}_{i,j})$$
$$= \prod_{k=1}^K \{\lambda_k \omega_i \exp(\boldsymbol{x}_{i,j}^T \boldsymbol{\beta}_k)\}^{dN_{i,j,k}} \exp\{-\Delta_k \lambda_k \omega_i \exp(\boldsymbol{x}_{i,j}^T \boldsymbol{\beta}_k) Y_{i,j,k}\},$$

where $i = 1, 2, \ldots, n$, $j = 1, 2, \ldots, m_i$, and $\Theta = \{\lambda_k, \boldsymbol{\beta}_k, k = 1, 2, \ldots, K\}$.

2.2 Prior

In the following description, we use $\theta(t)$ to denote either $\log \lambda_0(t)$ or one element in the p-dimensional vector $\boldsymbol{\beta}(t)$. Assume that the number of jumps P in $\theta(t)$ follows a discrete uniform distribution ranging from 1 to K. For a fixed P, the jump times $0 < \tau_1 < \tau_2 < \ldots \tau_p < \ldots < \tau_P = \tau_K$ are randomly selected from all time grids except the last one. Given P and the jump times, a hierarchical Markov-type process prior for $\theta(t)$ proposed by [28] is specified as follows:

$$\theta(\tau_1) \sim \mathcal{N}(0, a_0 \nu),$$
$$\theta(\tau_p)|\theta(\tau_{p-1}) \sim \mathcal{N}(\theta(\tau_{p-1}), \nu), \quad p = 2, 3, .., P,$$
$$\nu \sim \mathcal{IG}(\alpha_0, \eta_0),$$

where $a_0 > 0$ is a hyper-parameter that can be chosen as a large number to reflect higher uncertainty in the prior input, and $\mathcal{IG}(\alpha_0, \eta_0)$ denotes an inverse-gamma distribution with a shape parameter α_0 and a scale parameter η_0 such that the mean is $\eta_0/(\alpha_0 - 1)$. Similar priors have been used in generalized additive models [2, 6]. The gamma distribution, the most commonly used finite mean distribution, is used to model the frailty term $\omega_i, i = 1, \ldots, n$. For finite mean frailty distributions, we need the mean of the frailty distribution to be unity in order for the parameters of the model to be identifiable. Thus, we assume

$$\omega_i \overset{\text{i.i.d.}}{\sim} \mathcal{G}(\kappa^{-1}, \kappa^{-1}), \quad i = 1, 2, .., n,$$

where κ is the variance of the ω_i's and larger values of κ imply greater heterogeneity among clusters. Let $\eta = \kappa^{-1}$ for notational convenience. Vague hyper-priors for η are commonly used, such as the uniform distribution $\mathcal{U}(0, a)$ with a large a or the gamma distribution $\mathcal{G}(b, b)$ with b close to zero. In this chapter, a vague gamma prior $\mathcal{G}(0.001, 0.001)$ is used, which is denoted as $\pi_\eta(.)$. The joint prior density is proportional to

$$\pi_\eta(\eta) \prod_{i=1}^{n} \{\omega_i^{\eta-1} \exp(-\eta\omega_i)\} \frac{\eta_0^{\alpha_0}}{\Gamma(\alpha_0)} \nu^{-\alpha_0-1} \exp\left(-\frac{\eta_0}{\nu}\right) \nu^{-\frac{P}{2}} \exp\left\{-\frac{\theta(\tau_1)^2}{2a_0\nu}\right\}$$
$$\times \prod_{p\geq 2} \exp\left[-\frac{\{\theta(\tau_p) - \theta(\tau_{p-1})\}^2}{2\nu}\right].$$

2.3 Posterior Computation

The posterior samples are obtained under a Gibbs sampling framework based on the jth subject of the ith group observed in the kth time interval, where $i =$

$1, 2, \ldots, n$, $j = 1, 2, \ldots, m_i$, $k = 1, 2, \ldots, K$, and K is the total number of time grids. The parameters of interest include $\theta(t)$ and the frailty term ω_i's. The event indicators $dN_{i,j,k}$'s, the event time $T_{i,j}$'s, and the at-risk variables $Y_{i,j,k}$'s also need to be sampled. Let $D = \{dN_{i,j,k}, Y_{i,j,k}\}$, $\Theta = \{\theta(t)\}$, $W = \{\omega_i\}$. The Gibbs sampling algorithm draws D, Θ, ν, W, and η iteratively, where ν and η are hyper-parameters.

The first step is to sample the event time $T_{i,j}$, event indicators $dN_{i,j,k}$'s, and at-risk variables $Y_{i,j,k}$'s for augmented data, given Θ and W. This can be decomposed into two steps:

(I) Locate the grid interval for each event time. For a finite interval-censored subject, the event indicators $dN_{i,j,k}$'s follow a multinomial distribution with a size 1 and a probability vector $(e_{i,j,1}, e_{i,j,2}, \ldots, e_{i,j,k})$, where for $k = 1, 2, \ldots, K$,

$$e_{i,j,k} = \frac{p_{i,j,k}\boldsymbol{I}(\tau_k \in (L_{i,j}, R_{i,j}])}{\sum_{\tau_l \in (L_{i,j}, R_{i,j}]} p_{i,j,l}},$$

$$p_{i,j,k} = \begin{cases} \exp\left\{-\sum_{l=1}^{k-1} \Delta_l \lambda_l \omega_i \exp(\boldsymbol{x}_{i,j}^T \boldsymbol{\beta}_k)\right\} & \\ \quad - \exp\left\{-\sum_{l=1}^{k} \Delta_l \lambda_l \omega_i \exp(\boldsymbol{x}_{i,j}^T \boldsymbol{\beta}_k)\right\} & \text{if } k > 1, \\ 1 - \exp\left\{-\Delta_1 \lambda_1 \omega_i \exp(\boldsymbol{x}_{i,j}^T \boldsymbol{\beta}_1)\right\} & \text{if } k = 1. \end{cases}$$

Thus, if the observed interval $(L_{i,j}, R_{i,j}]$ only covers one time grid τ_k, then $dN_{i,j,k} = 1$ and all the other event indicators equal 0. Otherwise, if $(L_{i,j}, R_{i,j}]$ covers multiple time grids τ_k's, $dN_{i,j,k}$ is sampled from the multinomial distribution with the probability vector calculated based on these covered time grids τ_k's. In other words, the time interval $(\tau_{k-1}, \tau_k]$ with $dN_{i,j,k} = 1$ is sampled in this step.

(II) Within selected time grids, the exact time $T_{i,j}$ follows a doubly truncated exponential distribution on $(\tau_{k-1}, \tau_k]$ with a distribution function

$$F(u) = \frac{1 - \exp\{-\lambda_k (u - \tau_{k-1}) \omega_i \exp(\boldsymbol{x}_{i,j}^T \boldsymbol{\beta}_k)\}}{1 - \exp\{-\lambda_k \Delta_k \omega_i \exp(\boldsymbol{x}_{i,j}^T \boldsymbol{\beta}_k)\}}.$$

Then $T_{i,j}$ is sampled by the inverse distribution method, and the at-risk variables $Y_{i,j,k}$'s are calculated as defined above.

The next step is to sample each component of the baseline hazard $\log \lambda_0(t)$ and the regression coefficients $\boldsymbol{\beta}(t)$, given D and W. The reversible jump MCMC algorithm is applied here because the number of jumps P is random, and the dimension of the posterior distribution could vary from iteration to iteration. The probabilities of taking a birth, death, and update move are set as 0.3, 0.3, and 0.4 [29], respectively.

(I) Update move. In this step, both P and the jump times are fixed. The conditional posterior distribution of $\theta(\tau_p)$ given D, W, and all the other components in Θ is

$$\pi(\theta(\tau_p)|\Theta/\{\theta(\tau_p)\}, D, W) \propto \exp\left[-\frac{\{\theta(\tau_p)-\mu_p\}^2}{2\sigma_p^2}\right]$$
$$\times \exp\left\{-\sum_{i=1}^{n}\sum_{j=1}^{m_i}\sum_{k=1}^{K} \boldsymbol{I}(\tau_k \in (\tau_{p-1}, \tau_p])\Delta_k\lambda_k\omega_i \exp(\boldsymbol{x}_{i,j}^T\boldsymbol{\beta}_k)Y_{i,j,k}\right\},$$

where $\theta(\tau_p)$ is either $\log\lambda(\tau_p)$ or one component in $\boldsymbol{\beta}(\tau_p)$. The steps of computing μ_p and σ_p^2 can be found in Wang et al. [29]. Since it can be shown that the above function is log-concave, the adaptive rejection algorithm Gilks and Wild [9] is applied to sample $\theta(\tau_p)$.

(II) Birth move. A new jump time τ' is "born" in this move. This new τ' is randomly selected from the non-jump time grids.

(III) Death move. One of current jump time τ_p is removed, where the index p is uniformly selected from the current jump point set $\{1, 2, \ldots, P-1\}$. Details of birth move and death move are shown in the following sections.

2.3.1 Birth Move

Let $\{\tau'_p, p = 1, 2, \ldots, P+1\}$ and $\{\tau_p, p = 1, 2, \ldots, P\}$ denote new and current jump times, respectively. Assume $\tau'_p \in (\tau_{p-1}, \tau_p)$, then $\theta(\tau'_p)$ and $\theta(\tau'_{p+1})$ need to be sampled.

$$\theta(\tau'_p) = \pi_1\theta(\tau_{p-1}) + \pi_2\{\theta(\tau_p) + u\},$$
$$\theta(\tau'_{p+1}) = \pi_1\{\theta(\tau_p) - u\} + \pi_2\theta(\tau_{p+1}),$$

where weights are defined as

$$\pi_1 = (\tau'_p - \tau'_{p-1})/(\tau'_{p+1} - \tau'_{p-1}),$$
$$\pi_2 = (\tau'_{p+1} - \tau'_p)/(\tau'_{p+1} - \tau'_{p-1}),$$

where u is generated from a uniform distribution $\mathcal{U}(-\epsilon_0, \epsilon_0)$ and ϵ_0 is set to 1 in this study. Variable u here is an auxiliary variable to the old model, which helps balance out the one dimension increase of the proposed new model. When τ' is near the boundaries, set $\theta(\tau_0) = \theta(\tau_1)$ and $\theta(\tau_{P+1}) = \theta(\tau_P)$. Let $\theta = \{\theta(\tau_1), \theta(\tau_2), \ldots, \theta(\tau_P)\}$ and $\theta' = \{\theta(\tau'_1), \theta(\tau'_2), \ldots, \theta(\tau'_{P+1})\}$. The acceptance ratio can be computed with the posterior distribution $\pi(\theta'|\Theta/\{\theta'\}, \omega, \nu, D)$, the uniform density function π_u, and the Jacobian of the transformation,

$$R_{\text{birth}} = \frac{\pi(\theta'|\Theta/\{\theta'\}, \omega, \nu, D)}{\pi(\theta|\Theta/\{\theta\}, \omega, \nu, D)\pi(u)} \left| \frac{\partial\theta'}{\partial(\theta, u)} \right|.$$

The acceptance probability is defined as $\min\{1, R_{\text{birth}}\}$.

2.3.2 Death Move

One of the current jump times τ_p is removed, where the index p is uniformly selected from the current jump point set $\{1, 2, \ldots, P-1\}$. Then this can be treated as an inverse step of birth move. By using the same transformation function of the birth move, the expression of $\theta(\tau_p')$ can be computed as follows:

$$\theta(\tau_p') = \frac{1}{2}\left\{-\frac{\pi_1}{\pi_2}\theta(\tau_{p-1}) + \frac{1}{\pi_2}\theta(\tau_p) + \frac{1}{\pi_1}\theta(\tau_{p+1}) - \frac{\pi_2}{\pi_1}\theta(\tau_{p+2})\right\},$$

where the weights are defined as

$$\pi_1 = (\tau_p - \tau_{p-1})/(\tau_{p+1} - \tau_{p-1}),$$
$$\pi_2 = (\tau_{p+1} - \tau_p)/(\tau_{p+1} - \tau_{p-1}),$$

and the acceptance probability is $\min\{1, R_{\text{birth}}^{-1}\}$.

The hyper-parameter ν has a conjugate inverse-gamma prior, and the posterior distribution is also an inverse-gamma specified as

$$\nu|\Theta, D \sim \mathcal{IG}\left[\alpha_0 + \frac{P}{2}, \eta_0 + \frac{\theta(\tau_1)^2}{2a_0} + \sum_{p\geq 2} \frac{\{\theta(\tau_p) - \theta(\tau_{p-1})\}^2}{2}\right].$$

The conditional posterior distribution of η given W is

$$\eta|W \propto \left(\prod_{i=1}^{n} \omega_i\right)^{\eta-1} \eta^{n\eta} \frac{\exp(-\eta\sum_{i=1}^{n}\omega_i)}{\Gamma(\eta)^n} \pi_\eta(\eta),$$

that is, the conditional posterior distribution of η depends on the data only through W. The Metropolis–Hastings algorithm is implemented to evaluate the posterior distribution of η, where the acceptance rate is tuned to be around 25%. As mentioned before, a gamma distribution $\mathcal{G}(0.001, 0.001)$ is used as the prior $\pi_\eta(\cdot)$ for η in the following analysis.

The frailty ω_i is sampled as follows:

$$\omega_i|\Theta, D, \eta \sim \mathcal{G}\left(\eta + \sum_{j=1}^{m_i}\sum_{k=1}^{K} dN_{i,j,k}, \eta + \sum_{j=1}^{m_i}\sum_{k=1}^{K} \Delta_k\lambda_k \exp(\boldsymbol{x}_{i,j}^T\boldsymbol{\beta}_k)Y_{i,j,k}\right).$$

3 Bayesian Approach for Spatially Correlated Interval-Censored Data

Another common case in epidemiological and medical studies is to consider the correlation between observations based on geographic locations, *i.e.*, spatially correlated data.

3.1 Model Specification

Let $T_{i,j}$ denote the survival time for the jth subject in the ith cluster, where $i = 1, 2, \ldots, n$ and $j = 1, 2, \ldots, m_i$. Consider a Cox model with time-varying regression coefficients conditional on a Q-dimensional vector of covariates, $\mathbf{x}_{i,j}$, and the unobserved frailty random variable ω_i for the ith cluster. The hazard function can be written as

$$\lambda(t|\omega_i, \mathbf{x}_{i,j}) = \lambda_0(t) \exp(\mathbf{x}_{i,j}^T \beta(t) + \omega_i),$$

where $\lambda_0(.)$ is an unknown baseline hazard function common to all subjects, $\mathbf{x}_{i,j}$ is the $Q \times 1$ covariate vector for the jth subject in the ith cluster and $\beta(t)$ is the Q-dimensional regression coefficient function of main interest. The frailty ω_i can be either independent or correlated. Now, let us consider the model where $\beta(t)$ is time varying, $\omega_i{}'s$ are spatially correlated.

As shown in Sect. 2, the contribution of subject j in ith cluster to the observed data likelihood is

$$\Pr(T_{i,j} \in (L_{i,j}, R_{i,j}]|\omega_i, \mathbf{x}_{i,j}) = \Pr(T_{i,j} > L_{i,j}|\omega_i, \mathbf{x}_{i,j}) - \Pr(T_{i,j} > R_{i,j}|\omega_i, \mathbf{x}_{i,j}).$$

We assume that $\lambda_0(t)$ and $\beta(t)$ are left continuous step functions, where both the number and locations of the jumps are random and to be estimated. Let $k = 1, 2, \ldots, K$ denote all the ordered grids and $0 = \tau_0 < \tau_1 < \tau_2 < \ldots < \tau_K < \infty$ be the corresponding time points. Here we assume that the time points $(\tau_k, k = 1, 2, \ldots K)$ contain all potential jump points. The length of each time interval may be taken to be sufficiently small so that the hazard and coefficient functions can be appropriately estimated. Let $dN_{i,j,k}$ indicate whether or not the event time $T_{i,j}$ falls within the kth interval, i.e., $dN_{i,j,k} = 1(T_{i,j} \in (\tau_{k-1}, \tau_k])$. Let $Y_{i,j,k}$ be the at-risk variable defined as $Y_{i,j,l} = 1$ for $l < k$, $Y_{i,j,l} = 0$ for $l > k$, and $Y_{i,j,k} = (T_{i,j} - \tau_{k-1})/\Delta_k$ for $l = k$, where $\Delta_k = \tau_k - \tau_{k-1}$ is the width of the kth interval. Denote $\lambda_k = \lambda_0(\tau_k)$ and $\beta_k = \beta(\tau_k)$ as the baseline hazard function and the coefficient function evaluated at each time point. Thus, the augmented likelihood function for jth subject of ith cluster is

$$\ell_{i,j}\left(\Theta|\{dN_{i,j,k}, Y_{i,j,k}\}_{k=1}^{K}, \omega_i, \mathbf{x}_{i,j}\right)$$
$$= \prod_{k=1}^{K}\left\{\lambda_k \exp(\mathbf{x}_{i,j}^T\beta_k + \omega_i)\right\}^{dN_{i,j,k}} \exp\left\{-\Delta_k\lambda_k \exp(\mathbf{x}_{i,j}^T\beta_k + \omega_i)Y_{i,j,k}\right\},$$

where $i = 1, 2, \ldots, n$, $j = 1, 2, \ldots, m_i$, and $\Theta = \{\lambda_k, \beta_k, k = 1, 2, \ldots, K\}$. The conditional autoregressive (CAR) distribution is imposed for spatially correlated ω_i's. The general form of the CAR model is

$$\omega \propto \exp\left\{-\frac{1}{2}\omega^T\mathbf{V}\omega\right\},$$

where $\mathbf{V}$ is an $n \times n$ positive definite symmetric matrix. If we specify that $\mathbf{V}\cdot\mathbf{1} = \mathbf{0}$, then we get the intrinsic conditional autoregressive (ICAR) model [1]. Note that $\mathbf{V}$ is positive semi-definite, and the variance matrix $\mathbf{V}^{-1}$ no longer exists. An algebraic decomposition of the power term in CAR model is given by

$$\omega \propto \exp\left\{\frac{1}{2}\sum_{i<j}\mathbf{V}_{ij}(\omega_i - \omega_j)^2\right\}.$$

Since ω_i's are actually non-identifiable, in Bayesian implementation of this study, an identifying sum-to-zero constraint is imposed by centering the ω_i's around zero after each MCMC sampling iteration [3]. In practice, it is usually furthermore specified that $\mathbf{V} = \pi_\omega \cdot \mathbf{W}$, where π_ω is a precision parameter, $\mathbf{W}_{ii} = m_i$, $\mathbf{W}_{ij} = -1_{(i\sim j)}$, m_i is the number of neighbors for area i, and $i \sim j$ denotes that areas i and j are neighbors. Then we have

$$\omega \propto \exp\left\{-\frac{\pi_\omega}{2}\sum_{i<j}(\omega_i - \omega_j)^2 1_{(i\sim j)}\right\},$$

and it is also equivalent to

$$\omega_i|\omega_{-i} \sim \mathcal{N}(\bar{\omega}_{ii}, 1/(m_i\pi_\omega)),$$

where ω_{-i} is the set of all spatial frailties except the one for area i, $\bar{\omega}_{ii}$ is area i's neighbor mean of frailties, and $\mathcal{N}(\bar{\omega}_{ii}, 1/(m_i\pi_\omega))$ denotes a normal distribution with mean $\bar{\omega}_{ii}$ and variance $1/(m_i\pi_\omega)$. The conditional distribution above is to be used as a prior for ω_i in MCMC. Given π_ω, the prior for ω is as follows:

$$\omega \propto \pi_\omega^{(n-b)/2} \exp\left\{-\frac{\pi_\omega}{2}\sum_{i<j}(\omega_i - \omega_j)^2 1_{(i\sim j)}\right\},$$

where b is the number of disconnected groups of areas.

3.2 Prior Distributions

To simultaneously estimate time-varying coefficients and spatially correlated frailties, the specification of priors is shown as follows:

$$\begin{aligned}
\theta(s_1) &\sim \mathcal{N}(0, a_0\nu), \\
\theta(s_p)|\theta(s_{p-1}) &\sim \mathcal{N}(\theta(s_{p-1}), \nu), \qquad p = 2, 3, .., P, \\
\nu &\sim \mathcal{IG}(\alpha_0, \eta_0), \\
\omega_i|\omega_{-i} &\sim \mathcal{N}(\bar{\omega}_{ii}, 1/(m_i\pi_\omega)), \qquad i = 1, 2, \ldots, n, \\
\pi_\omega &\sim \mathcal{G}(0.01, 0.01).
\end{aligned}$$

The smoothness of $\theta(t)$ is also controlled by Markov-type process prior and reversible jump MCMC. The prior of frailties is based on ICAR model. The model can also be easily extended with other coefficient's priors with various degrees of smoothness or different frailties' priors to account for spatial correlation.

3.3 Posterior Inference

The posterior samples are obtained through MCMC sampling including a mixture of Gibbs sampling, Metropolis–Hastings, and the adaptive rejection algorithm. The computation is based on jth subject of the ith group observed in the kth time interval, where $i = 1, 2, \ldots, n$, $j = 1, 2, \ldots, m_i$, and $k = 1, 2 \ldots, K$. The parameters that need to be sampled include three parts: (1) the augmented event times T_{ij}'s, whose information is equivalent to those from our specially defined event indicator $dN_{i,j,k}$'s and at-risk variable $Y_{i,j,k}$'s; (2) the baseline λ_k, coefficients of covariates β_k; and (3) frailty terms ω_i's. Let $D = \{dN_{i,j,k}, Y_{i,j,k}\}$, $\Theta = \{\lambda_k, \beta_k\}$, and $\Omega = \{\omega_i\}$. The MCMC algorithm draws D, Θ and Ω iteratively.

3.3.1 Sample D

Since baseline hazards and regression coefficients are assumed to be piecewise constant, the sampling of augmented event time T_{ij} given Θ and Ω can be separated into two steps:

(1) Locate grid interval for each event time. For finite interval-censored subject j of ith group, event indicator $dN_{i,j,1}$,
$dN_{i,j,2}, \ldots, dN_{i,j,K}$ follows a multinomial distribution with size 1 and probability vector $(e_{i,j,1}, e_{i,j2}, \ldots, e_{i,j,K})$, where

$$e_{i,j,k} = \frac{p_{i,j,k}\mathbb{1}(\tau_k \in (L_{i,j}, R_{i,j}])}{\sum_{s_l \in (L_{i,j}, R_{i,j}]} p_{i,j,l}},$$

$$p_{i,j,k} = \begin{cases} \exp\left\{-\sum_{l=1}^{k-1} \Delta_l \lambda_l \exp(\mathbf{x}_{i,j}^T \beta_k + \omega_i)\right\} & \\ \quad - \exp\left\{-\sum_{l=1}^{k} \Delta_l \lambda_l \exp(\mathbf{x}_{i,j}^T \beta_k + \omega_i)\right\} & \text{if } k > 1 \\ 1 - \exp\left\{-\Delta_1 \lambda_1 \exp(\mathbf{x}_{i,j}^T \beta_1 + \omega_i)\right\} & \text{if } k = 1, \end{cases}$$

for $k = 1, 2, \ldots, K$. Thus, if the observed interval $(L_{i,j}, R_{i,j}]$ covers only one time grid τ_k, then $dN_{i,j,k} = 1$ and all other event indicators equal 0. Otherwise, if $(L_{i,j}, R_{i,j}]$ covers multiple time grids τ_k's, $dN_{i,j,k}$ is sampled from a multinomial distribution with probability vector calculated based on these covered time grids τ_k's. In other words, the time grid $(\tau_{k-1}, \tau_k]$ with $dN_{i,j,k} = 1$ is sampled in this step.

(2) Within selected time grids, the exact time $T_{i,j}$ follows a doubly truncated exponential distribution on $(\tau_{k-1}, \tau_k]$ with a distribution function

$$F(u) = \frac{1 - \exp\{-\lambda_k (u - \tau_{k-1}) \exp(\mathbf{x}_{i,j}^T \beta_k) + \omega_i\}}{1 - \exp\{-\lambda_k \Delta_k \exp(\mathbf{x}_{i,j}^T \beta_k + \omega_i)\}}.$$

Then $T_{i,j}$ will be sampled by an inverse distribution method, and $Y_{i,j,k}$ can be computed based on the aforementioned definition.

3.3.2 Sample Θ

This step is to sample each component of the baseline hazards and regression coefficients, given D and Ω. Suppose that $\beta(t)$ is time dependent, $\theta(t)$ is used to denote log baseline $\log(\lambda(t))$ and one element of $\beta(t)$. Reversible jump MCMC algorithm is applied here because the number of jumps P is random, and the dimension of posterior distribution could vary from iteration to iteration. The probability of taking a birth, death, and update move is set as 0.3, 0.3, and 0.4, respectively. For the update move, both P and jump times are fixed. The conditional posterior distribution of $\theta(s_p)$ given D, Ω and all other components in Θ is

$$(\theta(s_p)|\Theta/\{\theta(s_p)\}, D, \Omega) \propto \exp\left\{-\frac{(\theta(s_p) - \mu_p)^2}{2\sigma_p^2}\right\}$$
$$\times \exp\left\{-\sum_{i=1}^{n}\sum_{j=1}^{m_i}\sum_{k=1}^{K} \mathbb{1}(\tau_k \in (s_{p-1}, s_p])\Delta_k \lambda_k \exp(\mathbf{x}_{i,j}^T \beta_k + \omega_i) Y_{i,j,k}\right\},$$

for some jump time s_p. The steps for computing μ_p and σ_p^2 follow Wang et al. [28]. Since it can be shown that the above function is log-concave, an adaptive rejection algorithm [9] can also be applied to sample $\theta(s_p)$. For the birth move, a new jump time s' is "born" in this move. This new s' is randomly selected from non-jump time grids. In the death move, one of the current jump times s_p is removed, where the index p is uniformly selected from the current jump point set $\{1, 2, \ldots, P-1\}$. Details of the birth move and death move can be found in Zhang and Zhang [30].

3.3.3 Sample Ω

Suppose ω_i's are spatially correlated, the conditional posterior distribution takes the form

$$(\omega_i|\Theta, D, \pi_\omega, \omega_{-i}) \propto$$

$$\prod_{j=1}^{m_i}\prod_{k=1}^{K}\{\lambda_k \exp(\mathbf{x}_{i,j}^T\beta_k + \omega_i\}^{dN_{i,j,k}} \exp\{-\Delta_k\lambda_k \exp(\mathbf{x}_{i,j}^T\beta_k + \omega_i)Y_{i,j,k}\}\pi(\omega_i|\omega_{-i}),$$

where $\pi(\omega_i|\omega_{-i})$ denotes the prior in Sect. 3.2. Metropolis–Hastings algorithm can be applied to sample ω_i's. The precision parameter π_ω is sampled from $\mathcal{G}(0.01 + \frac{n-b}{2}, 0.01 + \frac{1}{2}\sum_{i<j}(\omega_i - \omega_j)^2\mathbf{1}_{(i\sim j)})$.

4 Illustrative Examples

In this section, two examples are provided to illustrate the methods introduced in the previous sections.

4.1 Dental Health Data

The dental health data from the Signal Tandmobiel project was conducted in Flanders (Belgium) to examine the oral health condition of Flemish primary schoolchildren. The children were divided into 15 strata, a combination of 3 educational systems (public, municipal, or private) and 5 provinces. Over 6000 children were recruited, which represented approximately 7% of the total target population in Flanders [27]. A total of 4468 of them were randomized and examined annually by 16 trained dentists using the standardized and widely accepted criteria recommended by the WHO. We focus on the time to the emergence of permanent tooth 24 (central incisor) in this chapter.

For the analysis, we considered the covariate *dmf* as a dichotomized variable that denotes the status of the primary predecessor of this tooth (0 = sound, 1 = decayed, missing, or filled). A random effect of province-by-gender was considered. Frailty is assumed to follow a gamma distribution with an equal shape and scale parameter η, which has a gamma hyper-prior $\mathcal{G}(0.001, 0.001)$. A total of 12,000 Gibbs samples was generated with a burn-in period of 2000 samples. The convergence of MCMC chains was checked by trace plots, autocorrelation plots, and Geweke's statistics.

Figure 1 presents the analysis results by applying the proposed method in Sect. 2. As tooth 24 does not emerge before age 5, the time scale in Fig. 1 is the time in years since age 5. The results include the point estimates and the corresponding 95% credible intervals. The positive estimate indicates that the children with a decayed primary predecessor have higher risks than those without, which is consistent with the results based on the iterative convex minorant algorithm Gòmez et al. [10]. However, there is an obvious trend of the coefficient estimate, and the effect becomes weaker over time. If the 95% credible interval includes 0, then one may conclude that the parameter is not significantly different from 0, and thus the effect is said to be statistically insignificant. As shown in Fig. 1, the credible interval of the *dmf* effect after "Year 11" contains 0, which indicates that the *dmf* effect becomes insignificant. Table 1 shows the frailty estimates. In general, girls have higher risk than boys. Specifically, in Antwerpen and Limburg, the two provinces in the north and adjacent to the Netherlands, the difference between girls and boys is larger than that in Vlaams Brabant and West Vlaanderen, the two provinces in the middle

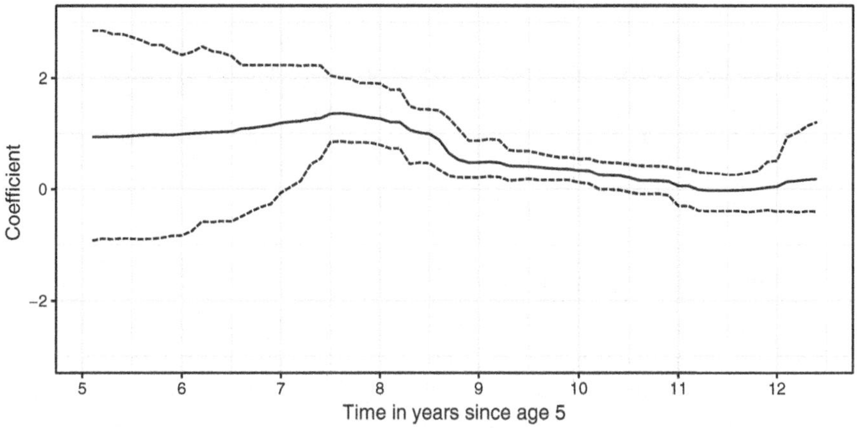

Fig. 1 Estimate of coefficients in children's dental health data. The black solid line is the posterior mean. The black dashed lines are 95% credible intervals

Table 1 Estimate of frailties with 95% credible intervals in the children's dental health data

	Antwerpen	Limburg	Oost Vlaanderen
Girls	1.18 (1.02, 1.35)	1.08 (0.92, 1.25)	1.19 (1.02, 1.36)
Boys	0.84 (0.72, 0.96)	0.81 (0.68, 0.93)	0.91 (0.78, 1.05)
	Vlaams Brabant	West Vlaanderen	
Girls	1.16 (0.98, 1.35)	1.06 (0.89, 1.23)	
Boys	0.93 (0.79, 1.08)	0.87 (0.73, 1.00)	

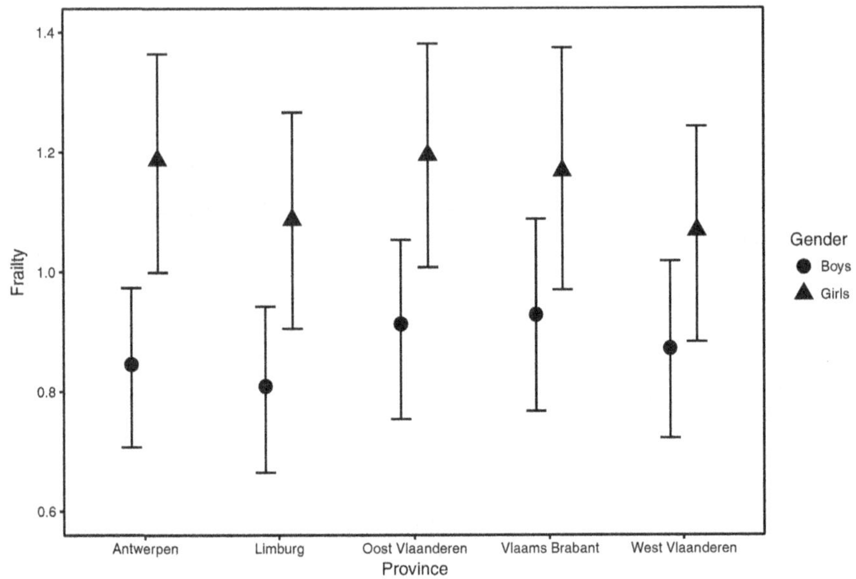

Fig. 2 Estimate of frailties with 95% credible intervals in the children's dental health data

of Belgium. Moreover, boys in Vlaams Brabant, where the capital city, Brussels, is located, have the highest risk compared to boys in other provinces (Fig. 2). The data can be found at https://www.tandfonline.com/doi/full/10.1080/01621459.2017.1356316 under "Supplemental" and the computational code is available from authors upon request.

4.2 Smoking Cessation Data

We applied the method in Sect. 3 on an aforementioned smoking cessation data. More details about the data can be found in Murray et al. [21]. In the full sample, a total of 5887 adult smokers were followed for 5 years. In this analysis, the event of interest is the time to smoking relapse, which is defined as the time from quitting to resuming smoking. Thus, a subset of 223 participants are included here who are known to have quit smoking at least once during the study period and have an identifiable Minnesota zip code of residence. The outcome of interest is the time to smoking relapse, which is interval censored since the subjects were only monitored at annual visits. The time scale has the study entry time as origin and the maximum of 5 years. The time to smoking relapse in this particular data set is either interval censored (64/223 or 29%) or right censored (159/223 or 71%). Two covariates are considered: gender (0 = Male, 1 = Female) and treatment (0 = usual care [UC]

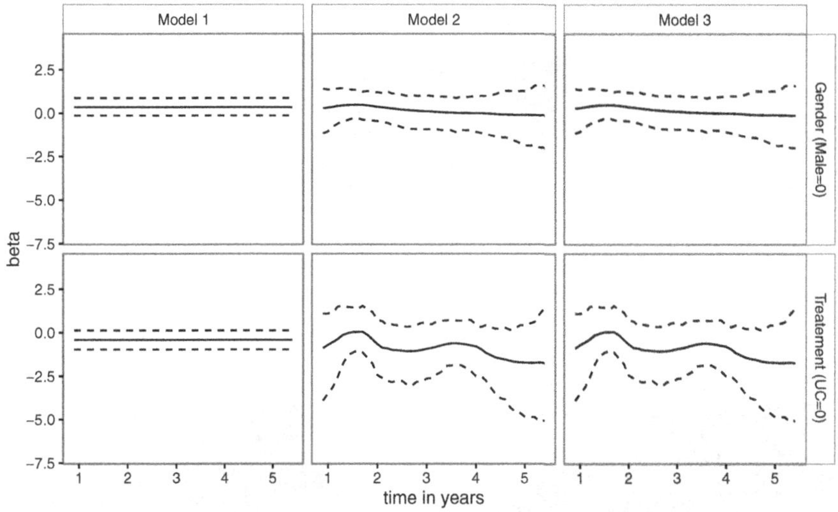

Fig. 3 Estimate of coefficients for smoking cessation data. Black solid line is posterior mean. Black dashed lines are 95% credible intervals. The effect difference in reducing relapse risk between smoking intervention and usual care is much smaller for the time around the two peaks (1.8 years and 3.8 years) than neighbor time periods

group that received no special antismoking intervention, 1 = smoking intervention [SI] group). Subjects from the same zip code area are treated as a spatial cluster.

Three models were used to fit the data to demonstrate the time-varying coefficients as shown below:

$$\text{Model 1} : \beta\ (t) \text{ is constant, } \omega_i\text{'s are spatially correlated.}$$
$$\text{Model 2} : \beta\ (t) \text{ is time varying, } \omega_i\text{'s are independent.}$$
$$\text{Model 3} : \beta\ (t) \text{ is time varying, } \omega_i\text{'s are spatially correlated.}$$

We ran 55,000 MCMC iterations, and the first 5000 iterations were discarded as the burn-in period. In Models 2 and 3, hyperparameter a_0 is fixed at 100 so that the coefficient for the first time grid is assigned a flat prior. The estimated coefficients with 95% credible intervals for all three models are presented in Fig. 3. From Model 1, the coefficient on gender (β_{gender}) has a posterior mean of 0.343 and 95% credible interval $(-0.175, 0.845)$, and the coefficient on treatment ($\beta_{\text{treatment}}$) has a posterior mean of -0.433 and 95% credible interval $(-0.991, 0.116)$. Although the credible intervals cover zero, the posterior means show that women are more likely to relapse than men, and smoking intervention is effective in reducing relapse risk. For Models 2 and 3, the coefficient for gender is close to a straight line, from which we can conclude that the effect is constant over time. However, the coefficient of treatment exhibits obvious trend, suggesting that the inference based on Model 1 could be misleading. Models 2 and 3 have similar trends for the estimates: it increases from a

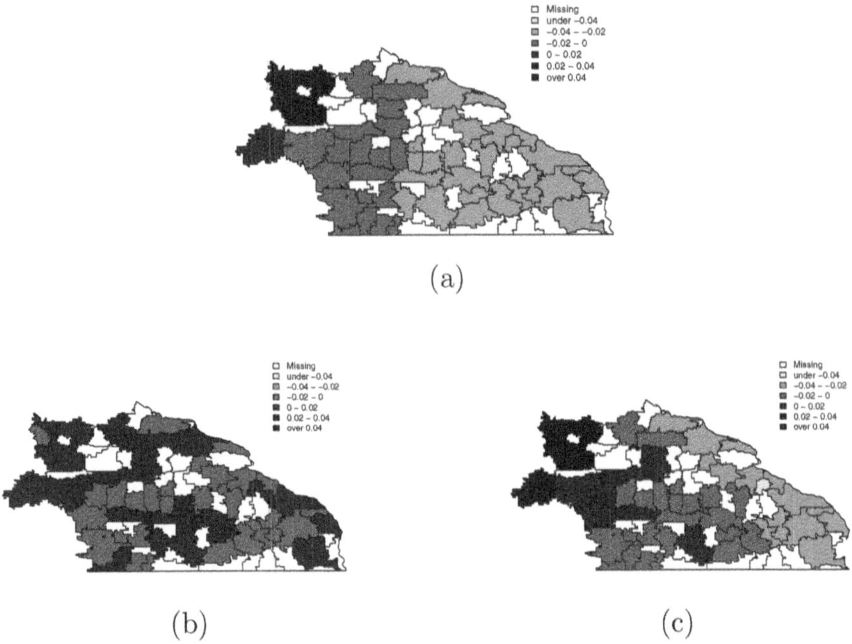

Fig. 4 Maps of posterior means for the spatial frailties ω_i over 51 zip code areas in southeast Minnesota based on Models 1, 2, and 3. The white areas are those zip codes without data

negative value to about zero around 1.8 years and then gradually approaches to -1 between Year 2 and Year 3. After that, the trend reaches the second peak around 3.8 years and ends with a downward curve.

Figure 4 maps the posterior means of spatial frailties (ω_i) for the smoking data using Models 3. It reveals that a few higher values of ω_i's occur in the northwest region, which happens to be close to the southern suburbs of Minneapolis. This indicates that higher risks of smoking relapse were observed in those regions. The LMPL from Model 3 (-200.8) is larger than LPML from Model 1 (-202.7) and Model 2 (-205.4), which indicates that Model 3 has better performance. The data can be found in Appendix, and the computational code is available from authors upon request.

5 Discussion and Remarks

Interval-censored survival data has been studied for decades. Examples of interval-censored data can be found in De Gruttola and Lagakos [4], Jewell et al. [15], Kim et al. [16], Sun [25], Shiboski and Jewell [23], Diamond et al. [5], Finkelstein [7],

Finkelstein andWolfe [8], Hoel and Walburg [13], Self and Grossman [22], Sun and Kalbfleisch [26], which discussed interval-censored data in AIDS, demographic, epidemiology, and medical science. In recent years, researchers have become interested in time-varying coefficients in time-to-event data. For example, several methods have been introduced for right-censored data, such as the partial likelihood approach in [31], histogram sieve procedures in [12], and the one-step estimation procedure for the cumulative parameter function in Martinussen and Scheike [19], Martinussen et al. [20]. Time-varying coefficients for interval-censored data, however, are much less developed. Kneib [18] introduced an extended geoadditive Cox model that estimates the nonlinear effects of covariates based on penalized splines. Sinha et al.[24] treated the unobserved exact time as latent variables and sampled from the full conditional posterior distribution via Gibbs sampling. The estimated curves in these approaches depend on a fixed number of knots, and the smoothness of the curves is controlled by the prior distribution or penalizing the difference between adjacent regression coefficients. In some recent studies, the reversible jump Markov chain Monte Carlo (MCMC) algorithm Green [11] was used for automatic knot selection. Kim et al.[17] used such an algorithm for a dynamic baseline hazard function. Wang et al. [28] proposed a Bayesian extension of the Cox model by applying an efficient reversible jump MCMC and putting dynamics on all coefficients as well as the baseline hazard, which were specified as piecewise constants. Zhang and Zhang [30] extended the Bayesian approach to spatially correlated interval-censored data.

In this chapter, Bayesian approaches for clustered interval-censored data and spatially correlated interval-censored data were discussed using Cox regression model with time-varying covariate effects. In order to capture the temporal nature of covariate effects more precisely, we have shown that it is important to consider the dependence structure for clustered outcomes. An important step in this procedure is to determine the number of jumps, which will affect the estimated smoothness of the estimated curves as well as effectiveness assessment. To this end, reversible jump MCMC was used to automatically select jumps during model fitting. The regression coefficients and the baseline hazard are piecewise constant and can be estimated, given the number of pieces and jump locations. A dynamic prior was specified to capture the time-varying coefficients.

The methods can be easily extended to other regression models or frailties' correlations. However, there are a few challenges with the current model. An immediate one is that the parametric assumption on frailties may not be valid. Nonparametric priors may be needed to relax the parametric assumption. In this chapter, Cox regression model was considered, and we may also think about other alternatives when Cox model assumptions are violated, such as proportional odds model, etc. Another future work direction could be multivariate or high-dimensional interval-censored data, which have a more complicated data structure.

References

1. Besag, J., Kooperberg, C.: On conditional and intrinsic autoregressions. Biometrika **82**(4), 733–746 (1995)
2. Brezger, A., Lang, S.: Generalized structured additive regression based on Bayesian P-splines. Comput. Stat. Data Anal. **50**(4), 967–991 (2006)
3. Carlin, B.P., Louis, T.A.: Bayes and empirical Bayes methods for data analysis. Stat. Comput. **7**(2), 153–154 (1997)
4. De Gruttola, V., Lagakos, S.W.: Analysis of doubly-censored survival data, with application to AIDS. Biometrics **45**, 1–11 (1989)
5. Diamond, I.D., McDonald, J.W., Shah, I.H.: Proportional hazards models for current status data: application to the study of differentials in age at weaning in Pakistan. Demography **23**(4), 607–620 (1986)
6. Fahrmeir, L., Lang, S.: Bayesian semiparametric regression analysis of multicategorical time-space data. Ann. Inst. Stat. Math. **53**(1), 11–30 (2001)
7. Finkelstein, D.M.: A proportional hazards model for interval-censored failure time data. Biometrics **42**, 845–854 (1986)
8. Finkelstein, D.M., Wolfe, R.A.: A semiparametric model for regression analysis of interval-censored failure time data. Biometrics **41**, 933–945 (1985)
9. Gilks, W.R., Wild, P.: Adaptive rejection sampling for Gibbs sampling. Appl. Stat. **41**, 337–348 (1992)
10. Gómez, G., Calle, M.L., Oller, R., Langohr, K.: Tutorial on methods for interval-censored data and their implementation in R. Stat. Model. **9**(4), 259–297 (2009)
11. Green, P.J.: Reversible jump Markov chain Monte Carlo computation and Bayesian model determination. Biometrika **82**(4), 711–732 (1995)
12. Higle, J.L., Sen, S.: Stochastic decomposition: an algorithm for two-stage linear programs with recourse. Math. Oper. Res. **16**(3), 650–669 (1991)
13. Hoel, D.G., Walburg, H.: Statistical analysis of survival experiments. J. Nat. Cancer Inst. **49**(2), 361–372 (1972)
14. Ibrahim, J.G., Chen, M.-H., Sinha, D.: Bayesian Survival Analysis. Wiley, London (2005)
15. Jewell, N.P., Malani, H.M., Vittinghoff, E.: Nonparametric estimation for a form of doubly censored data, with application to two problems in AIDS. J. Am. Stat. Assoc. **89**(425), 7–18 (1994)
16. Kim, M.Y., De Gruttola, V.G., Lagakos, S.W.: Analyzing doubly censored data with covariates, with application to AIDS. Biometrics **49**, 13–22 (1993)
17. Kim, S., Chen, M.-H., Dey, D.K., Gamerman, D.: Bayesian dynamic models for survival data with a cure fraction. Lifetime Data Anal. **13**(1), 17–35 (2007)
18. Kneib, T.: Mixed model based inference in structured additive regression. Ph.D. Thesis, LMU (2006)
19. Martinussen, T., Scheike, T.H.: A flexible additive multiplicative hazard model. Biometrika **89**(2), 283–298 (2002)
20. Martinussen, T., Scheike, T.H., Skovgaard, I.M.: Efficient estimation of fixed and time-varying covariate effects in multiplicative intensity models. Scand. J. Stat. **29**(1), 57–74 (2002)
21. Murray, R.P., Anthonisen, N.R., Connett, J.E., Wise, R.A., Lindgren, P.G., Greene, P.G., Nides, M.A., Group, L.H.S.R., et al.: Effects of multiple attempts to quit smoking and relapses to smoking on pulmonary function. J. Clin. Epidemiol. **51**(12), 1317–1326 (1998)
22. Self, S.G., Grossman, E.A.: Linear rank tests for interval-censored data with application to PCB levels in adipose tissue of transformer repair workers. Biometrics **42**, 521–530 (1986)
23. Shiboski, S.C., Jewell, N.P.: Statistical analysis of the time dependence of HIV infectivity based on partner study data. J. Am. Stat. Assoc. **87**(418), 360–372 (1992)
24. Sinha, D., Chen, M.-H., Ghosh, S.K.: Bayesian analysis and model selection for interval-censored survival data. Biometrics **55**, 585–590 (1999)

25. Sun, J.: A non-parametric test for interval-censored failure time data with application to AIDS studies. Stat. Med. **15**(13), 1387–1395 (1996)
26. Sun, J., Kalbfleisch, J.D.: Nonparametric tests of tumor prevalence data. Biometrics **52**, 726–731 (1996)
27. Vanobbergen, J., Martens, L., Lesaffre, E., Declerck, D.: The signal-Tandmobiel project a longitudinal intervention health promotion study in Flanders (Belgium): baseline and first year results. Eur. J. Paediatr. Dent. **2**, 87–96 (2000)
28. Wang, X., Chen, M.-H., Yan, J.: Bayesian dynamic regression models for interval censored survival data with application to children dental health. Lifetime Data Anal. **19**(3), 297–316 (2013)
29. Zhang, Y., Wang, X., Zhang, B.: Bayesian approach for clustered interval-censored data with time-varying covariate effects. Stat. Interface **12**(3), 457–465 (2019)
30. Zhang, Y., Zhang, B.: Semiparametric spatial model for interval-censored data with time-varying covariate effects. Comput. Stat. Data Anal. **123**(C), 146–156 (2018)
31. Zucker, D.M., Karr, A.F.: Nonparametric survival analysis with time-dependent covariate effects: a penalized partial likelihood approach. Ann. Stat. **18**, 329–353 (1990)

Bayesian Approach for Joint Modeling Longitudinal Data and Survival Data Simultaneously in Public Health Studies

Ding-Geng Chen, Yuhlong Lio, and Jeffrey R. Wilson

Abstract This chapter is aimed to overview the joint modeling through the harmonization of longitudinal data and time-to-event data with a Bayesian approach. We considered a randomized clinical trial in which both longitudinal data and survival data were collected to compare the efficacy and the safety of two antiretroviral drugs in treating patients who had failed or were intolerant of zidovudine (AZT) therapy. Using these data, we demonstrated the advantages of the Bayesian joint modeling over the classical approach of separately analyzing these types of data with Cox proportional hazard model and longitudinal linear mixed-effects model. We found that the Bayesian joint modeling can better address information loss on outcome-dependent missingness, which can preserve information from both longitudinal data and time-to-event data. The Bayesian joint modeling can produce unbiased estimates and retain higher statistical power for public health data analysis.

1 Introduction

In public health studies, we often collect different types of outcome data (i.e., responses) from each patient to address complex time-related research questions. A typical example is when researchers wish to assess the trajectories of time-varying phenomena (such as CD4 counts in HIV patients' progression over multiple years) and their connections to the time at which an event of particular interest

D.-G. Chen (✉)
College of Health Solutions, Arizona State University, Phoenix, AZ, USA

Department of Statistics, University of Pretoria, Pretoria, South Africa
e-mail: dinchen@asu.edu

Y. Lio
Department of Mathematical Sciences, University of South Dakota, Vermillion, SD, USA

J. R. Wilson
Department of Economics, Arizona State University, Phoenix, AZ, USA

Y. Lio et al. (eds.), *Bayesian Inference and Computation in Reliability and Survival Analysis*, Emerging Topics in Statistics and Biostatistics,
https://doi.org/10.1007/978-3-030-88658-5_16

occurred (e.g., death due to AIDS or dropout from the study). Traditionally, these different responses are often analyzed separately with a mixed-effects model (such as random-intercept and random-slope models) to estimate the longitudinal trends response, and a Cox-type survival model to analyze the time-to-event data (e.g., AIDS-related death, or censoring due to dropout and termination of study) to determine the hazard ratios [2, 23].

However, this traditional approach of analyzing the data independently has at least three potential problems. First, separate analyses of the responses fail to realize practical aspects of real-world situation, as it assumes that HIV patients' CD4 trajectories necessarily evolve in isolation from eventual AIDS-related death and censoring status. Second, separate analyses on a single outcome risks information loss from the other outcome response, resulting in biased and inefficient estimation of any intervention effectiveness [16]. Third, analysis of longitudinal outcomes handles missing values inaccurately when the analysis fails to incorporate available time-to-event data [2]. An optimal remedy to these challenges is to simultaneously model these responses using a joint-modeling approach. It produces more efficient estimates of treatment and intervention effectiveness.

Beginning in the early 1990s, HIV/AIDS clinical trials spurred the application of joint models in applied research because of the urgency to simultaneously understand the progression of CD4 lymphocyte count and its effect on patients' survival [10, 11, 18]. In recent times, clinical trials and observational studies widely use joint models. The increased usage is mainly due to advancements in statistical modeling techniques, the development of open-source software [13], and the fact that joint models provide "more powerful, accurate, efficient, and robust estimations" ([23], p. 1) compared to the classical approach of separate Cox and mixed-effect modeling [16, 17, 26]. Notwithstanding their increased use in health research, joint models are still emerging in statistical and biostatistical modeling.

This chapter is then aimed to further stimulate interest in joint modeling and to increase its application by providing an overview of the approach and its merits. A demonstration on how to use the approach to analyze data from public health clinical trials and intervention studies when longitudinal and time-to-event data is made available. To demonstrate the application in real-world public health settings, we re-analyze classical data from an HIV/AIDS study publicly available and used by many authors such as Goldman et al. [12] and Guo and Carlin [13].

2 Data and Preliminary Data Analysis

In this study, both longitudinal data and survival data were collected to compare the efficacy and safety of two antiretroviral drugs in treating patients who had failed or were intolerant of zidovudine (AZT) therapy. In these data sets, 467 HIV-infected patients met entry conditions (either an AIDS diagnosis or two CD4 counts of 300 or fewer, and fulfilling specific criteria for AZT intolerance or failure). The patients were randomly assigned to receive either didanosine (ddI) or zalcitabine (ddC). CD4 counts were recorded at study entry, and again at the 2-, 6-, 12-, and 18-month visits. The times to death were also recorded.

The longitudinal CD4 data is available in R library *JMbayes* as a built-in data frame named "*aids*" with 1408 observations on the following nine variables. The nine variables are (1) "patient" as patients identifier for a total of 467 patients, (2) "Time" as the time-to-death or censoring, (3) "death" as censoring indicator with 0 denoting censoring and 1 death, (4) "CD4" as the CD4 measure which is square-root transformed CD4 cells count to linearize the relationship between the CD4 measures and the associated "obstime", (5) "obstime" as the time points at which the CD4 cells count was recorded, (6) "drug" as a factor with levels *ddC* denoting zalcitabine and *ddI* denoting didanosine, (7) "gender" as a factor with levels *female* and *male*, (8) "prevOI" as a factor with levels *AIDS* denoting previous opportunistic infection (AIDS diagnosis) at study entry, and *noAIDS* denoting no previous infection, (9) "AZT" as a factor with levels *intolerance* and *failure* denoting AZT intolerance and AZT failure, respectively. Table 1 provides a sample of the data format from the first three patients with ten measures. For example, the first patient was censored (i.e., not dead with death = 0) at "Time" of 16.97 months. Patient #1 was observed at baseline, 6-month, and 12-month with the square root of CD4 counts of 10.68, 8.43, and 9.43, respectively. Patient #1 (gender is "male") was randomly assigned to "drug" of zalcitabine (i.e., ddC). Patient #1 previous opportunistic infected ("prevOI") and diagnosed with AIDS at study entry and was AZT *intolerance.*

For survival analysis, the first row of each patient in this data was selected to build a new data frame "*aids.id*", which has 467 rows for the 467 patients.

We illustrate the longitudinal trend of the CD4 measure by plotting a line graph for each of these 467 patients as shown in Fig. 1. In Fig. 1, the baseline CD4 measures are ranged from 0 to 20 with a similar range at 2-, 6-, 12-, and 18-month visits (i.e., "obstime"). An examination of the trend for each patient reveals that there is a reasonable linear relationship between CD4 measure and "obstime". These linear relations suggest different intercepts and different slopes across the 467

Table 1 Data format from the first three patients

Patient	Time	Death	CD4	obstime	Drug	Gender	prevOI	AZT
1	16.97	0	10.68	0	ddC	Male	AIDS	Intolerance
1	16.97	0	8.43	6	ddC	Male	AIDS	Intolerance
1	16.97	0	9.43	12	ddC	Male	AIDS	Intolerance
2	19.00	0	6.32	0	ddI	Male	noAIDS	Intolerance
2	19.00	0	8.12	6	ddI	Male	noAIDS	Intolerance
2	19.00	0	4.58	12	ddI	Male	noAIDS	Intolerance
2	19.00	0	5.00	18	ddI	Male	noAIDS	Intolerance
3	18.53	1	3.46	0	ddI	Female	AIDS	Intolerance
3	18.53	1	3.61	2	ddI	Female	AIDS	Intolerance
3	18.53	1	6.16	6	ddI	Female	AIDS	Intolerance

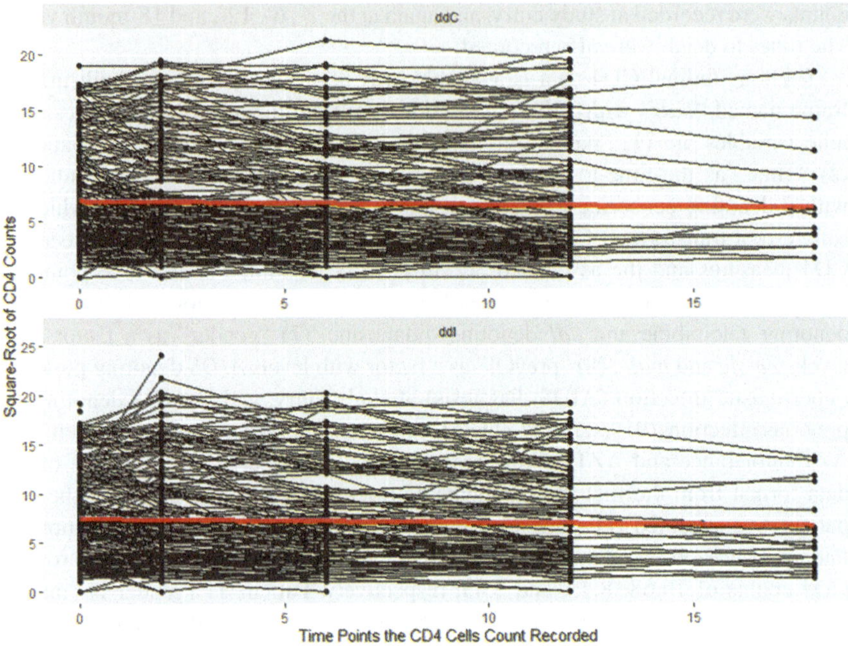

Fig. 1 Longitudinal trends for CD4 measures (square-root transformed CD4 counts) for the two drug treatments

patients. This relation suggests a linear mixed-effects model with random intercepts and random slopes to analyze the CD4 longitudinal measure data. In addition, there are missing values due to death and dropouts. There are information for 467 patients at baseline, for 368 patients at 2 months, for 310 patients at 6 months, for 226 patients at 12 months, and only for 34 patients at 18 months. These missing values are mostly missing not at random (MNAR) due to death and dropout and thus typical multiple imputation techniques cannot be directly applied. These longitudinal data should be analyzed with the survival model (i.e., "Time" to death or censoring) simultaneously with a joint-modeling framework.

3 Statistical Models

The development of joint modeling is to link time-dependent longitudinal observations (i.e., CD4 counts) time-to-event (i.e., time-to-death due to AIDS) to simultaneously assess drug effects in HIV patients. The impact of the joint modeling is motivated by the goal to produce a more efficient estimate than the separate modeling the continuous response or the time-to-event, as the longitudinal observations are time-dependent and measured with error as dropouts are missing not at random.

In the following subsections, an illustration of the use of joint modeling using AIDS data with three competing models are presented: (a) separate analysis of longitudinal continuous data on CD4 measures, (b) separate analysis of survival data on time-to-death due to HIV/AIDS, and (c) joint modeling of longitudinal continuous data and the analysis of survival data. We then present and juxtapose the three models' results to highlight the superiority of the joint model over the classical longitudinal continuous data model and survival data model in dealing with outcome-dependent missingness and retention of both longitudinal continuous data and survival data.

3.1 Separate Modeling of Longitudinal Continuous Data

The trend of the CD4 over time trajectories consists of $n = 467$ in the AIDS study. The observed response for patient i at time t is denoted by $y_i(t)$, $i = 1, \ldots$ n; and $t = 1, \ldots T_i$. These observed responses are continuous in nature where

$$y_i(t) = m_i(t) + \epsilon_i(t),$$

with $m_i(t)$ represents the true mean at time t for patient i, and $\epsilon_i(t)$ represents the random error, which is assumed to be $N(0, \sigma^2)$. The true mean, $m_i(t)$, is defined in a linear mixed-effects model as $x_i'(t)\beta + z_i'(t)b_i$ where

$$y_i(t) = m_i(t) + \epsilon_i(t) = x_i'(t)\beta + z_i'(t)b_i + \epsilon_i(t). \tag{1}$$

In Eq. (1), $x_i'(t)\beta$ is the fixed-effects component linked to the unknown fixed-effects parameter, β (e.g., such as drug effectiveness) and $z_i'(t)b_i$ is the between-patient random-effects component with a parameter of b_i. This mixed-effects model is common among public health researchers who model longitudinal continuous data. Such mixed-effects models are available in several R packages, primarily *nlme* [19] and *lme4* [1]. Extensive literature exists on model specifications and parameter estimation in mixed-effects models using the maximum likelihood estimation [13–15]. The syntax used to compute the linear mixed-effects model in the R statistical programming language and computing environment is as follows:

```
R> lmeFit.aids = lme(CD4 ~ obstime + drug, random = ~ obstime |patient, data
   = aids)
R> summary(lmeFit.aids)
```

3.2 Separate Modeling of Time-to-Event Data

In modeling the time-to-event data (time-to-death due to AIDS), let T_i denote the observed time ("Time" in Table 1) for the ith patient; δ_i ("death" in Table 1) is the censoring indicator that takes the value 1 if the patient is dead and 0 if otherwise. Therefore, the observed time-to-event data consist of the pairs $\{(T_i, \delta_i), i = 1, \ldots n\}$. The typical statistical approach to modeling time-to-event data is to use survival model with Cox proportional hazards regression [9], where the hazard function $[h(t)]$ consists of two parts. The first part focuses on the underlying baseline hazard function $[h_0(t)]$ to describe how the risk of event (death due to AIDS) per time unit changes over time at baseline levels of the covariates. The second part of the effect parameters, γ, describes how the hazard varies in response to explanatory covariates, w (drug effect and other covariates, etc.) where:

$$h\left(t|w\right) = h_0(t)\exp\left(w' \gamma\right). \tag{2}$$

The computation around this model can be obtained in R with the *survival* package [25]. The R code used for this Cox proportional hazards regression is:

R> survFit.aids = coxph(Surv(Time, death) ~ drug, x = TRUE, data = aids.id)
R> summary(survFit.aids)

3.3 Joint (Simultaneous) Modeling of Longitudinal Continuous Data and Time-to-Event Data

A joint model is proposed to address the effect on CD4 data simultaneous with the time-to-death due to HIV/AIDS. The joint modeling consists of the longitudinal continuous outcome, $y_i(t)$, for patient i at time t in Eq. (1) and the time-to-event data (T_i, δ_i), based on the hazard ratio in Eq. (2). The standard approach to achieve this joint modeling is to extend the hazard risk model in Eq. (2) to incorporate the history of longitudinal outcome from the time of enrollment to the time the child achieves permanency, which is denoted as $\Updownarrow(t) = \{m(u), 0 \leq u < t\}$, Therneau and Grambsch [24]. Thus, the full joint model is

$$h\left(t|\Updownarrow(t), w\right) = h_0(t)\exp\left(w' \gamma + \alpha m_i(t)\right). \tag{3}$$

The extra parameter α in Eq. (3) quantifies the effect of the underlying longitudinal CD4 outcome on the risk of death for every additional unit increase in the CD4 measure. In the R program output, the α parameter is labeled *Assoct*.

Parameter estimation on this joint modeling can be obtained using a semiparametric maximum likelihood estimation method [14, 15, 27], and implemented by Rizopoulos' [20, 21] with the R *JM* package.

A Bayesian perspective to estimate the parameters in the joint modeling was implemented by Rizopoulos [22] in his R package *JMbayes* for fitting the joint models under a Bayesian approach using Markov Chain Monte Carlo (MCMC) algorithms. This R package is useful in fitting a wide range of joint models both for longitudinal continuous and categorical responses. Under the Bayesian approach, the posterior distribution of the model parameters is derived under the assumptions that given the random effects both the longitudinal and event time process are assumed independent, and the longitudinal responses of each subject are assumed to be independent. The detailed theoretical derivation is illustrated by Rizopoulos [22]. In this chapter, we use the *JMbayes* package and the following syntax to demonstrate the joint model for the CD4 longitudinal continuous responses and the time-to-death for HIV/AIDS response for patients:

```
R> jointFit.aids <- jointModelBayes(lmeFit.aids, survFit.aids, timeVar =
   "obstime")
R> summary(jointFit.aids)
```

This R code runs MCMC for 20,000 iterations but can be changed to any other number of iterations for better convergence for the joint model with the R objects from executing the R codes for the linear mixed effects (i.e., *lmeFit.aids*) and Cox proportional hazards models (i.e., *survFit.aids*).

4 Results

4.1 Results from Separate Linear Mixed-Effects Model on CD4 Longitudinal Data

To analyze the longitudinal continuous CD4 data, an examination of the graphical relation between the CD4 measure and the number of months was made. Figure 1 shows that the CD4 measures have no easily determined pattern: Some patients have increasing CD4 measure, some have decreasing measure, and others have more no fixed pattern. However, a linear trend seemed reasonable, so we used the linear mixed-effects (LME) model in (1) with the R package *nlme* to investigate the longitudinal CD4 trend along with the observed time in months from the baseline to 18 months.

In using model selection to identify the best longitudinal model for these data, we fit four models:

- Model 1: random-intercept LME with interaction between "obstime" and "drug".
- Model 2 random-intercept LME without interaction between "obstime" and "drug".
- Model 3 random-intercept and random-slope LME with interaction between "obstime" and "drug".

Table 2 Model selection statistics for longitudinal linear mixed-effects models

Model	Random effects	Interaction	df	AIC	BIC	logLik	L.Ratio	p-value
1	Only intercept	Yes	6	7170.67	7202.16	−3579.34		
2	Only intercept	No	5	7168.85	7195.09	−3579.43	0.182	0.670
3	Intercept and slope	Yes	8	7135.44	7177.42	−3559.72		
4	Intercept and slope	No	7	7133.91	7170.65	−3559.96	0.476	0.490

- Model 4 random-intercept and random-slope LME without interaction between "obstime" and "drug".

As summarized in Table 2, we first compare the random-intercept LME models (i.e., Model 1 vs. Model 2). A comparison between Model 1 and Model 2 with the likelihood ratio chi-square test, we found that the Model 2 is not statistically significantly different from the Model 1. The difference in the likelihood ratio statistic is 0.182 and the p-value is 0.670. The AIC and BIC for the Model 2 are smaller than those in the Model 1. This means that Model 2 would be preferred based on the principle of model parsimony with less parameters (i.e., no interaction) among the random-intercept LME models.

Similarly, among the two random-slope LME models (i.e., Model 3 vs. Model 4), Model 4 is preferred due to non-significance of the likelihood ratio test, less AIC and BIC, as well as model parsimony as seen in Table 2.

To determine which model is preferred among the Model 2 and Model 4, we can get that the likelihood ratio statistic is 38.9373 (i.e., 2*(−3579.43-(−3559.96) = 38.9373) with two degrees of freedom (i.e., 7–5 = 2), which gives the p-value of <0.0001. This suggest that the Model 4 (i.e., random-slope LME without interaction) is a better fit than the Model 2 (i.e., random-intercept LME without interaction). In addition, the AIC and BIC for Model 4 (i.e., AIC = 7133.91 and BIC = 7170.65) are smaller than those for Model 2 (i.e., AIC = 7168.85 and BIC = 7195.09), which further confirmed that the random-slope LME model without "obstime" and "drug" interaction is the best model among the four LME models to fit the longitudinal CD4 measure data.

The results for the best LME model (i.e., Model 4 in Table 2) for the longitudinal CD4 measure is presented in Table 3 (left side, titled "Separate linear mixed-effects model"). With this Model 4, the estimated intercept parameters $\hat{\beta}_0 = 6.918$ ($SE = 0.308$; $p < 0.001$), slope parameter for time trend $\hat{\beta}_1 = -0.149$ ($SE = 0.015$; $p < 0.001$), and the slope parameter for the "drug" effect $\hat{\beta}_2 = 0.549$ ($SE = 0.433$; $p < 0.205$). In summary with the separate longitudinal LME modeling, we found a statistically significant overall declining trend for CD4 measure for these 467 patients. However, the "drug" effect is not statistically significant to the CD4 measures.

The mixed-effects model treats missing values from the longitudinal CD4 as missing at random. This is an unreasonable assumption as these missing values originate from the HIV/AIDS patients which could be a result of death or dropout. Those missing CD4 responses are not missing at random as we know their missing

Table 3 Summary of the results from the two separate models and the joint models

	Separate modeling of longitudinal and survival data			*Joint modeling*		
	Separate Cox proportional hazards regression model			*Survival component*		
	Coef.	*SE*	P-value	Coef.	*SE*	P-value
Drug(ddI)	0.210	1.234	0.151	0.328	0.003	0.089
	Separate linear mixed-effects model			*Longitudinal component*		
	Coef.	SE	P-value	Coef.	SE	P-value
Intercept	6.918	0.308	<0.001	6.949	0.008	< 0.001
obstime	−0.149	0.015	<0.001	−0.227	0.001	< 0.001
Drug(ddI)	0.549	0.433	0.205	0.497	0.011	0.264

mechanism on when they died, and therefore treating them as missing at random in this mixed-effects longitudinal model is erroneous and can produce biased estimates.

4.2 Results of Separate Cox Proportional Hazards Regression

Of the 467 patients, there are 237 randomly assigned to 'drug = ddC' and 230 to 'drug = ddI'. There are 88 deaths of the 237 patients in ddC and 100 deaths of the 230 patients in ddI. The time-to-death data is analyzed using Cox proportional hazards regression in Eq. (2) to determine the drug effects. We found it statistically non-significant with an estimated log hazard rate of 0.210 ($SE = 1.234$, $p = 0.151$), which is presented in Table 3 (left side, titled as "Separate Cox proportional hazards regression model"). The estimated survival function can be seen in Fig. 2 and it can be seen that the estimated survival functions for these two drugs are very close together without much difference.

4.3 Results of Joint Modeling of Longitudinal CD4 and Time-to-Death

The joint modeling of longitudinal responses of CD4 measure and time-to-death data involves integrating the models in (3) and (4). The model is used to test the hypothesis that the CD4 measures are associated with time-to-death, as it pertains to the type of drug.

The parameters of the joint model can be estimated through MCMC for 20,000 iterations with the R objects from the linear mixed-effects (*lmeFit.aids*) and Cox proportional hazards models (*survFit.aids*). A graphical representation of the MCMC runs for the longitudinal component of joint modeling are displayed in

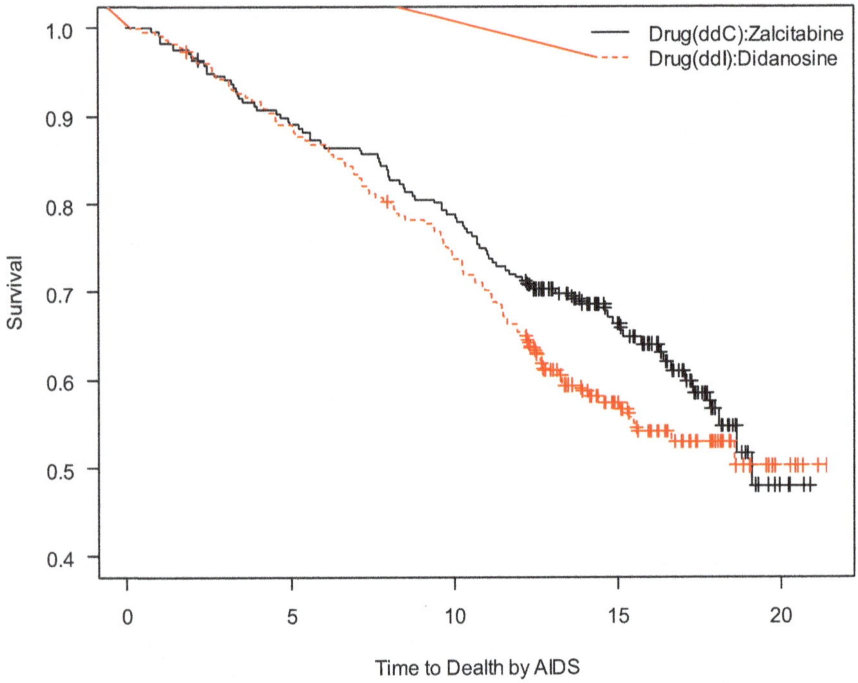

Fig. 2 Estimated survival functions for the two drug treatments

Fig. 3. Similar plots are available for other parameters. Figure 3 demonstrates convergence in the MCMC series.

The estimated parameters for the joint longitudinal component and survival component are summarized in Table 3 (right side). The standard errors are smaller than in the separate models. This suggests that the joint model presents more efficient estimates. As a result, the drug effect parameter estimateis more statistically significant.

In particular, the posterior estimates in the joint model for the association parameter "Assoct" is -0.294 (SE $= 0.003$, p-value < 0.001) and 95% Bayesian credible interval is (-0.378, -0.207). This result provides strong evidence of an association between the two submodels (longitudinal component on CD4 measure and time-to-death due to HIV/AIDS). This indicates that a patient's survival status is significantly related to the longitudinal characteristics of the CD4 which are specified at the initial CD4 level and the rate of CD4 changes. This finding is clinically logical since higher CD4 counts are typically linked with better health status and patients with a more rapid decline in CD4 counts would be expected to have a poorer health condition and less survival probability.

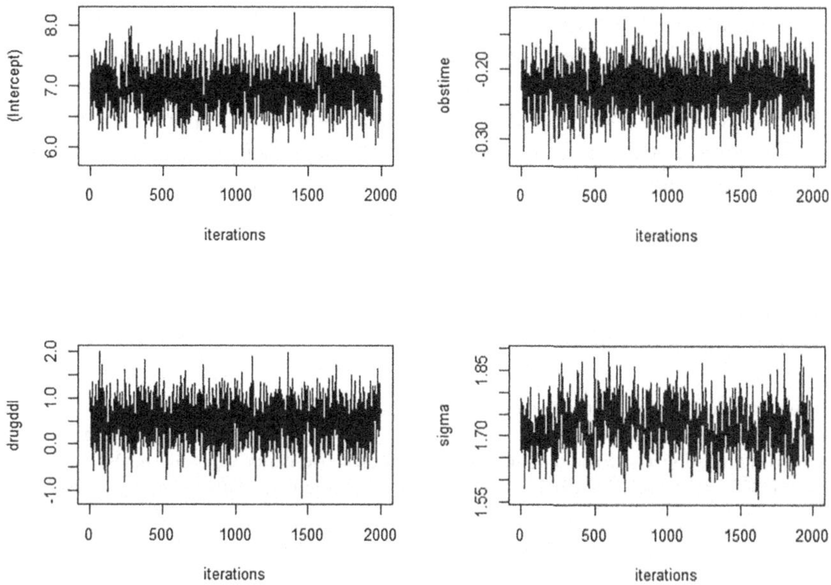

Fig. 3 MCMC illustration for the parameters in the longitudinal CD4 component

5 Conclusions and Recommendations

In this chapter, data from an HIV/AIDS are used to demonstrate the merits of the joint modeling of longitudinal continuous data and time-to-event data simultaneously. The joint-modeling approach has several advantages over separate modeling, both fundamentally and practically.

Fundamentally, the joint-modeling framework incorporated time-to-event data into the observed longitudinal CD4 measurements to mitigate the impact of missing CD4 values due to patient death/dropout. Historically, when applying mixed-effects modeling, the death/dropouts in longitudinal data are treated as missing at random, thus justifying the need for multiple imputations. However, such an approach is flawed in these data, and the failure to detect and address such errors leads to biased estimates and, in some cases, wrong conclusions for public health policymakers and practitioners. We present a joint-modeling framework that is more logically consistent with study designs that dually track time-to-event and longitudinal outcome data while addressing missing data.

Practically, the joint-model framework has higher statistical power to detect an effect or a relationship when one truly exists in survival models [2, 21, 23]. In the analysis of the HIV/AIDS data, the efficiency of the joint-modeling framework was evident in the incorporation of the longitudinal measures and the survival model. The joint modeling of data increases the statistical power to detect the predictive role of CD4 trajectories in understanding the survival structure of time-to-death due to

AIDS. Such higher statistical power has cost implications in that greater efficiency requires smaller sample sizes.

Given the benefits of the joint-modeling framework, we recommend that when designing clinical trials and public health intervention studies to understand treatment effects on time-to-event data, researchers should incorporate longitudinal data. The joint models properly handle outcome-dependent missingness, but they also potentially allow researchers to achieve higher statistical power even when sample sizes are small. Researchers should endeavor to collect time-to-event data so that the missing data from longitudinal measurements can be addressed and statistically modeled. Joint modeling is in the direction of emerging data pooling and harmonization practices, where Bayesian approaches are commonly used to incorporate multiple data sources [3–8].

Acknowledgments This work is based on the research supported partially by the National Research Foundation of South Africa (Grant Number 127727) and the South African National Research Foundation (NRF) and South African Medical Research Council (SAMRC) (South African DST-NRF-SAMRC SARChI Research Chair in Biostatistics, Grant Number 114613).

References

1. Bates, D., Maechler, M.: lme4: Linear mixed-effects models using S4 classes. R package (Version 0.999375–34). http://CRAN.R-project.org/package=lme4 (2010)
2. Brombin, C., Di Serio, C., Rancoita, P.M.: Joint modeling of HIV data in multicenter observational studies: a comparison among different approaches. Stat. Methods Med. Res. **25**(6), 2472–2487 (2016). https://doi.org/10.1177/2F0962280214526192
3. Chen, D.G.: Incorporating historic control information with empirical Bayes. Comput. Stat. Data Anal. **54**, 1646–1656 (2010)
4. Chen, D.G., Ho, S.: From statistical power to statistical assurance: it's time for a paradigm change in clinical trial design. Commun. Stat. Simul. Comput. **46**(10), 7957–7971 (2017)
5. Chen, D.G., Ting, N., Ho, S.: Informative priors or non-informative priors? A Bayesian re-analysis of binary data from macugen phase III clinical trials. Commun. Stat. Simul. Comput. **46**(6), 4535–4546 (2017). https://doi.org/10.1080/03610918.2015.1122049
6. Chen, D.-G., Fraser, M.W.: A Bayesian approach to sample size estimation and the decision to continue program development in intervention research. J. Soc. Soc. Work Res. **8**(3), 457–470 (2017). https://doi.org/10.1086/693433
7. Chen, D.-G., Fraser, M.W., Cuddeback, G.S.: Assurance in intervention research: a Bayesian perspective on statistical power. J. Soc. Soc. Work Res. **9**(1), 159–173 (2018). https://doi.org/10.1086/696239
8. Chen, D., Testa, M.F., Ansong, D., Brevard, K.C.: Evidence building and information accumulation: Bayesian paradigm cohesive for child welfare intervention research. J. Soc. Soc. Work Res. **11**(3), 1–16 (2020). https://doi.org/10.1086/711376
9. Cox, D.R.: Regression models and life-tables. J R Stat Soc Ser B Methodol. **34**(2), 187–220 (1972). https://doi.org/10.1111/j.2517-6161.1972.tb00899.x
10. De Gruttola, V., Tu, X.M.: Modelling progression of CD4-lymphocyte count and its relationship to survival time. Biometrics. **50**(4), 1003–1014 (1994). https://doi.org/10.2307/2533439
11. Faucett, C.L., Thomas, D.C.: Simultaneously modelling censored survival data and repeatedly measured covariates: a Gibbs sampling approach. Stat. Med. **15**(15), 1663–1685 (1996). https://doi.org/10.1002/(SICI)1097-0258(19960815)15:15<3C1663::AID-SIM294>3E3.0.CO;2-1

12. Goldman, A., Carlin, B., Crane, L., Launer, C., Korvick, J., Deyton, L., Abrams, D.: Response of CD4+ and clinical consequences to treatment using ddI or ddC in patients with advanced HIV infection. J. Acquir. Immune Defic. Syndr. Hum. Retrovirol. **11**, 161–169 (1996)
13. Guo, X., Carlin, B.P.: Separate and joint modeling of longitudinal and event time data using standard computer packages. Am. Stat. **58**(1), 16–24 (2004). https://doi.org/10.1198/0003130042854
14. Henderson, R., Diggle, P., Dobson, A.: Joint modelling of longitudinal measurements and event time data. Biostatistics. **1**(4), 465–480 (2000). https://doi.org/10.1093/biostatistics/1.4.465
15. Hsieh, F., Tseng, Y.K., Wang, J.L.: Joint modeling of survival and longitudinal data: likelihood approach revisited. Biometrics. **62**(4), 1037–1043 (2006). https://doi.org/10.1111/j.1541-0420.2006.00570.x
16. Ibrahim, J.G., Chu, H., Chen, L.M.: Basic concepts and methods for joint models of longitudinal and survival data. J. Clin. Oncol. **28**(16), 2796–2801 (2010). https://doi.org/10.1200/JCO.2009.25.0654
17. Li, S.: Joint modeling of recurrent event processes and intermittently observed time-varying binary covariate processes. Lifetime Data Anal. **22**(1), 145–160 (2016). https://doi.org/10.1007/s10985-014-9316-6
18. Pawitan, Y., Self, S.: Modeling disease marker processes in AIDS. J. Am. Stat. Assoc. **88**(423), 719–726 (1993). https://doi.org/10.1080/01621459.1993.10476332
19. Pinheiro, J., Bates, D., DebRoy, S., Sarkar, D. R.: nlme: linear and nonlinear mixed effects models. R package (Version 3.1–149). http://CRAN.R-project.org/package=nlme (2009)
20. Rizopoulos, D.: JM: an R package for the joint modeling of longitudinal and time-to-event data. J. Stat. Softw. **35**(9), 1–33 (2010). https://doi.org/10.18637/jss.v035.i09
21. Rizopoulos, D.: Joint models for longitudinal and time-to-event data: With applications in R. Chapman & Hall/CRC Biostatistics Series, Boca Raton (2012)
22. Rizopoulos, D.: The R Package JMbayes for fitting joint models for longitudinal and time-to-event data using MCMC. J. Stat. Softw. **72**(7), 1–46 (2016). https://doi.org/10.18637/jss.v072.i07
23. Roustaei, N., Ayatollahi, S.M.T., Zare, N.: A proposed approach for joint modeling of the longitudinal and time-to-event data in heterogeneous populations: An application to HIV/AIDS's disease. *BioMed Research International*. **2018** (2018)
24. Therneau, T., Grambsch, P.: Modeling Survival Data: Extending the Cox Model. Springer, Cham (2000)
25. Therneau, T., Lumley, T.: "Survival": survival analysis including penalised likelihood. R package (Version 2.35–8). http://CRAN.R-project.org/package=survival (2009)
26. Wu, L., Liu, W., Yi, G.Y., Huang, Y.: Analysis of longitudinal and survival data: joint modeling, inference methods, and issues. J. Probab. Stat. **2012**(640153), 1–17 (2012). https://doi.org/10.1155/2012/640153
27. Wulfsohn, M.S., Tsiatis, A.A.: A joint model for survival and longitudinal data measured with error. Biometrics. **53**(1), 330–339 (1997). https://doi.org/10.2307/2533118

Index

Y. Lio et al. (eds.), *Bayesian Inference and Computation in Reliability and Survival Analysis*, Emerging Topics in Statistics and Biostatistics,
https://doi.org/10.1007/978-3-030-88658-5

N

O

P

Q

R

The manufacturer's authorised representative in the EU is Springer Nature Customer Service Centre GmbH, Europaplatz 3, 69115 Heidelberg, Germany. If you have any concerns regarding our products, please contact ProductSafety@springernature.com

Printed and bound by CPI Group (UK) Ltd, Croydon, CR0 4YY
22/09/2026
02220954-0001